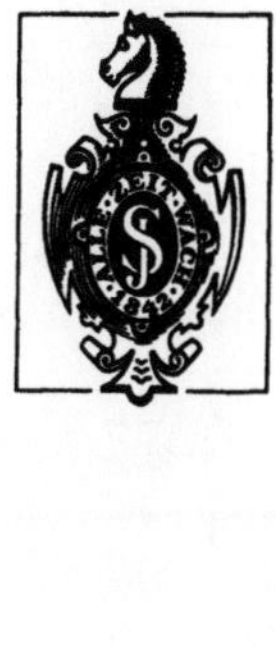
1842

Fang Zhi-yang Sheng Zhi-yong
Li Ngao Ge Sheng-de (Eds.)

Modern Treatment of Severe Burns

With 115 Figures, Some in Color, and 44 Tables

Springer-Verlag
Berlin Heidelberg New York
London Paris Tokyo
Hong Kong Barcelona
Budapest

Fang Zhi-yang, Prof. M.D.
PLA Research Institute of Trauma-Burn Surgery
Changhai Hospital, Second Military Medical University
174 Changhai Road, Shanghai 200433, PR China

Sheng Zhi-yong, Prof. M.D.
Trauma-Burn Center
Postgraduate Military Medical College of PLA
Beijing 100037, PR China

Li Ngao, Prof. M.D.
PLA Research Institute of Burn
Third Military Medical University
Chongqing 630038, PR China

Ge Sheng-de, Prof. B.S., M.D.
PLA Research Institute of Trauma-Burn Surgery
Changhai Hospital, Second Military Medical University
174 Changhai Road, Shanghai 200433, PR China

ISBN-13: 978-3-642-76625-1 e-ISBN-13: 978-3-642-76623-7
DOI: 10.1007/978-3-642-76623-7

Library of Congress Cataloging-in-Publication Data
Modern treatment of severe burns/Fang Zhi-yang... [et al.] (eds.).
p.cm. Includes bibliographical references and index.
ISBN-13: 978-3-642-76625-1
1. Burns and scalds-Treatment. I. Fang, Zhi-yang.
[DNLM: 1. Burns-therapy. W0 704 M689] RD96.4M57 1992
617.1'106-dc20 DNLM/DLC 91-5148

Softcover reprint of the hardcover 1st edition 1992

Typesetting: Thomson Press (India) Ltd., New Delhi, India
24/3130-5 4 3 2 1 0-Printed on acid-free paper.

Contents

List of Contributors*

Fang Zhi-yang, M.D., Professor of Surgery
PLA Research Institute of Trauma-Burn Surgery
Changhai Hospital, Second Military Medical University
174 Changhai Road, Shanghai 200433, PR China

Ge Sheng-de, B.S., M.D., Professor of Surgery
PLA Research Institute of Trauma-Burn Surgery
Changhai Hospital, Second Military Medical University
174 Changhai Road, Shanghai 200433, PR China

Huang Wen-hua, M.D., Professor of Surgery
PLA Research Institute of Burn
Third Military Medical University
Chongqing 630038, PR China

Li Ngao, M.D., Professor of Surgery
PLA Research Institute of Burn
Third Military Medical University
Chongqing 630038, PR China

Liu Shi-kang, M.D., Associate Professor of Surgery
PLA Research Institute of Trauma-Burn Surgery
Changhai Hospital, Second Military Medical University
174 Changhai Road, Shanghai 200433, PR China

Sheng Zhi-yong, M.D., Professor of Surgery
Trauma-Burn Center
Postgraduate Military Medical College of PLA
35 Fu-Cheng Road, Beijing 100037, PR China

Tang Sheau-shi, M.D., Professor of Surgery
Reijin Hospital, Shanghai Second Medical University
197 Reijin Er Road, Shanghai, 200020, PR China

---

* Includes only first-named author.

Wang Shi-liang, M.D., Professor of Surgery
PLA Research Institute of Burn
Third Military Medical University
Chongqing 630038, PR China

Wang Wen-zheng, M.D., Professor of Surgery
PLA Research Institute of Trauma-Burn Surgery
Changhai Hospital, Second Military Medical University
174 Changhai Road, Shanghai 200433, PR China

Yang Zong-chen, M.D., Professor of Surgery
PLA Research Institute of Burn
Third Military Medical University
Chongqing 630038, PR China

Zhu Zhao-ming, M.D., Professor of Surgery
Trauma-Burn Center
Postgraduate Military Medical College of PLA
35 Fu-cheng Road, Beijing 100037, PR China

1 Introduction

Fang Zhi-yang

1.1 History of Traditional Treatment of Burns in China

China is a country of ancient culture. The treatment of burn injury was documented more than 1500 years ago. As early as the Eastern Jin Dynasty, the *Handbook of Prescriptions for Emergencies* written by Ge Hong (281–341 A.D.) and in the Southern Qi Dynasty (479–502 A.D.) Liu Juan-Zi's *Remedies Left Over by Ghosts*, a book dealing mainly with diagnosis and treatment of traumatic wounds, are the earliest known monographs on "external diseases" in China. They record the treatment of burns with topical agents such as the preparation of a lard ointment of the liquid extract of *Angelica anomalea* Lallem, *Gardenia jasminoides* Ellis, *Glycyrrhiza uralensis* Fisch, *Radia salviae miltiorrhizae*, and the white cortex of willow. These herbs are found to be astringents and antibiotics. During the Sui Dynasty, a doctor of the Imperial Medical Academy (550–630 A.D.), Chao Yuan-fang, was authorized by imperial decree to compile the book *General Treatise on the Etiology and Symptomatology of Diseases* (610 A.D.), the first book on etiology and symptomatology in China. This book with its valuable descriptions has been an authoritative and important reference for medical students for more than 1000 years. Chao Yuan-fang suggested that the burn wound surface must not be infected, and considered that infection could aggravate the depth of burn wound, resulting in the involvement of tissues under the muscles. Valuable information was mentioned in *Qian Jin Fang* (*Essential Prescriptions Worth a Thousand Gold*) written in 652 A.D. by Sun Simiao, a well-known physician (581–682 A.D.) of the Tang Dynasty. The suggested methods consisted of combinations of internal medication using Chinese herbs, such as antipyretics and antidotes for toxic substances, and external application of extract of the mixture of *Gardenia jasminoides* Ellis, *Scutellaria* root, and swallowwort root for clearing the wound surface. In the book *The Medical Secrets of an Official* compiled by Wang Tao (752 A.D.), local application of Chinese herbs for crust formation was an important part of the treatment. Cineole, which consisted of insoluble tannic acid, was frequently used. These ancient methods are still in use as popular prescriptions in present-day clinical practice in China, and they are relatively effective for mild burn wounds.

In the Ming Dynasty, Xue Yi, a well-known court physician, revised and annotated *The Essentials of External Diseases* (1545 A.D.), emphasizing that programs both of internal and external treatment were necessary for burns. The frequently used medicinal herbs were the compound decoctions for the purposes of regulating "vital energy and blood", strengthening the "spleen and stomach", and promoting pus discharge and tissue repair.

Advances in medical practice during the Qing Dynasty led to the recognition that burn wound, especially in severe cases with extensive burns, was a generalized disease with internal damage of the *Zang-Fu*(viscerae), and emphasized that internal and external management should be combined in the treatment of burns.

During the years 1665–1838 A.D., many dissertations dealing with the "fire poison attacking the interior viscera" suggested that the knowledge of promoting host defense required decoctions of medicinal herbs used for antipyretic and detoxifying effects.

However, due to the slow advance of medical sciences and technology, many lives of severely burned patients have been lost in the past. The only basis for treatment has been the "principle of *Bian Zheng Lun Zhi*", which is a symptomatic treatment guided by diagnosis based on overall analysis of the cause and nature of the burns, symptoms and signs, location of burned area, and patient's physical condition according to the basic theories of traditional Chinese medicine. Nevertheless, many drugs prepared from the Chinese medicinal herbs have demonstrated their actions of promoting immunity and inhibition of pathogenic organisms. Investigations into these actions will be continued [1].

1.2 Modern Treatment of Severe Burns in China

Burn surgery was developed as a new speciality within the sphere of surgery in 1958, and the methods of burn therapy have been developed in the main metropolises such as Beijing, Shanghai, and Chongqing, and popularized in most parts of China. Since then large burn institutes or trauma-burn institutes have been established where clinical and laboratory research and teaching have been carried out.

In major burns with extensive third-degree wounds, a large amount of skin autograft is needed. Usually it is not readily available due to limited skin donor sites. A method of intermingled transplantation using autograft and allograft (the "Chinese method") was developed in the 1960s in China. More recently the microskin grafting technique has been developed, which has a wound coverage area 8- to 18-fold that of the donor site [2]. Skin grafting using cultured epithelial cells for the treatment of a small area of third-degree burn is under clinical trial. The problem of delayed resuscitation of the patient with extensive burns remains unsolved. Severe burn shock often induces multiple organ failure, i.e., dysfunction of the liver, kidney, and lung. Recent evidence suggests that complement activation associated with burn injury is related to production of chemotactic peptides, which cause stimulation of circulating neutrophils. Activation of the neutrophils leads to the production of toxic free oxygen radicals. Therefore, free radical scavenger might be indicated in the early postburn stage.

Sepsis is one of the major causes of death in patients with severe burns. An increased susceptibility to infection of burned patients associated with loss of the skin barrier is apt to result in local and/or systemic infection, which seems to be related to acquired immunodeficiencies. Administration of hyperimmunoplasma induced by endotoxin has successfully resulted in controlling burn wound sepsis caused by *Pseudomonas aeruginosa.*

Antimicrobial agents which are effective against *Pseudomonas aeruginosa* are selected by performing drug sensitivity tests. Silver aspartate and silver nicotinate have proved effective. Both of the drugs together with silver 2-sulfhydryl-4-nitropyridine-*N*- oxide, a proved potent drug, and the recently synthesized pipemidic acid and silver pipemidate were used as effective topical cream. More recently the silver salt of norfloxacin has been demonstrated by Ge Sheng-De et al. [3] as a new antimicrobial agent for *Pseudomonas aeruginosa* infection.

It is well known that pulmonary complications following inhalation injury are the major threats to the survival of burned patients. Commonly the pulmonary function of the patients progressively deteriorates to form ARDS (adult respiratory distress syndrome), which is an important cause of early death in burned patients with inhalation injury. Experimental models of steam and smoke inhalation injuries in rabbits, dogs, and sheep with chronic lung lymph fistulae have been developed for laboratory studies. In addition to blood gas study, a series of bacteriological, immunological, and biochemical tests, along with examinations with X-ray and fiber optic bronchoscopy, were performed on the dog model. The research work was carried out by pathologists, pathophysiologists, biochemists, and bacteriologists in the Burn Research Institute of the Third Military Medical College of the People's Liberation Army. The etiology of ARDS was studied by teamwork.

Statistical data from 48978 burned patients collected from 283 army hospitals between 1958 and 1978 have been analyzed [4]. The incidence of burns caused by fire and scald, chemical agents, and electricity were 87.59%, 6.55%, and 3.72%, respectively, and burns to the neck and upper and lower extremities were found in 81.18%, 57.27%, and 13.20% of patients, respectively.

The incidence of burn shock was 10.85%, and the incidence of patients with or without third-degree burns was 25.75% and 5.25%, respectively. The total survival rate was 95.1%, with an overall mortality of 4.9%.

1.3 Statistical Analysis of Severely Burned Patients

From 1958 through 1987, a total of 3204 patients with severe burns [adults: total burns covering more than 50% of total body surface area (TBSA) or third-degree (3°) burns covering more than 30% of TBSA; children: total burns over 30% TBSA or 3° burns over 20% TBSA] were admitted to the following institutions: Changhai Hospital, Trauma–Burn Research Institute, Second Military Medical College, Shanghai; Southwest Hospital, Burn Research Institute, Third Military Medical College, Chongqing; Ruijin Hospital, Burn Research Institute, Second

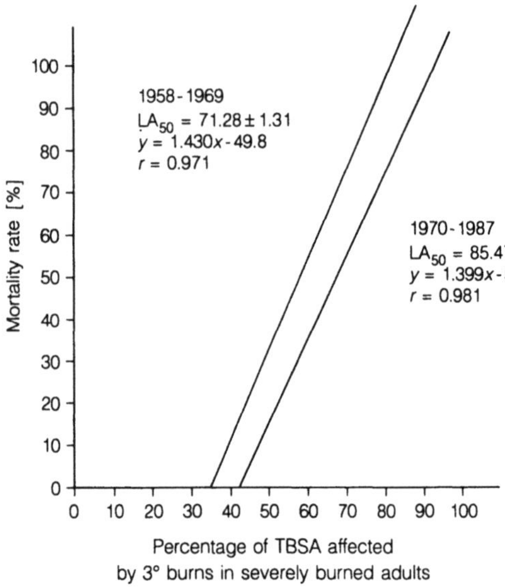

Fig. 1.1. Graph derived from linear regression equations of proportion of TBSA affected by 3° burns in adults. The regression coefficients of mortality and proportion of TBSA affected are statistically significant

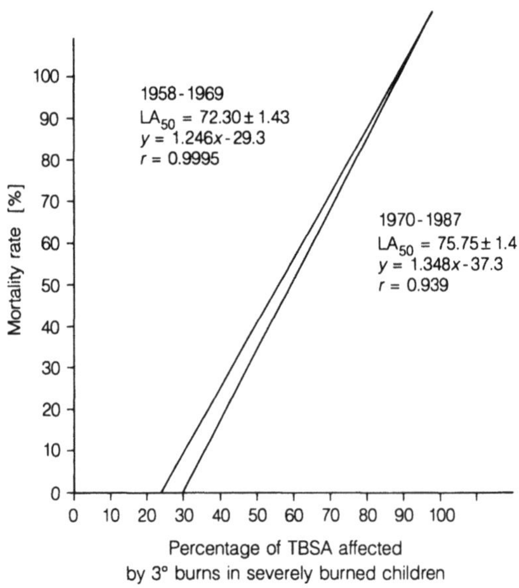

Fig. 1.2. Graph derived from linear regression equations of proportion of TBSA affected by 3° burns in children. The relationship between mortality and total burn area is statistically significant

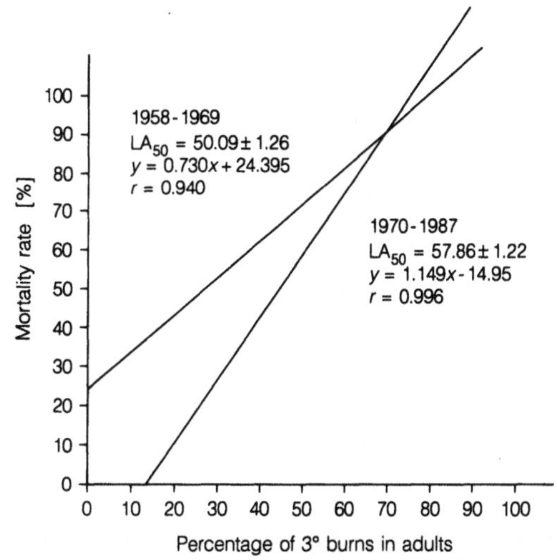

Fig. 1.3. Linear graph derived from a linear regression equation of extent of 3° burns in adults. There is a statistically significant association between mortality and 3° burns

Table 1.1. Causes of severe burns in adults

Cause	Flame	Hot liquid	Chemical	Electric	Miscellaneous	Total
No. of cases	1324	290	219	54	251	2138
%	61.93	13.56	10.24	2.53	11.74	100

Table 1.2. Causes of severe burns in children

Cause	Flame	Hot liquid	Chemical	Electric	Miscellaneous	Total
No. of cases	374	611	59	7	15	1066
%	35.08	57.32	5.53	0.66	1.41	100

Medical University, Shanghai; 304th Hospital, Trauma Centre, Postgraduate Medical College, Beijing. There were 1323 cases between 1958 and 1968, and 1881 cases between 1970 and 1987. The causes of burns are listed in Table 1.1 and 1.2. The LA_{50}, the percentage of TBSA burned that results in a fatal outcome for 50% of the patients, is shown for the periods 1958–1969 and 1970–1987 in Figs. 1.1–1.3 and Tables 1.3–1.6.

Table 1.3. Deaths among severely burned adults in relation to the proportion of TBSA covered by burns

Period	Total burns (% TBSA) (3° burns)	50–69 (30–49)	70–89 (50–69)	90+ (70+)
1958–1969	No. of cases	353	202	147
	Deaths	91	85	122
	Mortality rate (%)	25.78	42.08	82.99
1970–1987	No. of cases	651	447	308
	Deaths	88	143	214
	Mortality rate (%)	13.52	31.99	69.48
1958–1987	No. of cases	1004	649	455
	Deaths	179	228	336
	Mortality rate (%)	17.83	35.13	73.85

Table 1.4. Linear regression equation of proportion of TBSA burned and mortality in severely burned adults

Period	Linear regression equation	Correlation coefficient	LA_{50} (%)
1958–1969	$y = 1.430x - 49.8$	0.971	71.28 ± 1.31
1970–1987	$y = 1.399x - 59.6$	0.981	85.47 ± 1.22
1958–1987	$y = 1.401x - 55.77$	0.976	82.41 ± 1.21

Table 1.5. Deaths among severely burned children in relation to the proportion of TBSA covered by burns

Period	Total burns (% TBSA) (3° burns)	30–49 (20–29)	50–69 (30–49)	70+ (50+)
1958–1969	No. of cases	420	137	64
	Deaths	47	49	37
	Mortality rate (%)	11.19	35.77	57.81
1970–1987	No. of cases	328	96	51
	Deaths	29	18	32
	Mortality rate (%)	8.84	18.75	62.75
1958–1987	No. of cases	748	233	115
	Deaths	76	67	69
	Mortality rate (%)	10.16	28.75	60.00

Table 1.6. Linear regression equation of proportion of TBSA burned and mortality in severely burned children

Period	Linear regression equation	Correlation coefficient	LA_{50} (%)
1958–1969	$y = 1.246x - 29.3$	0.9995	72.30 ± 1.43
1970–1987	$y = 1.348x - 37.3$	0.939	75.75 ± 1.41
1958–1987	$y = 1.246x - 29.3$	0.989	73.50 ± 1.42

References

1. Cheng GJ (1975) Introduction. In: The combined therapy of the traditional Chinese and western medicine for burns (in Chinese). Anhui Medical College, p. 1–2
2. Zhang ML, Tsao DS, Zheng ZD (1987) The use of microskin grafting in extensive burns (in chinese). Chin J Plast Surg Burns 3: 100–102
3. Ge SD, Tu SZ, Fang ZY et al. (1987) The effect of pyridone acid derivative to topical antibiotics on the prevention and treatment of *Pseudomonas aeruginosa* infection following burns (in Chinese). Chin J Plast Surg Burns 3: 10–13
4. Li N, Li ZZ, Lei ZH (1984) An analysis of 48,978 burn patients (in chinese). Med J Chin PLA 9: 401–407

2 Emergency Care, Triage, and Transportation

Wang Shi-liang and Li Ngao

Method of rescue, initial care, and transportation are extremely important in saving the life of burn victims. Proper medical sorting and planned organization for burn disasters are of paramount importance.

2.1 Emergency Care

The aim of emergency care is to remove the causes of injury and deliver preliminary aid in an expeditious manner.

2.1.1 Removal of the Causes of Burn

In a group of 5506 cases, the commonest cause of burn was heat (Table 2.1). In the case of flame burn, the fire should be extinguished by pouring water or smothering with blankets, coats, or rugs (inflammable materials such as plastics and nylon should not be used). The flame can also be put out by rolling on the ground. The victim should not run or remain standing, otherwise facial burn and/or inhalation injury will occur. Clothes soaked with hot fluid or chemicals should be removed immediately. Jumping into a nearby pond or river, if present, is encouraged.

All chemical burn wounds should be irrigated continuously with copious amounts of water as early as possible to remove the caustic agents. Priority in water irrigation should be given to the eyes. Generally, neutralizing agents are not needed if irrigation is thorough and complete, and it is usually a waste of precious time to search for a proper neutralizing agent. In the case of injury due to certain special chemicals such as hydrofluoric acid, neutralizing agent should be employed. We have made up a mixture named "immersion mixture of calcium and magnesium," especially for the purpose of neutralizing hydrofluoric acid [1]. It consists of calcium chloride, magnesium sulfate, and sodium bicarbonate.

Disconnection of the electric current as quickly as possible is the most urgent step for rescuing electrically injured victims. Mouth to mouth respiration and/or external cardiac massage should be instituted early, if the victim is apneic and/or the arterial pulse is not palpable in the carotid or femoral region.

Table 2.1. Causes of burns in 5506 cases

	Thermal injury								Chemical burns				Electrical burns	Others
Cause	Boiling water	Flames	Hot liquid	Gasoline flame	Molten metals	Gun-powder explosion	Steam	Gas explosion	Acid	Alkali	Phosphorus	Toxic agent		
Percentage	39.74	17.91	8.85	6.28	5.21	3.12	2.99	2.92	3.01	1.53	0.46	0.33		
Total					87.02					5.33			2.59	5.06

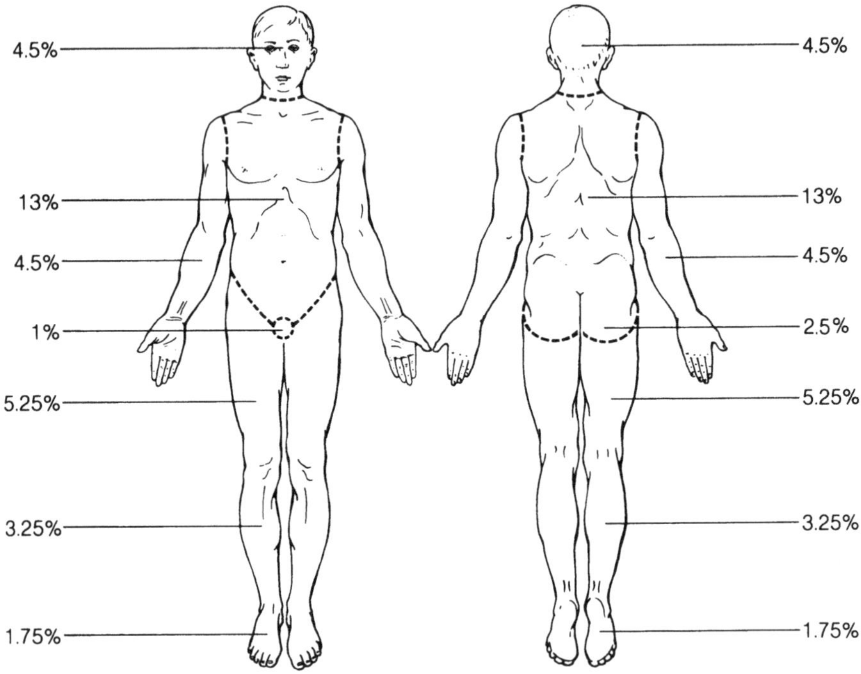

Fig. 2.1. The "Chinese rule of nine" for estimating percentage of TBSA burned

2.1.2 Primary Care

Life-threatening complications such as massive hemorrhage, asphyxia, open pneumothorax, and serious poisoning should be treated immediately. Then the victim should be moved from the scene of the accident and transported to the nearest medical facility. In the meantime, the proportion of total body surface area (TBSA) affected and the depth of burn should be estimated. Usually the "Chinese rule of nine" [2] is preferred (Fig. 2.1). Attention must be paid to the search for possible inhalation injury and associated injuries such as fractures, soft tissue trauma, and visceral injury, for their clinical features are often concealed by the presence of severe burns of the body surface and are thereby overlooked. Sedatives or narcotics are often administered to combat pain as part of the antishock treatment. The drugs commonly used are morphine, pethidine (Dolantin, Hoechst), sodium barbiturate, etc.

In the case of burn shock, such drugs are better given intravenously because drugs given by other routes would not be readily absorbed. Pain can be relieved by cryotherapy, i.e., the burn area is placed under running cold water, immersed in cold water, or covered with a cold compress for at least 0.5–1 h. There is no unanimity regarding the cold water temperature although a temperature of 5°–15° C is usually preferred. Cryotherapy is not advisable for patients with extensive burns or shock, for most of them would not stand the chilling, and the shock might be worsened.

Burn wounds should be covered and protected from further contamination and injury by any available dressings, such as first aid dressings, standard burn dressings, triangular bandages, clean sheets, or even clean clothes. Colored or unsterile topical drugs should not be used. Colored drugs will change the appearance of burn wound and make further identification difficult. Open wounds must be bound and fractures splinted.

Fluid resuscitation should be started as early as possible. In the case of minor and moderate burns, patients may be allowed to drink soup, rice water, milk, or any salt-containing fluid. However, plain water should be restricted in order to avoid the danger of water intoxication. Burn beverage tablets have proved effective; each tablet contains sodium chloride 0.3 g, sodium bicarbonate 0.15 g, and phenobarbital 0.03 g and is dissolved in 100 ml water or other liquid. Burn beverage tablets are used particularly in mass burn casualties after a conflagration or other disaster. However, i.v. fluids should be started early with larger burns or in patients who have shown signs and symptoms of circulatory decompensation such as nausea, vomiting, restlessness, rapid pulse, low blood pressure, and low urinary output.

In extensive burns, badly soiled burns, burns complicated by fractures, major soft tissue injury, and internal organ trauma, administration of antibiotics is mandatory.

The extent and depth of burn, concomitant injuries, and disposition of patients should be recorded in detail so as to facilitate further treatment.

2.2 Triage

It is well known that triage is important in times of war and after major disasters. Well-organized and properly directed triage will facilitate rescue procedures and reduce the incidence of burn complications and, of course, mortality. The effect of triage depends not only on the severity of the burn injury, but also the number of victims, the environment of the scene, as well as the available facilities and personnel.

A group of 420 adult burn patients admitted to our institute were divided into four groups according to the severity of the burn injury, i.e., the proportion of total body surface area (TBSA) covered by total burns or third-degree (3°) burns (Tables 2.2, 2.3) [2] (a) total burns < 30% TBSA, 3° burns < 10% TBSA; (b) total 30%–49% or 3° 10%–19%; (c) total 50%–69% or 3° 20%–29%; (d) total ≧ 70% or 3° ≧ 30%.

As shown in Tables 2.2 and 2.3, differences exist among these groups not only in the incidence of shock and sepsis, but also in the mortality rate. In 1970, a classification of adult burn patients into four categories was approved during the Chinese National Burn Conference: (1) minor: partial-thickness burns < 10% TBSA; (2) moderate: total burns 11%–33% of TBSA or 3° burns < 10% of TBSA;

Table 2.2. Incidence of shock, sepsis, and mortality in 420 adults with burns

Extent of burns (% TBSA)	0–29	30–49	50–69	70–100
Number of patients	187	85	63	85
Number with shock (%)	5(2.6)***	29(34.1)**	36(57.1)***	73(85.9)
Number with moderate and severe shock (%)	0(0)***	8(9.4)	13(20.6)***	53(63.6)
Number with sepsis (%)	5(2.6)**	9(10.6)***	23(37.1)***	56(73.7)
Number of deaths (%)	0(0)*	2(2.2)***	18(28.6)***	64(77.7)

* $p < 0.05$.
** $p < 0.01$ between the two adjacent groups.
*** $p < 0.005$.

Table 2.3. Relationship between 3°-BSA and incidence of sepsis and mortality in 420 adults with burns

Total extent of burns		Extent of 3° burns (% TBSA)				
		0–9	10–19	20–29	30–39	40–
0%–29% TBSA	Number of patients	41	2	0	–	–
	Sepsis cases	2	2	0	–	–
	Number of deaths	0	0	0	–	–
30%–49% TBSA	Number of patients	30	7	1	2	0
	Sepsis cases	1	3	1	2	0
	Number of deaths	1	0	0	0	0
50%–69% TBSA	Number of patients	18	12	5	3	2
	Sepsis cases	4	7	2	3	2
	Number of deaths	5	4	3	2	1

(3) severe: total burns 31%–50%, 3° 11%–20%, or total burns < 30% but complicated by one of the following: (a) occurrence of shock, (b) combined injury and/or intoxication (severe trauma, chemical poisoning, etc.), (c) moderate or severe inhalation injury (i.e., involving respiratory tract below the level of larynx), (d) deep burns of special regions, such as hand, face, and perineum; (4) extremely severe: total burns > 50% or 3° > 20%.

Of course, factors such as patient's age, preexisting disease, and patient's general condition should also be taken into account. As a rule, this classification is the basis for triage. However, triage may vary according to the site and the available facilities and medical personnel, especially in a major disaster or in time of war.

Table 2.4. Comparison of incidence of severe shock and survival rate in burns patients treated near the scene of the accident and after long-distance transportation

	Treated near scene of accident	Treated after long-distance transportation
Number of patients	27	23
Mean total extent of burns (% TBSA)	60.5	57.5
Mean extent of 3° burns (% TBSA)	18.1	15.3
Mean age (years)	24.3	23.4
Number of cases with severe shock	17 (62.9%)*	21 (91.3%)
Number of patients who	22 (81.4%)*	12 (52.2%)

*$p < 0.05$.

2.3 Transportation

After rescue and primary care, patients should be transported from the scene of the accident to a nearby hospital or clinic for further treatment. However, because of the markedly increased incidence and severity of shock and possible death after rough transportation, especially over a long distance, such transfers should be carefully deliberated and well planned. If facilities are available, as a general rule, patients are moved to a clinic as near as possible. If shock is already threatening the patient's life, treatment is better instituted in a medical station at the site of the accident and transportation postponed until the patient's general condition has improved sufficiently. Sometimes, even though patients could be taken to a well-equipped hospital at a distance, treatment would be difficult and very much handicapped by the poor general condition of the patients, who might die from irreversible shock, fulminating invasive infection, and/or multi-organ failure in spite of intensive therapeutic treatment. In 1961, there were 50 male casualties after a large fire. They were dispatched to two hospitals; 23 of them were sent to a better equipped hospital 150 km away, and 27 were admitted to the nearest medical facility, only 5 km from the scene of disaster. As shown in Table 2.4, the severity of burn injury in these two groups of patients was similar. The mean total burn area was 60.5% and 57.5% TBSA and the 3° burn area was 18.1% and 15.3% TBSA respectively. The mean ages were similar, 24.3 and 23.4 years respectively. Nevertheless, the outcomes diverged significantly. The incidence of severe shock was 62.9% vs 91.3% and survival rate 81.4% vs 52.2% ($p < 0.05$) in these two groups.

This experience greatly improved our understanding of transportation tactics in emergency care for burns. We concluded that patients with severe burns, particularly those with profound shock, should not be allowed to be transported over long distances during the first 2 days after injury. It is better to treat the victims in the vicinity of the disaster, and transport them after the shock stage when their general condition permits.

2.3.1 Best Time for Transportation

The best time for transportation of burn patients depends upon the causes and extent of burns, general condition of the patient, and method and facilities of transportation. In the past it was thought that the peak hypovolemia occurred 6–12 h after the burn injury, and therefore it was suggested that the patient should be transported before 6 h after the injury. However, clinical practice and experimental studies indicated that the time that burn shock reaches its peak varies. Usually, the more severe the burns, the earlier the burn shock. With extremely severe burns it might occur as early as within 1–2 h postinjury, especially in those patients who have superimposed combined injuries or additional trauma as a result of improper rescue technique. We analyzed a group of 420 cases of adults admitted to our burn institute within 72 h postburn, and found that the incidence of severe shock clearly varied with burn size and admission time (Tables 2.2, 2.4).

1. Group I: there were 187 burn patients (44.3%) with total burns covering less than 29% TBSA, of whom only 5 (2.6%) showed mild shock and none displayed severe shock. Incidence of shock in this group bore a relationship to admission time.
2. Group II: 85 patients (20.1%) with total burns covering 30%–49% TBSA showed severe shock. Most of them were admitted after 8 h postburn.
3. Group III: 63 patients (15.4%) with total burns to 50%–69% of TBSA showed severe shock. In this group, the incidence of severe shock rose to 13.3% and 27.7% in patients who were admitted within 2 and 4 h postburn, respectively. However, most were admitted 4–24 h post burn, accounting for 40% of the cases in the present group. Shock had not been demonstrated in patients admitted 24 h after injury, because early fluid replacement and emergency care were initiated in the vicinity of the accident site and also during the transportation.
4. Group IV: 85 burn patients (20.1%) with total burns to 70%–100% of TBSA carried a 63.6% incidence of severe shock. In this group, as shown in Fig. 2.2, the incidence of severe shock rose to 70.5% even in the patients admitted within 2 h postburn, with a peak incidence of up to 100% when the admission time was delayed 4–8 h after the burn, and still remained high at 40% though the admission time was 24–48 h. No shock occurred in those admitted after 48 h postburn, and their primary care, including fluid replacement therapy, was given before the admission even though the amount of fluid administered was far from adequate.

Considering the above data, we propose the following guidelines for time of transportation.

1. In the case of burns to less than 29% of TBSA the patient can be transported at any time after injury.
2. It is better to transport patients with burns to 30%–49% TBSA to the hospital for definitive treatment within 8 h postburn.

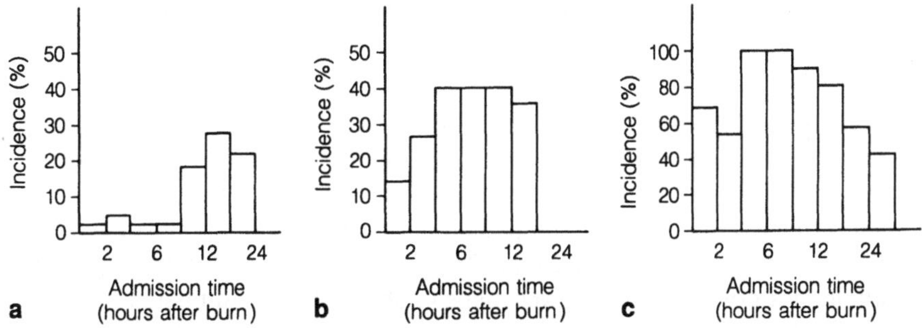

Fig. 2.2 a–c. Distribution of incidence of severe shock in adults with different extent of burns and admission time. **a** 30%–49% TBSA; **b** 50%–69% TBSA; **c** 70%–100% TBSA

3. It is desirable to send patients with burns to 50%–69% of TBSA to the medical facility for definitive treatment within 4 h postinjury. Primary care and fluid therapy may be given in the vicinity of the disaster and the patients may be transported 24 h after the burn when their general condition has stabilized.
4. For patients with burns to 70%–100% of TBSA, it seems obligatory to transport them to the referral hospital within 1–2 h after the burn. Otherwise treatment would be better instituted in the nearest medical facility, and transportation only allowed when the patients' general condition permits, usually 48 h after injury.
5. In severely burned patients, fluid replacement should be started early and continued during the whole journey, especially if a long journey is expected.

A similar experience of the early medical care given in the Los Alfaques disaster in 1978 was reported by Arturson [3]. He made a comparative study between a group of 58 patients taken to Barcelona and another group of 82 patients taken to Valencia, and it was found that the main reason for the significantly greater mortality in the latter group of patients was lack of medical treatment during the journey. In contrast with this group, the patients in the former group received adequate medical treatment en route to the hospital.

Of course, besides the extent of the burn, the best time for transportation is also influenced by other factors such as the patient's general condition, the severity of supervening shock, modes and means of transport and medical facilities, and personnel. If severe shock has supervened, no matter what the extent and depth of the burns are, antishock therapy must be instituted and transportation postponed until the hemodynamic status becomes stable.

2.4 Primary Care Before and During Transportation

The initial treatment which is provided before transportation is extremely important in combating shock and preventing other complications, and in stabilizing the general condition of the patient during transportation. In group of 148 patients with burns to over 50% of TBSA, the incidence of shock before admission was as follows:

1. Twenty (32.7%) of the 61 patients who received initial replacement therapy before admission developed severe shock, while 43 (49.5%) out of 87 patients receiving no fluid replacement had severe shock ($p < 0.05$).
2. Thirty-eight (35.5%) of the 108 patients who received analgesics or sedatives before admission developed shock; 28 (70.0%) of 40 patients receiving neither analgesics nor sedatives showed signs of shock during admission ($p < 0.05$).
3. Of the 63 patients whose wounds were covered by various dressings before admission, 14 (22.2%) exhibited shock; and 53 (62.3%) of the 85 patients without wound dressings showed signs of shock on admission ($p < 0.005$).

Of course, there are many factors affecting the development of shock, but these common and simple measures employed in primary care of burns have certainly been shown to reduce both morbidity and mortality following major burns.

2.4.1 Analgesia and Sedation

Generally, Dolantin (or Demeral or Lydol), morphine, or Dolantin and promethazine (Phenergan, Wyeth) injected intramuscularly are indicated to alleviate the pain. In the case of burns, however, the analgesics or sedatives should be given intravenously in the noncompensating circulation, as they may not be promptly absorbed when the intramuscular route is used. If the burn is associated with craniocerebral trauma, sodium phenobarbital may be used instead of morphine or Dolantin. A lytic cocktail such as chlorpromazine or acepromazine should be restricted before or during the transportation in order to prevent postural hypotension.

2.4.2 Local Care

The wound should be covered with a clean sheet, sterile dressing, or artificial skin to minimize contamination, relieve pain, and protect the wound from further damage.

2.4.3 Fluid Replacement Therapy

As stated above, oral burn beverage (0.3 g sodium chloride and 0.15 g sodium bicarbonate in each tablet, one tablet/100 ml water) or other salt-containing drinks can be given in the case of minor or moderate burns. Because ileus and vomiting are common complications in severe and extremely severe burns, intravenous fluids should be administered early instead of oral fluids.

Occasionally, continuous administration of intravenous fluids is not practical during transportation, and "stage infusion" is recommended (see Sect. 2.5 below).

2.4.4 *Antibiotic Prophylaxis*

Prophylactic antibiotics are given to those patients with severe or extremely severe burns and badly soiled burns.

2.4.5 *Tracheostomy*

It is difficult to perform tracheostomy during transportation; therefore, it is better performed in patients with signs and symptoms of existing or possible airway obstruction due to inhalation injury or severe head, face, and neck burns before transportation.

2.4.6 *Indwelling Urinary Catheter*

An indwelling urinary catheter should be inserted and secured in patients with burns involving more than 30% TBSA before transportation in order to observe urinary output hourly, which is an essential parameter for the evaluation of the circulatory state and also for guidance of the fluid therapy.

2.4.7 *Means of Transport*

Transportation may be achieved by any vehicle available, such as stretcher, ambulance, boat, train, or airplane. Helicopter transportation is now increasingly being used. If an aircraft is used, it is better to lay the patient transversely across the cabin to protect him or her from the hazard of postural hypotension during takeoff and landing. If a car or ambulance is used, violent shaking or rocking should be avoided. Loading the vehicle with sandbags is a method of eliminating a bumpy ride.

2.4.8 *Combined Injuries and Poisoning*

Burns combined with fractures, soft tissue injuries, or internal organ damage are not uncommon. Hemostasis and splinting should be promptly performed. Poisoning due to inhalation injury or chemical burns should of course be treated before transportation.

Table 2.5. Amount of fluid given each time in stage infusion

Extent of burns (% TBSA)	Amount of each infusion (ml)
30–49	1000–1500
50–69	1500–2000
70 +	2000–2500

2.5 Stage Infusion

Stage infusion is the therapeutic method of choice for treating victims who must be evacuated from the scene of disaster and can receive neither resuscitation at the scene nor continuous intravenous infusion during transportation. The patient receives an intravenous infusion in stages, at each of several brief stops spread over the whole journey. We compared two groups of patients with a similar extent of burns, 30%–80% TBSA. One group (46 cases) received stage infusion during long-distance transportation to our hospital; the other (39 cases) received no infusion but traveled only a short distance. Obviously, patients in these two groups were subjected to quite different amounts of jolting during transportation. However, the incidence of shock on admission, the response to initial replacement therapy, the quantity and quality of infusion fluid, and the survival rate of the patients were all about the same. This illustrates the therapeutic effect of stage infusion, which can thus be recommended as a method of giving fluids during transportation, if continuous intravenous infusion is impossible at all. For further verification of the effect of stage infusion, an animal experiment was performed, which demonstrated that in dogs with full-thickness burn (50% TBSA) shock could be prevented or ameliorated by using stage infusion. The incidence of shock in this group of dogs did not differ significantly from that in another group of dogs suffering from the same extent of burn injury but receiving continuous intravenous infusion. At the same time, no complications such as heart overload, brain edema, or lung edema were found as a result of rapid intravenous infusion as a part of stage infusion. Therefore, we consider that stage infusion is not only effective but also fairly safe. The guidelines are as follows:

1. Dosage and duration: the amount of fluid required is calculated on the basis of percentage of body surface burned (Table 2.5). Each divided portion of infusion lasts about 2–3 h.
2. Type of fluid: balanced salt solution [for simplicity, using two-thirds isotonic saline solution and one-third isotonic lactate (M/6) or bicarbonate (1.25%) solution] is employed in most cases. In addition, 5%–10% dextran and colloids can be given if available. The ratio of balanced salt solution and colloids could be 2:1 or 1:1. Oral water or intravenous fluids of 5%–10% dextrose in water could be given correspondingly. Simple water or dextrose

solution without salt supplement should be strictly prohibited in order to prevent water intoxication.

3. Interval between infusions: after each infusion, the patient can usually be transported for a distance of 50–100 km (depending on the speed of the ambulance) or for about 2 h.

References

1. Chen GX, Wang SL, Li Ao et al. (1989) Emergency care of hydrofluoric acid burns using "immersion mixture of calcium and magnesium". Abstract of 12th burn and plastic surgery conference of PLA, Dec 1988, Guang Zhou, China, p 95
2. Burn Research Institute of the 3rd Military Medical College (ed) (1977) The treatment of burns. People's Health Publisher, Beijing, pp 1–11, 90–103
3. Arturson G (1981) The Los Alfaques disaster: a boiling-liquid, expanding-vapor explosion. Burns 7(4): 233–251

3 Initial Fluid Replacement Therapy

Fang Zhi-yang

Burn injury, particularly that resulting from extensive deep burns, is considered as a systemic disease rather than as skin damage alone. The pathophysiological changes resulting from major burns have an extensive and profound influence on almost every organ system of the victim. It is clear that the functional alterations in the organ systems make the clinical picture of burns patients more complicated.

3.1 Pathophysiological Response of Shock Stage in Severe Burns

The stress caused by severe burns induces serious pathophysiological changes when the "homeostasis" of the host is disturbed. The physician should be familiar with the body's response. In the early postburn course, or the burn shock stage, extracellular fluid loss into the interstitial space of the wound and its surroundings, even in remote areas, due to increase of capillary permeability, is the basic component of early burn hypovolemic shock. Another component of burn shock has been identified 48–72 h postburn, i.e., an increase in the concentration of fibrinogen polymers in the accumulated edematous fluid. These polymers have a molecular weight ranging from 700 000 to 1 000 000. This component probably produces mechanical obstruction of the lymphatics and venules, which drains the accumulated edematous fluid.

The increased microvascular permeability may be induced by direct heat and the release of chemical mediators, e.g., histamine, 5-hydroxytryptamine, kinins, prostaglandins, and leukotrienes, which either initiate or modulate the increased permeability of the vascular endothelium. The heat-damaged protein activates the complement and coagulation system.

Recently, it has been found that the arachidonic acid cascade from the phospholipids is involved. In the production of the prostaglandins, thromboxane is also produced, and it has the effect of inducing dermal ischemia, which is opposite to that of prostacyclin (PGI_2). The cascade is shown in Fig. 3.1.

3.1.1 Plasma Volume and Cardiac Output

Dogs sustaining a 45%–49% third-degree flame burn without fluid therapy showed a sharp drop in cardiac output, which slightly preceded the decrease in plasma volume and increase in hematocrit (Fig. 3.2). Blood volume decreased to

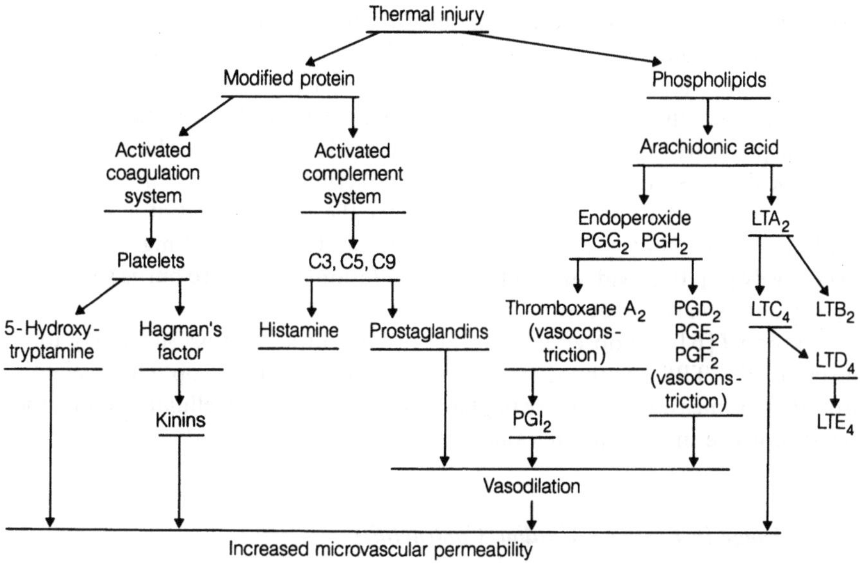

Fig. 3.1. Agents which may participate in acute-phase response leading to increased microvascular permeability and vasoconstriction (dermal ischemia). (Modified from [1, 2])

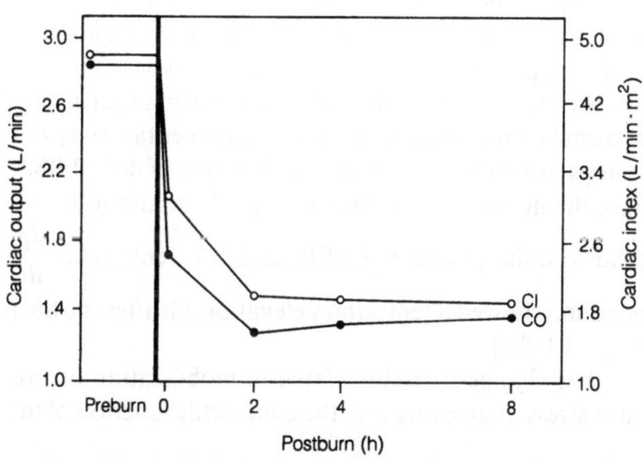

Fig. 3.2. Cardiac output and cardiac index alterations in dogs during burn shock after thermal injury

46%–77% and plasma volume to 48.8%–61.89% of normal values 2 h after the burn injury [3]. In flame injuries involving third-degree (3°) burns to 45.5% ± 3.2% of total body surface area (TBSA), the peripheral blood pressure dropped to 100 mmHg, and in the meantime the femoral vascular volume decreased to one-half its normal value, as measured with an electromagnetic flowmeter. This result indicated that the peripheral blood pressure does not represent the vascular flow volume during early burn shock [4]. Plasma leakage usually reaches its peak level 4–6 h postburn. Experimental burns in rats (3° burns 20% TBSA) showed that the increase in vascular permeability reached its peak level 1 h postburn and then gradually decreased 3–6 h later. The amount of plasma leakage estimated by the radioimmune serum albumin (RISA) method in the area of the latissimus dorsi muscle below the burn wound at 1,3, and 6 h postburn was 593.5 ± 29.51, 120.4 ± 71.8, and $58.5 \pm 27.6\,mg^{-1}\ 100\,s^{-1}$ respectively [5]. It is evident that fluid resuscitation after severe burns should be carried out as early as possible.

Moncrief [6] also observed that the cardiac output of dogs sustaining total burns of 50% TBSA without transfusion showed a sharp drop which slightly proceded the measured decrease in plasma volume and extracellular volume, and the abrupt rise in hematocrit value.

3.1.2 Change in Postburn Cardiac Contractility

The alteration in mechanism of cardiac muscle is a basic change during burn shock, but myocardial contractility has rarely been studied. Most of the medical literature has reported that the cardiac output decreases immediately after the burn injury and usually precedes the decrease in plasma volume. The mechanism of the decrease in cardiac output has been considered to be the effect of myocardial depressing factor (MDF) on the myocardium, as reported by Baxter [7]. But this hypothesis could not be confirmed experimentally by B.A. Pruitt (1989, personal communication). In an experimental study of myocardial contractility in dogs, we discovered that with 3° burns of 40% TBSA without fluid resuscitation, the mean survival time was 4–5 h; continuous measurement of left ventricular systolic pressure (LVSP) and left ventricular $\frac{dp}{dt}\max \Big/ \mathrm{IP}$ (isovolumetric pressure) showed a temporary elevation 1 h after the burn, followed by a decrease (Figs. 3.3–3.5).

The changes may be related to mobilization of circulatory functions under burn stress, suggesting that the contractile function of the myocardium decreased in the cardiac isovolumetric contraction phase. The value of $\frac{dp}{dt}\max \Big/ \mathrm{IP}$ decreased earlier than that of LVSP, and the time of beginning of shock and therapy, and the effect of pre- and postload, may be excluded. This suggests that the course of burn shock is closely related to myocardial function of contractility, which appeared to be a sensitive and early parameter of the changes in cardiac contractility, in addition to peripheral resistance and circulatory volume. The rebound of $\frac{dp}{dt}\max \Big/ \mathrm{IP}$ in the later stage may be related to the greater decrease in isovolumetric pressure than in $\frac{dp}{dt}\max$. These changes not only involve the cardiac contractility

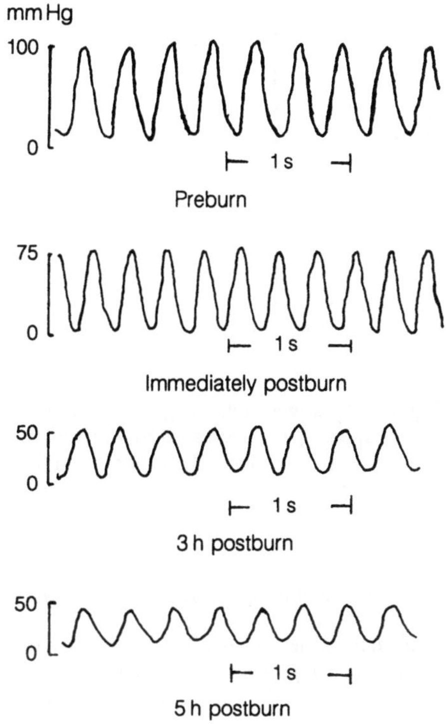

Fig. 3.3. Changes in left ventricular systolic pressure in rabbits after thermal injury

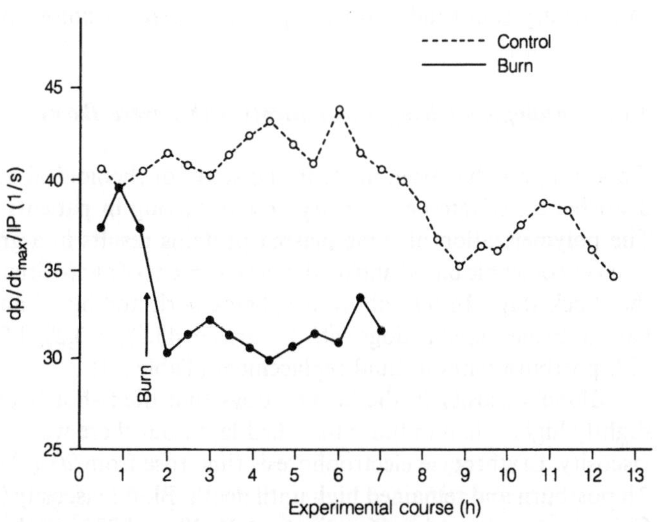

Fig. 3.4. Comparison of $\frac{dp}{dt}\max \Big/ \text{IP}$ changes between burned and control dogs

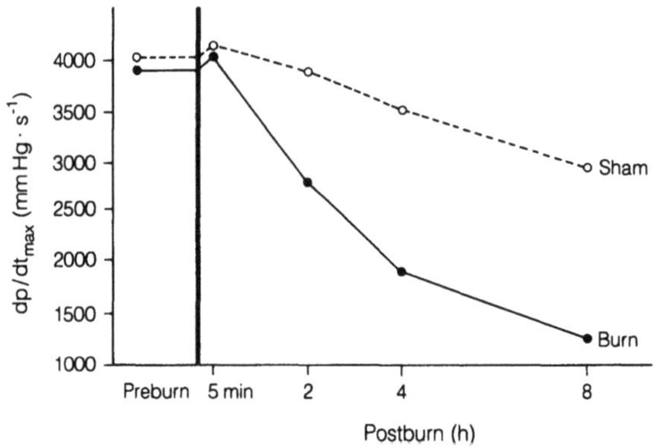

Fig. 3.5. Changes in dp/dt_{max} in dogs during burn shock after thermal injury. Range and rate of dp/dt_{max} was decreased by 400 mmHg/s per hour postburn in the burned group, and was decreased by 50 mmHg/s per hour in the control group (dogs subjected to a sham burn procedure)

but also the diastolic function. The $\frac{dp}{dt}$max value decreases to 80%–60% of the mean preburn value 2–5 h after burn injury, and at the same time the L_4 value also decreases [8,9]. Liu and Fang [9] and Cheng et al. [10], in experiments with dogs sustaining 3° burns to 45% of TBSA and rabbits suffering 3° burns to 20% of TBSA measured LVSP, $\frac{dp}{dt}$, and $p-\frac{dp}{dt}$ loop after treatment with hypertonic Ringer's solution. The results suggested that this therapeutic regimen markedly improved cardiac contractility in the treated group. The decrease in cardiac contractility is not induced by negative cardiac chromotropic effects.

3.1.3 Rheological Changes in Patients with Severe Burns

Good progress has been made in the study of rheological abnormalities in the disturbances of microcirculatory flow occurring in patients with severe burns. The polymerization of some plasma proteins results in a great increase in the viscosity of whole blood and further impairment of microcirculation, especially in the shock stage. In our laboratory, hematocrit and blood and plasma viscosity have been measured in dogs with 3° burns to 45.5% ± 3.2% TBSA at 2, 4, 6, 8, and 10 h postburn without fluid replacement (Table 3.1).

Blood viscosity in the burned dogs that died shortly after the injury was slightly higher than in those that died later, but there was no change in plasma viscosity. Erythrocyte electrophoresis time rose from 20 ± 2.91 s to 23 ± 1.7 s at 2 h postburn and remained high until death. Blood viscosity (SDZ-3 viscometer, China) was measured in 16 patients at 24, 48, and 72 h postburn. They sustained total burns to 69.03% TBSA (range, 35%–100%) and 3° burns to 18.7% TBSA,

Table 3.1. Rheological changes after severe burns in dogs without fluid replacement

	Preburn	Postburn (h)				
		2	4	6	8	10
Hematocrit	46.35 ± 5.68	(a) 56.50 ± 6.89	55.6 ± 4.78	58.3 ± 8.73		
		(b) 54.00 ± 2.15	59.0 ± 2.65	58.7 ± 3.51	60.30 ± 5.51	63.3 ± 4.18
Blood viscosity (P)	5.97 ± 0.99	(a) 9.10 ± 2.98	8.58 ± 0.94	11.5 ± 6.52		
		(b) 7.13 ± 0.86	8.80 ± 1.04	8.70 ± 0.37	9.10 ± 1.25	8.50 ± 1.14
Plasma viscosity (P)	1.71 ± 0.18	(a) 1.85 ± 0.28	1.82 ± 0.29	2.09 ± 0.15		
		(b) 1.73 ± 0.12	1.73 ± 0.20	1.63 ± 0.06	1.80 ± 0.17	1.80 ± 0.48

(a) 3° burns to 45.9% ± 3.05% of TBSA, died within 6 h, $n = 7$.
(b) 3° burns to 45.3% ± 3.51% of TBSA, died within 12 h, $n = 3$.

and the results were 6.33 ± 0.83 P, 6.30 ± 1.60 P, and 5.85 ± 0.70 P respectively. The values returned to normal 7 days and 14 days postburn. These results showed that even with routine fluid resuscitation within 72 h after injury the blood viscosity remained high [10].

Blood viscosity changes are minimized by prompt and complete blood volume restoration. In our experiment the increase in blood viscosity is more or less related to inadequate replacement and low-speed infusion. It is paralleled by the changes in hematocrit to some degree. Mao Ning et al. reported that leukocyte adhesiveness in the venules was markedly reduced after injection of 20% *Lugusticum Wallichii* Franch (LWF) in burned rabbits [11].

3.1.4 Changes in Endogenous Opioid Substances

A decade ago the opioid receptors and their native ligands and the endogenous opioid peptides were discovered. To date, over ten opioid peptides with different molecular weights have been isolated from biological tissues and demonstrated to have opioid actions in vitro and in vivo [12].

Recently, there have been many reports dealing with the importance of these endogenous opioid substances in the regulation of the activity of the cardiovascular system. In the course of development of burn shock, these substances are most likely to be involved.

3.1.4.1 Enkephalin Content in Rat Brain After Scalding

Leu-enkephalin Content in Regional Brain Tissue. Immediately after the burn, the leu-enkephalin (LEK) content is reduced in the hypothalamus, corpus striatum, and lower brain stem, but is increased in the thalamus ($p < 0.05$), compared with the controls. The LEK content in the four aforementioned areas is reduced 1 h after the burn, especially in the hypothalamus ($p < 0.01$) and lower brain stem ($p < 0.05$). Three hours postburn the difference in LEK content between burned rats and controls is not statistically significant.

Effect of Burn of the Met-enkephalin Content. Immediately after the burn, MEK content in the corpus striatum and hypothalamus is reduced by 86% ($p < 0.01$) and 55% ($p < 0.05$) of the control value, respectively. An hour after the burn, the MEK content in the hypothalamus is still at a lower level ($p < 0.01$) while 3 h after the burn, the MEK content is reduced only in the corpus striatum ($p < 0.01$), but, in contrast, increased in the lower brain stem ($p < 0.01$) [13].

3.1.4.2 Dynorphin B Content in Hypothalamus and Pituitary in Severely Scalded Rats

In 1982 Goldstein and Udlenfried isolated dynorphin B from the brain tissue. Wang Chang-Hai et al. showed [14] that dynorphin B content of the brain of burned rat 30 min after 3° burn to 20% TBSA burn was greatly increased in the pituitary and the hypothalamus, about 9.89- and 14.72-fold over controls, respectively. Two hours later the dynorphin B level in the pituitary and the hypothalamus decreased.

3.1.4.3 β-Endorphin Level in Burned Rats and Patients

The ir-β-endorphin content in plasma and the pituitary was increased about 10.8- and 30.3-fold, respectively, at 2 h after scalding, but it was reduced significantly in the hypothalamus. Six and 24 h after the injury, the ir-β-endorphin level in plasma, pituitary, and hypothalamus was increased markedly [15]. These results suggest that endogenous opioid substances are important factors in the pathophysiological course during the early stages of burn shock.

3.1.4.4 Opioid Antagonists in Burn Shock

The use of naloxone has provided crucial evidence supporting the role of an endogenous opioid system in the pathogenesis of experimental shock and spinal injury. Numerous antidotal chemical studies have also indicated that this opioid antagonist has therapeutic effects on circulatory function in septic and cardiogenic shock.

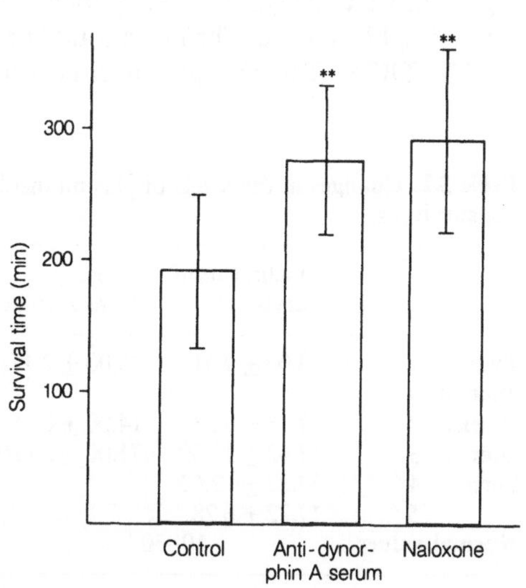

Fig. 3.6. Effect of antidynorphin A serum and naloxone on survival time in scalded rats.** $p < 0.01$

Recently some investigators have reported the use of opioid antagonists such as naloxone, dynorphin A antiserum, and β-endorphin antiserum, for the treatment of burn shock, For example, Lin Bao-Cheng et al. [16] observed that naloxone significantly improved cardiovascular function, blood pressure, and respiratory rate, prevented a fall in body temperature, and prolonged survival time of burned rats after injection of 50 μg/77 μl naloxone/saline into the lateral ventricle. Gao Guang-Cheng et al. [17] reported that after injection of naloxone or dynorphin A antiserum via the caudal vein immediately postburn, the survival time (Fig. 3.6), blood pressure, and ECG pattern (P-R, QRS, ST) of rats were significantly improved.

3.1.5 Endocrine Changes in Severely Burned Patients

The hypothalamus, adrenal cortex, and medulla form an integrated system in response to stress. Burn injury is known to initiate a series of endocrine and metabolic changes.

It has been shown that the circulating or urinary catecholamine level was significantly increased on the day of admission or 2 days after the burn and at 3 and 4 weeks following burn injury. At 5 weeks postburn the levels declined to normal. In our cases changes in urinary epinephrine content were more marked than changes in norepinephrine 2 days after the burn [18, 19]. Plasma cortisol, renin, and angiotensin II levels were found to be significantly elevated, and the elevations in cortisol and renin were more pronounced until the end of the 4- to 5-week period following the burn. The high level may have lasted for such a long period because other associated complications contributed to the increase.

In our study, 20 patients with total burns covering a mean 55.9% ± 18.7% of TBSA (range, 25%–94%) and mean 3° burns of 32.5% ± 22.87% TBSA (range, 0%–65%) were analyzed. Three patients died 2 or 3 weeks postburn and the remaining 17 survived. The mean total burns area of those who died was 90.6% ± 8.7% TBSA. The changes in circulating levels of plasma cortisol, renin,

Table 3.2. Changes in the levels of plasma insulin and fast blood sugar in survivors and nonsurvivors

		Insulin (μu/ml)$\bar{X}$ ± SE		Fast blood sugar (mg/dl)$\bar{X}$ ± SE	
		Survivors	Nonsurvivors	Survivors	Nonsurvivors
Two days after burn		33.00 ± 9.51	33.00 ± 2.47	167.13 ± 11.09	209.00
Weeks after burn	2	27.73 ± 6.23	14.00 ± 0.25	138.93 ± 9.13	113.00
	3	43.42 ± 11.69	71.00 ± 25.10	153.75 ± 23.34	386.00
	4	33.22 ± 12.63	–	155.60 ± 25.73	200
	5	17.22 ± 6.28	–	120.94 ± 13.86	220
Normal values		10–30		80–120	

Table 3.3. Changes in the levels of plasma cortisol, renin, and angiotensin in survivors and nonsurvivors

	Cortisol (μg/ml)$\bar{X} \pm SE$		Renin (ng/ml)$\bar{X} \pm SE$		Angiotensin (pg/ml)$\bar{X} \pm SE$	
	Survivors	Nonsurvivors	Survivors	Nonsurvivors	Survivors	Nonsurvivors
Two days after burn	40.82 ± 7.67	66.25 ± 11.93	6.51 ± 2.54	0.29	155.39 ± 45.76	142.00
Weeks after burn 2	40.57 ± 6.86	39.75 ± 9.81	5.82 ± 1.55	1.72	30.09 ± 6.35	14.00
3	42.87 ± 5.36	51.75 ± 1.14	5.06 ± 1.02	0.62	95.40 ± 27.60	180.00
4	20.33 ± 4.55	24.45 ± 8.15	2.27 ± 0.39	0.30	52.40 ± 10.44	—
5	31.33 ± 9.36	87.50	3.51 ± 0.40	—	79.91 ± 13.65	—
Normal values	12.00 ± 2.00		0.53 ± 0.47		26.0 ± 10.0	

Table 3.4. Changes in the levels of urine catecholamine, epinephrine, and norepinephrine in survivors and nonsurvivors

	Catecholamine (μg/24 h urine)$\bar{X} \pm SE$		Epinephrine (μg/24 h urine)$\bar{X} \pm SE$		Norepinephrine (μg/24 h urine)$\bar{X} \pm SE$	
	Survivors	Nonsurvivors	Survivors	Nonsurvivors	Survivors	Nonsurvivors
Two days after burn	57.77 ± 19.07	–[a]	18.22 ± 5.82	–[a]	39.47 ± 13.70	–[a]
Weeks after burn 2	38.57 ± 8.83	20.33 ± 1.59	20.88 ± 6.42	8.57 ± 1.47	23.60 ± 5.32	11.76 ± 2.60
3	32.46 ± 8.21	26.88	8.74 ± 1.21	3.84	22.46 ± 7.22	23.04
4	39.85 ± 8.64	8.60	12.96 ± 3.56	4.30	25.09 ± 7.00	4.30
5	20.71 ± 3.99	–	15.42 ± 5.77	–	22.18 ± 6.22	–
Normal value range	28.70 ± 9.10		7.60 ± 5.30		20.50 ± 7.10	

[a] No urine collected.

angiotensin II, insulin, and fasting blood sugar and the changes in urinary catecholamine were compared between the surviving and nonsurviving patients. The results are shown in Tables 3.2–3.4. The nonsurvivors showed a continuous rise in plasma levels of cortisol, angiotensin II, insulin, and blood sugar, but a decline in plasma renin levels at the end of week 4. Other workers have demonstrated markedly elevated plasma cortisol levels with suppressed insulin levels in nonsurviving burn patients [20]. In contrast, the plasma insulin levels were elevated at the end of week 3 in our investigation. Goodall et al. [21] demonstrated subnormal catecholamine in nonsurviving burn patients, believed to be due to adrenal insufficiency. This result concurs with that of our investigation.

3.2 Fluid Resuscitation

There are still many disputes regarding immediate fluid replacement in the acute phase of severe burns. Plasma and electrolyte solutions have been recommended as essential fluids in the routine formulae, e.g., the Evans, Brooke, and Parkland formulae.

3.2.1 Colloid Solution

The advantages of fluid resuscitation using colloid solution have been documented. Cardiac output is significantly better, and pulmonary vascular resistance and lung water do not increase to the level that is seen in patients receiving crystalloid solution. The use of plasma as the main fluid resuscitation solution helps to maintain important immunoproteins and antibodies close to normal levels. The antibacterial defense mechanism is, therefore, less impaired and consequently the incidence of burn wound infection and sepsis is significantly reduced.

3.2.1.1 Comparison Between Shock and Nonshock Burns

The amounts of colloid and crystalloid solution used in fluid resuscitation in shock and nonshock adult burns patients are compared in Table 3.5 [22].

In a group of children with burns of 40% TBSA the amount of colloid and crystalloid in the nonshock group was 1.3504 ± 0.1739 ml (mean $\pm$ SD) and in the shock group 2.038 ± 0.1796 ml. The ratio of colloid to crystalloid was 1:1.38 in the former and 1:0.85 in the latter group. A fluid formula was introduced as a clinical guide: First 24 h: $2° + 3°$ burns (% TBSA) × body weight (kg) × 1.5 ml (colloid + crystalloid) + 2000–3000 ml (daily water requirement).

If total burns cover $\geqq 70\%$ TBSA or 3° burns cover $\geqq 50\%$ TBSA the colloid to crystalloid ratio is 1:1, and if total burns cover $< 70\%$ TBSA ratio is 1:2. Half of

Table 3.5. Fluid resuscitation in adult burns patients

Extent of burns (% TBSA)	Nonshock (ml $\bar{X} \pm SD$)	Shock (ml $\bar{X} \pm SD$)	p
40%–59%	1.0626 ± 0.0811	1.4640 ± 0.1738	<0.05
60%–100%	1.2487 ± 0.0641	1.6480 ± 0.2996	<0.01

Colloid:crystalloid = 1:1.

Table 3.6. Fluid resuscitation regimes during shock

	Colloid (ml/kg/1% TBSA)		Lactated Ringer's solution (ml/kg/1% TBSA)	5% dextrose in water (ml)
	Whole blood	Dextran		
First 24 h	0.3	0.3	0.6	2000
Second 24 h	0.15	0.15	0.3	2000

the total amount is to be given in the first 8 h with the remainder during the following 16 h.

3.2.1.2 Modified Early Fluid Resuscitation Formula

A modified early fluid resuscitation formula using colloid and crystalloid solution was introduced by Guo and Sheng [23]. It uses fresh whole blood and dextran instead of plasma as colloid. In the first 24 h, 0.3 ml whole blood, 0.3 ml dextran, and 0.6 ml lactated Ringer's solution per kilogram body wt. for each percent TBSA are given. The daily basic requirement of water is given by infusion of 5% dextrose in water in the amount of 70 ml/kg body w. In the second 24 h the amount of whole blood, dextran, and lactated Ringer's solution given is half that in the first 24 h. Daily water requirement is maintained. The remaining principles of the fluid resuscitation regimen are the same as those in the first 24 h (Table 3.6).

In order to confirm the advantage of whole blood transfusion, Guo Zhen-Rong has carried out a series of clinical and experimental studies. From the data, it is concluded that the use of whole blood during burn shock does not increase hemoconcentration or viscosity (Fig. 3.7). Platelet adherence and aggregation do not significantly change (Fig. 3.8), so whole blood does not influence hemorheological variables. It also corrects anemia, hypoproteinemia, and oncotic pressure (Figs. 3.9–3.10), improves myocardial contractility and acid-base balance, reduces tissue edema (Figs. 3.11–3.12), and improves host defense. The results in both patients and dogs indicate that the use of whole blood for fluid resuscitation in burn shock is beneficial.

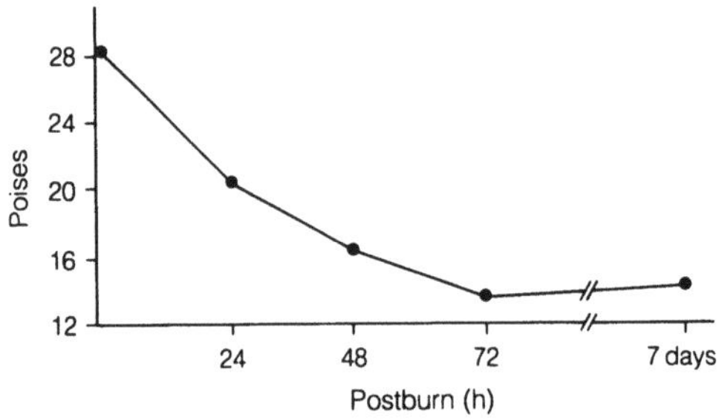

Fig. 3.7. Sequential changes in blood viscosity (in poises) of 22 burn patients at a shear rate of 10

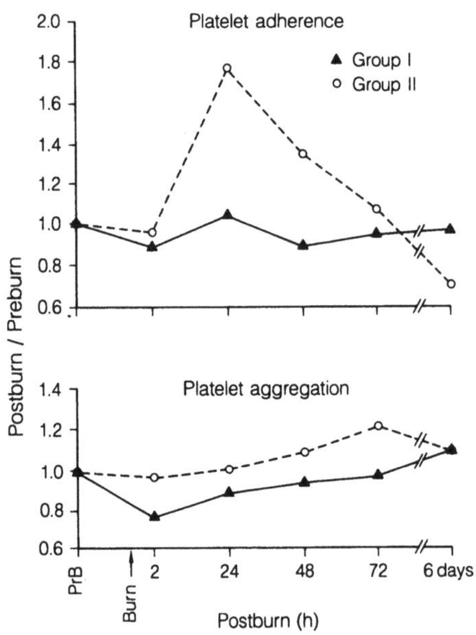

Fig. 3.8. Sequential changes in platelet aggregation and platelet adherence (expressed as a ratio of postburn/preburn values). *PrB*, preburn

3.2.2 Fluid Formula Using Hypertonic Solution

Forty years ago, Fox (1968) [24] treated his burned patients with slightly hypertonic (1/6 *M*) electrolyte solution or lactic solution (167 m mol Na) until the urine pH was neutral or highly alkaline and the blood pH was in the normal range. The mixture of 500 ml isotonic lactate Ringer's solution and 80 ml M sodium lactate equal 250 mmol hypertonic lactate Riger's solution was used as a rule. The hypertonic solution used by Monafo [25] contained 300 mmol/l sodium, 200 mmol/l lactate, and 100 mmol/l chloride, and it was

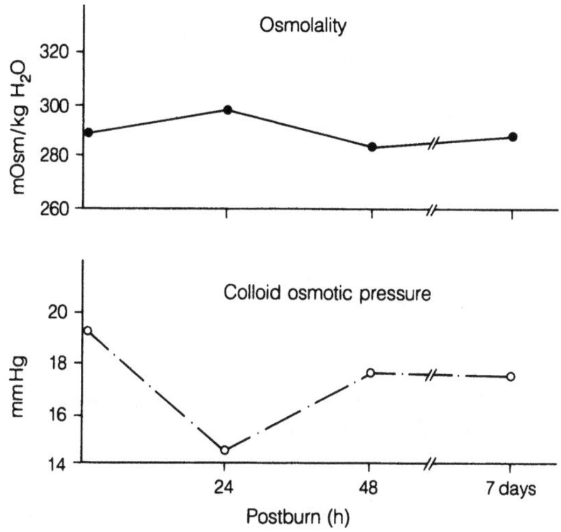

Fig. 3.9. Changes in serum colloid osmotic pressure and osmolality in 31 patients

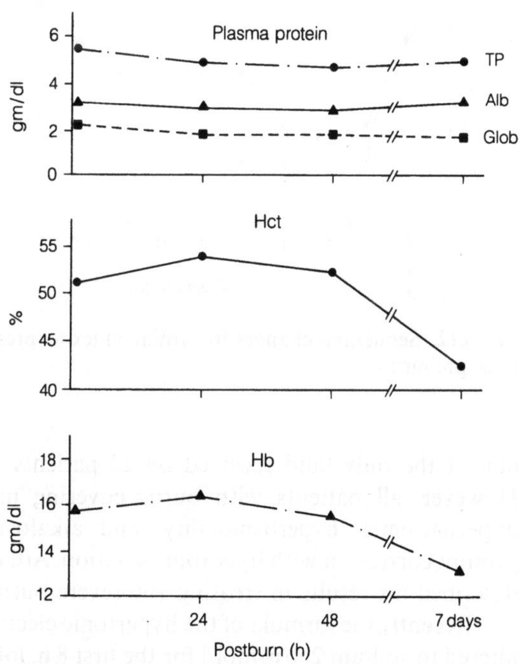

Fig. 3.10. Changes in homoglobin, hematocrit, and plasma protein in 293 burn patients. *TP*, total protein; *Alb*, albumin; *Hct*, hematocrit; *Glob*, globulin; *Hb*, hemoglobin

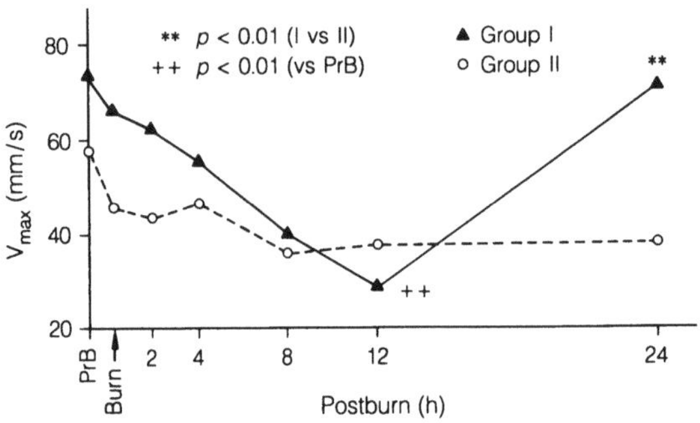

Fig. 3.11. Sequential changes in V_{max} after burn. V_{max}, maximum velocity of myocardial contraction; *PrB*, preburn

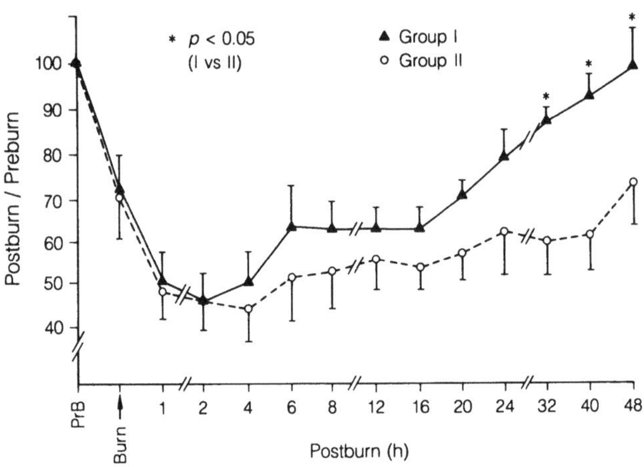

Fig. 3.12. Sequential changes in cardiac index (expressed as ratio of postburn/preburn). *PrB*, preburn

almost the only fluid received by 23 patients with 22%–95% TBSA burned. However, all patients with burns covering more than 65% TBSA showed hypernatremia, hyperosmolality, and alkalosis, which sometimes required prompt correction with hypotonic solution. After his initial publication, Monafo described his results in treating 106 severe burns patients in 1973 [26].

Recently the formula of the hypertonic electrolyte solution therapy has been altered to sodium 250 mmol/l for the first 8 h, followed by a solution containing sodium 220 mmol/l for the second 8 h, a solution containing sodium 190 mmol/l for the third 8 h, and finally a solution containing sodium 150 mmol/l for the next day.

Eight male and two female patients with burns involving mean TBSA 46% (range, 30%–55%) and 3° burns affecting mean TBSA 30% (range, 0%–45%) were

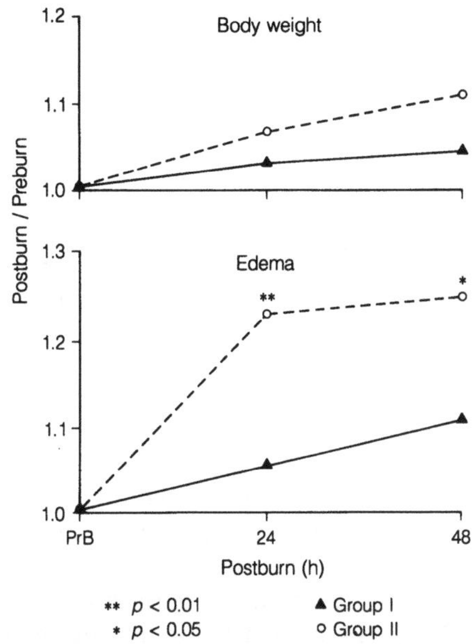

Fig. 3.13. Sequential changes in tissue edema and body weight (expressed as ratio of postburn/preburn). *PrB*, preburn

entered into our clinical trial. The average infusion rate was 1.52 ml/kg per 1% TBSA burned, with sodium 0.60 mmol/kg per 1%, in the first 24 h, and 1.24 ml/kg per 1%, with sodium 0.2 mmol/kg per 1%, in the second 24 h. Urinary output was 62.4 ml/h for the first 24 h and 93.1 ml/h in the second 24 h. Plasma sodium was slightly increased or maintained in the normal range. There was only one case with plasma osmolality elevated to 343 mOsm/kg H_2O, when the serum normal range. There was only one case with plasma osmolality elevated to 343 mOsm/kg, when the serum sodium level was as high as 176 mmol/l. The hypertonic electrolyte solution was then discontinued and the patient recovered. All patients taking part in the clinical trial survived [27].

The mechanism of action of sodium is based on the fact that it is the main extracellular cation responsible for maintenance of extracellular volume. Postburn alteration of water and electrolytes leads to a tendency toward hyponatremia, as mentioned earlier, and hypoalbuminemia. The changes in permeability of the capillary wall make leakage of water and electrolytes and osmotic imbalance inevitable (Starling's law). Administration of hypertonic lactated solution may improve the capillary osmotic pressure, which tends to draw water from the cells into the functional extracellular fluid, thereby lowering tissue edema, increasing the extracellular volume, and resulting in a better therapeutic effect. The hypertonic sodium tends to lower aldosterone secretion and causes osmotic diuresis (Fig. 3.13).

The addition of albumin (12.5 g/l) to hypertonic crystalloid solution (240 mmol/l sodium) has been employed with success by Jelenko et al. (1979)

Table 3.7. Comparison of hypertonic solution and lactated Ringer's solution: infusion volume, urinary output, and body weight change

	Hypertonic group (HG)	Balanced Ringer's group (BG)	Control group (CG)
Influsion volume (ml) in first 24 h	343.6 ± 26	627.5 ± 62.9	
Na^+ (mmol/kg/% BSA)	1.0	1.0	
Urine volume (ml/kg/h)	2.060 ± 0.50*	2.81 ± 0.59**	0.69 ± 0.6
Diuretic index	0.381 ± 0.092*	0.286 ± 0.065	
Body weight (kg)	+ 5.0 ± 0.3*	+ 10.7 ± 0.2	

*$p < 0.05$; **$p < 0.01$.

[28], and a controlled clinical trial with this solution demonstrated rapid, effective fluid resuscitation with minimal edema formation.

Experimental studies with rabbits were carried out to clarify the mechanism of fluid resuscitation in burn shock. Twenty-four rabbits were given 3° burns of 30% TBSA by immersion in water at 100°C water for 25 s. The animals were divided into three groups of eight: the hypertonic salt solution group (HG), balanced salt solution group (BG), and no fluids (control group). In the HG, the electrolyte contents were Na^+ 240 m mol/l, K^+ 3 m mol/l, Mg^{2+} 3 m mol/l, Ca^{2+} 4 m mol/l, Cl^- 100 m mol/l, and lactate 150 m mol/l, while in the BG the electrolyte contents were Na^+ 130 mmol/l, K^+ 3 mmol/l, Cl^- 83 mmol/l, and lactate 53 mmol/l. The infusion started 30 min after the burn with Na^+ 1 mmol/kg per 1% TBSA burned in the first 24 h. One half of the calculated total fluid volume was given in the first 8 h postburn, and the other half was given in the next 16 h (Table 3.7). Plasma and intraerythrocyte concentrations of Na^+ and K^+ were determined before burn and at 4, 12, and 24 h postburn. The results are shown in Fig. 3.14.

Plasma and intraerythrocyte Na^+ levels decreased in all groups in the early postburn hours. In the CG the plasma Na^+ level decreased continuously but the intraerythrocyte Na^+ level increased gradually. In the BG, however, both plasma and intraerythrocyte Na^+ levels increased gradually. Moreover, in the BG both plasma and intraerythrocyte Na^+ levels returned to normal by the end of the first postburn day [29]. The therapeutic effect of early fluid resuscitation with hypertonic salt solution was assessed by analyzing the mechanism of electrolyte regulation of the renal epithelial cell membrane through determination of $Na^+ - K^+$ ATPase activity. The postburn $Na^+ - K^+$ ATPase activity of the membrane decreased by 70% ($p < 0.01$) of its normal value in the controls, but only by 20%–30% in the HG and the BG ($p < 0.05$) (Fig. 3.15).

It is, therefore, obvious that kidney function is relatively satisfactory when hypertonic salt solution is used in early fluid resuscitation after burns.

Recently Mehokenus et al. [30] reported that, according to the Fox formula, a solution of sodium 224 mmol/l was given to burned piglets (25–30 kg) after an

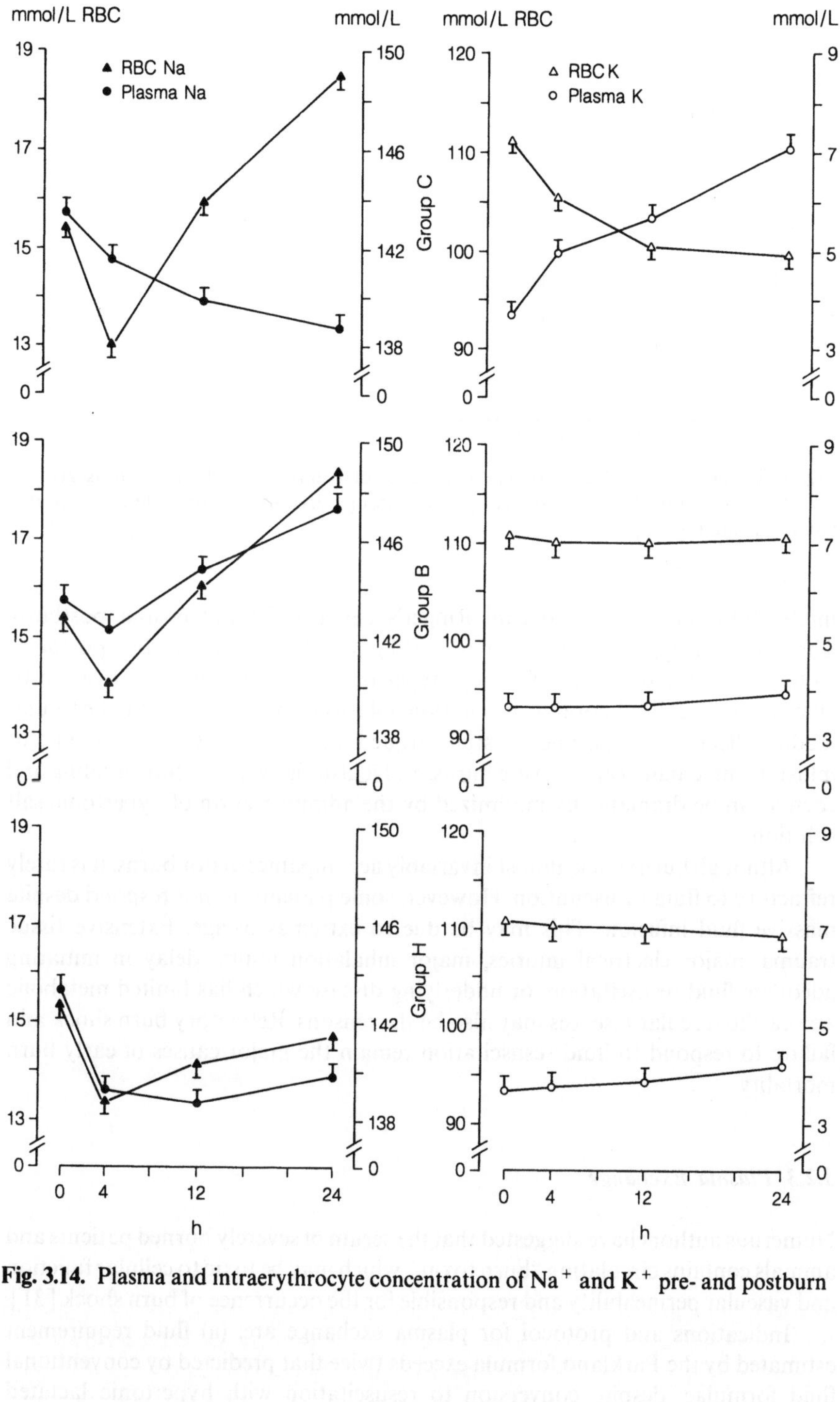

Fig. 3.14. Plasma and intraerythrocyte concentration of Na^+ and K^+ pre- and postburn

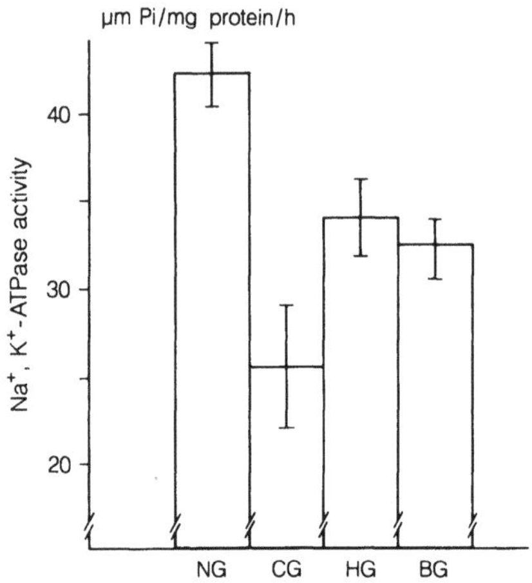

Fig. 3.15. Na^+-K^+-ATPase activity of renal tubular epithelial cells in various groups. *NG*, normal groups; *CG*, control group (burn group); *HG*, hypertonic saline group; *BG*, balanced saline group

initial bolus infusion of 1000 ml Ringer's between 30 and 60 min postburn. Thereafter the hypertonic solution of 1 ml/kg per 1% was given 2–24 h postburn. In terms of hemodynamic efficiency, hypertonic salt solution has proved to be efficient as a colloid-contained solution infusion, in spite of a smaller fluid-loading effect. This experimental study argued the importance of an initial bolus infusion immediately after severe burns, and it also showed that fluid loading and edema can be dramatically minimized by the administration of hypertonic salt solution.

Although burn shock almost invariably accompanies major burns, it is rarely refractory to fluid resuscitation. However, some patients do not respond despite massive fluid infusion. This may be due to extremes of age. Extensive tissue trauma, major electrical injuries, major inhalation injury, delay in initiating adequate fluid resuscitation, or underlying disease which has limited metabolic and cardiovascular reserves may also be the reasons. Refractory burn shock and failure to respond to fluid resuscitation remain the major causes of early burn mortality.

3.2.3 Plasma Exchange

Numerous authors have suggested that the serum of severely burned patients and animals contains circulating "burn toxin," which may be toxic to cellular function and vascular permeability and responsible for the occurrence of burn shock [31].

Indications and protocol for plasma exchange are: (a) fluid requirement estimated by the Parkland formula exceeds twice that predicted by conventional fluid formulae, despite conversion to resuscitation with hypertonic lactated sodium solution, (b) massive myoglobinuria associated with failure to respond to fluid resuscitation failure (c) failure to respond to fluid resuscitation, with persistent lactic acidemia, depressed mental status, and arterial hypotension.

The plasma exchange procedure involved plasmapheresis in adult patients by simultaneously replacing milliliter for milliliter 1.5 times the patient's calculated blood volume with type-specific fresh frozen plasma. The blood volume for adult males was estimated to equal approximately 7% of their total body weight in kilograms. For females and children the estimated blood volume was 6% of their body weight. Fluid resuscitation with Ringer's lactate solution was continued throughout the course of plasma exchange and modified with the guidance of urine output [32].

Completion of fluid resuscitation after burn shock is defined by:

(a) ability of the patient to maintain adequate urine output for two consecutive hours at a given rate of fluid infusion; (b) resolution of lactic and metabolic acidosis; and (c) stable vital signs, such as recovery of mental states. The plasma exchange therapy is then discontinued.

Maintenance fluid requirements are increased in patients with major burns and are predicted by the following formulae:

Evaporative water loss from wound = (25 + % TBSA) × (BSA m^2) ml/h.

Other maintenance fluid requirements (urine, stool, respiratory loses, etc.) = (62.5 ml) × (TBSA m^2) ml/h.

Thus, total maintenance fluid requirements equal evaporative + insensible loss = (87.5 + % TBSA) × (BSA m^2) = ml/h (BSA = body surface calculated from the nomogram Dubois).

Plasma exchange may provide a potential alternative for fluid resuscitation in burn shock by returning the altered internal environment toward normal. The mechanism of action of plasma exchange involves the removal of circulating toxic factors or replacement of specific deficiencies such as coagulation factors, serum transport of binding protein, opsonic protein, complement, immunoglobulin, fibronectin, and other components.

3.3 Complications of Fluid Resuscitation

Complications may occur in the fluid resuscitation stage after severe burns. The most common complications encountered are hyper- or hyponatremia, acidosis, and acute renal failure.

3.3.1 Hypernatremia or Hyponatremia

Hypernatremia is commonly seen in burns patients who have received hypertonic saline solution. The clinical response to this kind of fluid deficit is loss of body weight, increase in serum sodium and chloride above 150 mmol/l and

110 mmol/l, respectively, an increase in serum and urine osmolality, elevated blood urea nitrogen (BUN), and a reduction in urinary sodium. When serum sodium increases to a level of 170–180 mmol/l, delirium, convlsion, and death may ensue.

Treatment by replacement of extracellular fluid deficit, using 5% dextrose in water in adult patients, increases urinary output and facilitates the return of serum sodium and chloride to normal.

Hyponatremia rarely occurs in extensive burns of adults during burn resuscitation, but occurs more frequently in children, when they rapidly receive electrolyte-free or hypotonic solution. It is quickly induced, and may result in convulsion due to water intoxication. Treatment consists of restriction of 5% dextrose in water and the administration of a limited volume of 3%–5% sodium chloride. The amount of sodium given should not exceed 20 g, and the sodium must be administered at a slow rate over a 6- to 12-h period.

3.3.2 Acidosis

Acid-base imbalance with metabolic acidosis is most frequently seen in severe burn patients in the early postburn period. It appears that when the arterial pH falls below 7.35 and there is significant decrease of base excess, there may be a state of metabolic acidosis. Inadequate tissue perfusion is the most common cause of metabolic acidosis, which has a profound effect on the cardiovascular system, producing a decreasing myocardial contractility, and a decreased response of myocardium and peripheral circulation to catecholamine, predisposing the patient to cardiac arrhythmias.

Treatment consists of correction of peripheral perfusion, maintaining adequate oxygen saturation, the administration of sodium bicarbonate with 7.5% solution in an amount to correct the base deficit by ml 7.5% $NaHCO_3 = 0.77 \times$ body wt. (kg) $\times$ 5 mmol, or Tris buffer (0.3 *M*).

3.3.3 Acute Renal Failure

Renal damage is often seen in major burns, but it is less common in current clinical practice, particularly in burn centers where the appropriate early fluid resuscitation can be carried out. Acute renal failure (ARF) appears to be an early postburn complication due to fluid loss and hypovolemic shock, severe hemoglobinuria and myoglobinuria, and other toxic agents, and its incidence varies from 1.3% to 38% depending on the cause of renal damage. Mortality is high once the diagnosis has been established.

The pathological changes of ARF can occur in the glomerulus, the tubule, or both. The damage can be worsened by hypovolemia from fluid loss and by hemorrhage, hemoglobinuria, and myoglobinuria from hemolysis and unremoved devitalized muscle and nephrotoxic agents, particularly antibiotics with nephrotoxicity.

Oliguria is the most common clinical criterion of the diagnosis of ARF and is a symptomatic diagnosis in itself.

Differential diagnosis between oliguria and ARF can be carried out by further determination of specific gravity and osmolarity of urine, the ratio of urine osmolarity to plasma osmolarity, urine urea to plasma urea, and urine creatinine to plasma creatinine, urine sodium, fractional excretion of sodium (FeNa), α-glucosidase, leucine aminopeptidase (LAP), and serum and urine β_2-microglobulin.

Urine sodium concentration is by itself an index of distal tubular function response to aldosterone. Serum creatinine concentration reflects the efficiency of glomerular filtration.

The enzyme α-glucosidase (with a molecular weight of 200 000) is specific for the epithelium of the proximal renal tubule. Increased urinary concentration of α-glucosidase indicates that the lesion is located in the proximal tubule. Of similar significant is the increased urinary concentration of leucine aminopeptidase. This enzyme is in fact present, although not exclusively, in the epithelium of the proximal renal tubule, while β_2-microglobulin, a serum protein of 11 000 daltons, is completely filtered by the glomerulus and then almost completely reabsorbed (99%) by the proximal tubule. An increased amount of β_2-microglobulin in the urine is suggestive of proximal tubule damage, while an increased serum concentration reflects a decreased glomerular filtration rate [33].

In addition to the tubule damage, a glomerular lesion can also be assumed on the basis of increased serum β_2-microglobulin in conjunction with low creatinine clearance and proteinemia of the mixed type (Table 3.8).

In clinical practice, caution should be exercised in making a diagnosis during early fluid resuscitation in burn shock. It is often the case that the fluid volume calculated by the fluid formula turns out be inadequate for various reasons, such as delayed administration or associated injury with fluid or blood loss. More fluid should then be infused to meet the patient's needs. In practice, if oliguria is

Table 3.8. Differential diagnosis: oliguria versus acute renal failure (ARF)

	Oliguria	ARF
Urine specific gravity	1.015	1.010
Urine osmolarity	>500	<300
Osmolality (urine/plasma)	2–5:1	1:1
Urea (urine/plasma)	>8	<3
Creatinine (urine/plasma)	>40	<20
Urine sodium (mmol/l)	<10	>30
FE_{NA} (%)	$<3\%$	$>5\%$
α-Glucosidase (μg/l)	Normal	Increased
Leucine aminopeptidase (LAP) (μg/l)	Normal	Increased
β_2-Microglobulin (μg/l)	Normal	Increased

FE_{Na}, excreted fraction of filtered sodium.

accompanied by changes of vital signs indicating hypovolemic shock, more fluid is prescribed. If oliguria persists in spite of improvement in the vital signs, additional fluid is mandatory; usually 1000 ml or more, including colloidal and balanced electrolyte solutions, should be infused within 30 min, followed by 5% glucose solution. When necessary, diuretics such as furosemide or sodium ethacrynate are prescribed. Mannitol is not a diuretic agent of choice because of the potential occurrence of solute nephrosis. If oliguria is not relieved, or is even followed by anuria, i.e., when every effort at treating oliguria fails, the diagnosis of ARF is made, and the treatment should proceed accordingly.

The universal homeostatic response of severely burned patients is the release of arginine vasopressin (AVP) to restore volume with less water retention. The AVP rcsponsc savcs valuablc volumc at thc cxpcnsc of fluid tonicity in the presence of free water administration. Administration of 5% glucose in water as free water, as reported, will rapidly lower body fluid tonicity, and renal edema will ensue, resulting in ARF.

Additional solutions of crystalloids and Ringer's lactate to increase urinary output will lead to further edema formation in the kidney as well.

It must be remembered that in fluid resuscitation in severely burned patients, fluid formulae can only be used as general guidelines. The volume of fluid to be infused must be individually assessed in accordance with the patient's requirements in order to avoid the occurrence of multiple system organ failure, including ARF.

3.4 Study of Combined Treatment in Severe Burns

Burn shock is a very complex pathophysiological course which consists of many clinical problems to be treated. Although fluid replacement therapy is of primary importance for the treatment of hypovolemia, additional combined treatment may also play an important role in treating many pathophysiological changes induced by some chemical mediators or metabolites. Therefore, combined treatment of early burns with fluid as the main component is recommended.

3.4.1 Modulation of the Arachidonic Acid Cascade

3.4.1.1 Aspirin-Like Drugs

The aspirin-like drugs, i.e., indomethacin and phenylbutazone, inhibit bioconversion of arachidonic acid to endoperoxides. Treatment with indomethacin (20 mg/kg twice daily) in scald injury results in marked suppression of increased lymph flow. The transcapillary transport is reduced, but the functional ultrastructure of the blood-lymph barrier is not altered by indomethacin treatment [34].

3.4.1.2 Inhibition of Thromboxane Biosynthesis

The specific thromboxane synthetase inhibitors, i.e., imidazole, methimazole, and dipyridamole, decrease the adhesiveness of thrombocytes and leukocytes and abolish the vasoconstrictive effects of thromboxane. Progressive dermal ischemia is therefore reduced [35]. Recently, it has been reported that Dazmegrel for intramuscular injection in burned guinea pigs does not improve the dermal ischemia [36]. Pretreatment with Dazoxiben (5 mg/kg, i.v.) in traumatized dogs markedly decreases thromboxane concentration in plasma and prevents circulatory failure [37].

3.4.1.3 Scavengers

Of interest in this respect is the blockage of oxygen-free radicals by so-called scavengers. The polymorphonuclear neutrophil (PMN) is a potential source of oxygen-free radicals which are produced in connection with the respiratory burst of these phagocytic cells. The cytoplasm of the leukocytes is protected from oxygen-free radical damage by the presence of the so-called scavenger, superoxide dismutase (SOD) and catalase. If the oxygen-free radicals leak into the interstitial space, damage to cell membranes is likely to occur. The following interventions have been found useful experimentally in limiting tissue injury from oxygen-free radicals in rats, guinea pigs, and rabbits with thermal injury [38].

1. Removal of $O_2^{\overline{\cdot}}$ by superoxide dismutase
2. Removal of H_2O_2 by catalase
3. Use of scavengers: sodium benzoate, dimethyl sulfoxide (DMSO), vitamin E, and coenzyme Q_{10}
4. Removal of iron by apolactoferrin or deferoxamine

There are now strong hints in studies of thermal injury that oxygen radicals produced from autostimulated phagocytic cells play a critical role in resulting complications.

3.4.1.4 Steroids

The steroids express antiinflammatory activity by means of a complex series of cellular responses. They can decrease release of arachidonic acid from phospholipids, and can also inhibit the formation of leukotrienes. Nevertheless, despite these potential therapeutic advantages, adverse side effects of steroids, e.g., suppression of the immune response, limit their use as anti-inflammatory agents.

3.4.2 Glucose-Insulin Potassium Therapy

Glucose-insulin-potassium (GIK) therapy, as an adjunctive treatment, may show effects on cardiac and renal function in the early phase of severe burns. In early postburn patients, within 48 h after burns, infusion of 1 L of 10% of glucose in water containing 2.5 IU insulin and 30 ml 10% potassium chloride, results in a prominent and continued elevation of cardiac index (CI) due to elevated stroke volume index (SVI) and left ventricular stroke work index (LVSWI). It is postulated that GIK infusion has a beneficial effect in improving myocardiac contractility and inner layer myocardial blood supply, as measured by means of radiomicrospheres in burned rabbits [39]. This therapy also produces a remarkable increase in urine volume during burn shock.

3.4.3 Administration of RA-642

RA-642 is a pyrimidine derivative (2,2-[4,8-bis(diathylamino)-pyrimido-[5,4-*d*] pyrimidine-2,6-diyl) di-(2-methoxyethyl) imius] diethanol) which has vasodilating and central hypertensive potency effects, as reported by Kadats et al. [40]. Yin Ming et al. [41] recently reported the effects of the administration of RA-642 in differential doses to burned animals. The survival time was prolonged significantly in mice when RA-642 was administered (7.5 mg/kg i.p.). In the cat model (i.v. 0.25 mg/kg per hour), it maintained LVSP, $\frac{dp}{dt}$ max and (dp/dt) P and L_0 at 24 ± 3 kPa, 484 ± 193 kPa, and 24 ± 8 and 28 ± 17 colony-forming units (CFUs), respectively, at 8 h postburn. The values were significantly higher than those of the control group. Cats treated with RA-642 had a lower blood lactate level (1.4 ± 1.0 vs. 3.8 ± 1.6 mmol/l) and lower plasma β-glucuronidase activity than the animals in the control group. It is suggested that RA-642 may be of value as a therapeutic agent for burn shock.

3.4.4 Administration of Fructose-1, 6-Diphosphate and Dichloroacetate

During the early postburn period there is a disorder in cellular metabolism associated with acid-base imbalance. Deprivation of high-energy phosphate compounds results in fluid and electrolyte maldistribution, and biochemical and cellular structural changes, with an irreversible fatal outcome. So it is necessary to improve cellular metabolism and to increase the production of high-energy phosphate compounds. Effects of fructose-1, 6-diphosphate (FDP) and sodium dichloroacetate (DCA) administration on energy metabolism and intracellular pH of the hearts in severely burned rats were studied using the ^{31}P nuclear magnetic resonance (NMR) technique [42]. Favorable effects of combined administration of FDP (350 mg/kg) and DCA (70 mg/kg) have been observed during experimentally induced burn shock in small animals. It seems that the imbalance state of myocardiac energy metabolism after severe burn can be corrected by treatment with FDP. Intracellular acidosis can also be partly corrected after FDP administration, but is never restored to normal levels. Nevertheless, more favorable effects can be obtained by administration of FDP plus DCA. Not only can intracellular pH return to normal levels, but there are also some favorable effects on myocardiac energy metabolism owing to the correction of intracellular pH. Accumulation of lactic acid during shock contributes to intracellular acidosis, which inhibits the activity of phosphofructokinase (PFK), this preventing the transfer of fructose-6-phosphate to fructose-1,6-diphosphate. FDP bypasses the inhibitory effect of acidosis on PFK by stimulating pyruvate kinase, and DCA reduces lactate levels through its effect on PDH and diverting pyruvate to the tricarboxylic acid cycle. Another favorable effect of FDP administration is the conservation of ATP and the increase in the net yield of ATP from glycolysis. It has also been demonstrated that FDP enriches red blood cells with a phosphorylated intermediate (2,3-DPG), which shifts the oxyhemoglobin dissociation curve to the right. Decreased oxygen hemoglobin affinity permits oxygen release and its utilization for cellular metabolism, which is enhanced by DCA administration. DCA can be of little value during hypoxia when the pyruvate level is low and little mitochondrial NAD^+ is present. But an enhanced glycolytic rate by FDP will enrich cellular pyruvate. Through its effect on oxyhemoglobin dissociation and increasing the oxygen partial pressure, FDP may improve tissue hypoxia and increase the mitochondrial NAD^+ level.

3.5 Intensive Care in Early Treatment of Burns

The treatment of extensive burns, particularly the early shock stage, in aged patients, and burns complicated by severe inhalation injury and cranial injury, usually requires intensive care. Hence, it is necessary to establish an intensive care unit in burn centers.

3.5.1 Clinical Signs

Generally speaking, vital signs such as consciousness, body temperature, especially core temperature, respiratory rate, pulse, and hourly urine volume are recorded.

3.5.2 Hemodynamic Monitoring

Extensive burns can affect cardiovascular function considerably. Therefore, hemodynamic monitoring is of great importance in a burn intensive care unit. Functions of the cardiovascular system are measured with a better under-

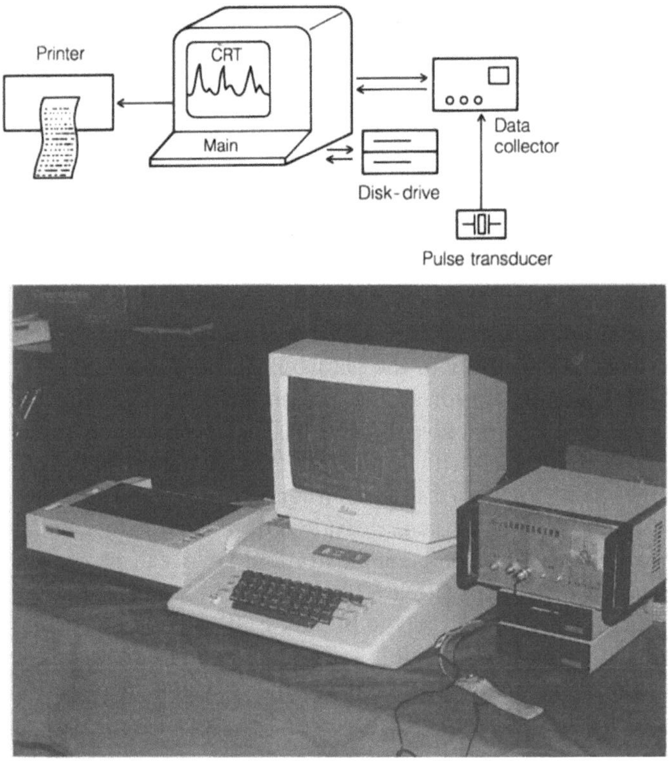

Fig. 3.16. Microcomputer-based hemodynamic monitoring system with a sphygmogram

standing of the severity of burns, there is a better observation of the hemodynamic status, and a better policy of emergency burn treatment can be formed.

The invasive technique of monitoring central venous pressure (CVP), pulmonary artery pressure (PAP), and pulmonary arterial wedge pressure (PAWP), using a Swan-Ganz catheter with the thermodilution or dye-dilution method, is rather cumbersome. Besides, this monitoring technique increases the risk of infection, embolization, and cardiac complications.

Noninvasive techniques such as impedance measurement or the ultrasonic Doppler technique are unsuitable for patients with chest or back burns, and in addition technical errors are inevitable. The authors [43] have developed a noninvasive hemodynamic monitoring system which consists of a pulse transducer, a data collector, a cathode ray tube, a printer, and a disk drive (Figs. 3.16–3.18).

The transducer is fixed to some specific area on the body surface, where pulsation of an underlying artery, particularly the radial artery, is measured. The femoral or carotid artery can also be used.

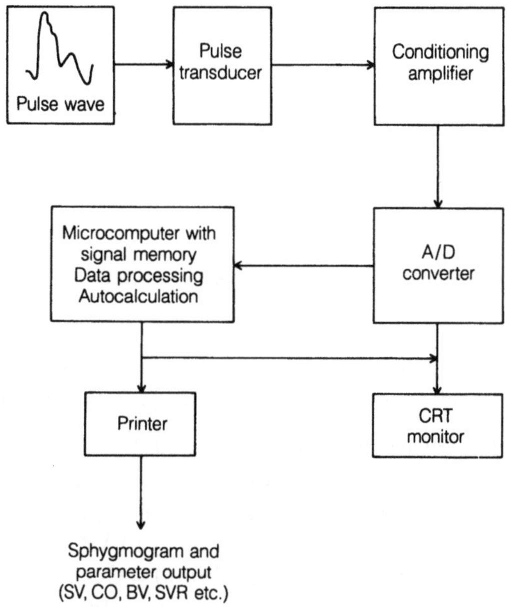

Fig. 3.17. Functional structure of the sphygmography monitoring system

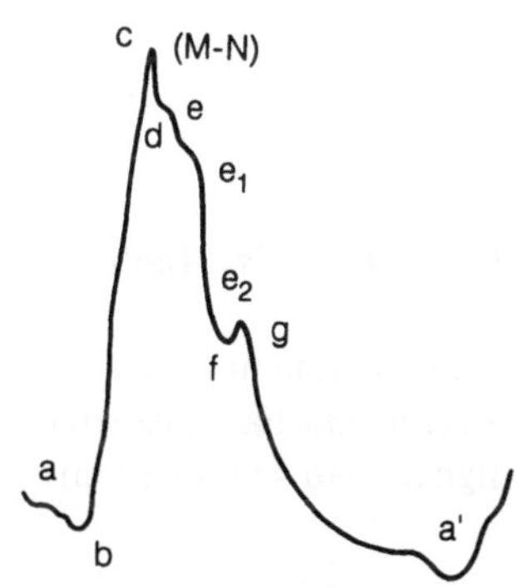

Fig. 3.18. Nomenclature of each characteristic point of the sphygmogram: *a*, atrial pressure wave; *b*, opening of aortic valve; *c*, peak systolic pressure; *d*, decreasing pressure during aortic dilatation; *e*, peak of tidal wave; e_1, beginning diastole of left ventricle; e_2, closure of aortic valve; *f*, start of steady descending stage of arterial pressure; *g*, peak of returned tidal wave

This newly developed system for sphygmography is designed on the basis of biorheology and physiology. An equation has been developed for working out a sphygmogram curve to calculate the stroke volume (SV, in milliliters):

$$SV = SA \cdot r / ASR$$

where SA is the integral pressure of the pulse cycle, translated from sphygmogram and blood pressure, *r* is the calibration constant (determined by making a

Table 3.9. Comparison of the sphygmography and thermal dilution methods for determining cardiac output

No. of patients	Cardiac output (l/min)			
	Sphygmogram		Thermal dilution	
	Mean	SD	Mean	SD
49	5.024	1.120	4.568	0.834

Correlation analysis: $r = 0.882$; $F = 164.8$; $p < 0.001$.

simultaneous measurement using an independent method), and ASR is arterial specific resistance. Consequently, it can be established that:

HR (heart rate, beats/min) = 60/T
CO (cardiac output, l/min) = SV × HR/1000
MAP (mean arterial pressure, mmHg) = SA/T + DBP
SW (stroke work, G, M) = SV × MAP × 0.0144
MW (minute work, kg, M/min) = CO × MAP × 0.0144
SVR (systemic vascular resistance, dyn · cm^3/s = 79.96 × MAP/CO

Cardiac output was determined using the sphygmogram in 12 patients simultaneously with the thermal dilution method using the Swan-Ganz catheter. The results are shown in Table 3.9.

3.5.3 Blood Gas Analysis

In the treatment of extensive burns and severe inhalation injury, it is necessary to correct acid-base disturbance. When PaO_2 is lower than 70 mmHg and $PaCO_2$ higher than 45 mmHg, artificial ventilation may be applied.

3.5.4 Extravascular Lung Water

A system has been developed for the determination of extravascular lung water in cases of inhalation injury and fluid overloading.

3.5.5 Renal Function Monitoring

1. Serum or plasma osmolarity
2. Biochemical determination of serum and urine electrolytes and blood and urine protein metabolites

3.5.6 Analysis of Various Substances

Various substances in the blood such as fibronectin, norepinephrine and epinephrine, cortisol, blood sugar, insulin, antidiuretic hormone, and vasopressin are determined in the early period after burn injury.

References

1. Arturson G (1979) Microvascular permeability to macromolecules in thermal injury. Acta Physiol Scand [Suppl] 463: 111–122
2. Arturson G (1985) The pathophysiology of severe thermal injury. J Burn Care Rehabil 6: 129–146
3. Chang ZD (1960) Experimental fluid resuscitation study on burn in the dog. Selected paper of scientific technique in Shanghai no 72
4. Fang ZY, Ge SD (1984) Experimental research for burn shock in dogs. J Exp Surg 1: 78–80
5. Fang ZY, Chen YL, Liu SK et al. (1980) Research of burn shock, III. effect of cimetidine on vascular permeability after thermal injury in rats. Acad J 2nd Milit Med Coll 1: 5–9
6. Moncrief JA (1979) Replacement therapy. In: Artz CP, Moncrief JA, Pruitt BA (eds) Burns, a team approach. Saunders, Philadelphia, pp 169–191
7. Baxter CR, Cook WA, Shires ST (1966) Serum myocardial depressment factor in burn shock. Surg Forum 17: 1
8. Chen ZD, Fu WZ, Yu KD et al. (1982) The changes of cardio-contractility of dogs during burn shock. Acad J 2nd Milit Med Coll 3 [Suppl]: 6–16
9. Liu SK, Fang ZY (1990) Alteration of the hemodynamics on myocardial contractility during severe burned dog. (in press)
10. Cheng JG, Fu WJ, Cheng ZD (1988) Effect of different crystalloid fluid infusion on myocardial contractility during early stage of burn shock. Chin J Appl Physiol 4: 188–192
11. Mao N, Don TC (1982) The effect of *Lugusticum Wallich* Franch (LWF) on microcirculatory rheology in burned rabbits. Acad J 2nd Milit Med Coll 3 [Suppl]: 1–5
12. Holady WG, John W (1983) Cardiovascular effects of endogenous opiate system. Annu Rev Pharmacol Toxicol 23: 541–594
13. Zhu YX, Lin BC, Song CY et al. (1983) The effect of burn on the content of enkephalin in rats brain, In: Yang ZJ, Shong ZY, Shi JX (eds) The treatment and research in burns. Science Press, Bejing, pp 237–303
14. Wang CH, Zhu YX (1987) Effect of burn on the immunoreactive dynorphin B content in the hypothalamus. Acad J 2nd Milit Med Coll 8: 9–13
15. Hu S, Wang MU (1988) Effect of thyrotrophin releasing hormone and β-endorphin in scalded rat. Med J Chin PLA 13: 180–185
16. Lin BC, Song CY (1985) Effect of naloxone for burn shock in rats. Chin J Appl Physiol 1: 212–215
17. Gao GC, Zhu XY, Wang CH et al. (1988) Effect of antiserum of dynorphin A and large dose of naloxone for treatment of burn shock in rats. Chin J Exp Surg 5: 19–23
18. Fang ZY, Cheng YL (1985) Relationship between endocrine changes and clinical course of severe burns. Chin J Plast Burns 1: 6–9
19. Chansauria JPN, Sinha JK, Mathur AK et al. (1980) Hormonal and associated metabolic alterations following burn injury: part I, relationship to degree of burn. Burns 7: 10–15

20. Wilmore DN (1974) Catecholamines, mediator of hypermetabolic response to thermal injury. Ann Surg 180: 653–699
21. Goodall MC, Stone C, Haynes BW (1975) Urinary output of adrenaline and noradrenaline in severe burns. Ann Surg 145: 479–487
22. Ge SD, Wang W (1964) Early fluid replacement in severe burns. Ann 2nd Milit Med Coll 25: 95–98
23. Guo ZY, Sheng ZY, Zhu ZM et al. (1989) The use of blood in burn shock—clinical and experimental study. J Burn Care Rehabil 10: 226–231
24. Fox CL Jr (1968) The role of alkaline sodium salt solution in the treatment of severe burns. Ann NY Acad Sci 150: 823–826
25. Monafo WW (1970) Treatment of burn shock by the intravenous and oral administration of hypertonic lactated saline solutions. J Trauma 10: 575–586
26. Monafo WW, Chunrasakal H, Ayvasion VH (1973) Hypertonic sodium solution in the treatment of burn shock. Am J Surg 126: 778–783
27. Ge SD, Fang ZY, (1982) Hypertonic solution in treatment of burn shock. Acad J 2nd Milit Med Coll 2: 65–68
28. Jalenco A, Williams JB, Wheelar ML et al. (1979) Studies in shock and resuscitation. I. use of a hypertonic, albumin containing fluid demand regimen (HALED) in resuscitation. Crit Care Med 7: 157–167
29. Xia ZF, Fang ZY, Ge SD et al. (1987) Effect of hypertonic solution in treatment burned rabbits on erythrocyte Na^+ and K^+, and Na^+–K^+ ATPase activity in renal tubular. Chin J Exp Surg 4: 65–69
30. Mehrkenus HH, Linder KH, Ahnefeld FW et al. (1987) Fluid resuscitation with hypertonic salt solutions in experimental burn shock. Burns 13: 53–56
31. Kremer H, Allgöwer M, Craf M et al. (1981) The present studies of research in burn toxin. Intensive Care Med 7: 71–76
32. Jones JV (1980) Plasmapheresis: current research and success. Heart and Lung 9: 671–674
33. Yu H, Cooper EH (1983) Urinary protein profiles after burn injury. Burns 9: 339–349
34. Arturson G, Jonsson CE (1973) Effects of indomethacin on the trans-capillary leackage of macromolecules and the efflux of prostaglandins in paw lymph following experimental scalding injury. Ups J Med Sci 78: 181–188
35. Delbeccaro EJ, Robson HC, Heggers JP et al. (1980) The use of specific thromboxane inhibitors to preserve the dermal microcirculation after burning. Surgery 87: 137–141
36. Wang SL, Ligao , Alexander JW et al. (1988) The effect of the thromboxane synthetase inhibitor Dazmegrel (UK 38485) on blood perfusion of burned skin: symposium of burn and plastic surgery. Acad J 3rd Milit Med Coll 8:306–310
37. Howard HH (1986) Inhibition of thromboxane biosynthesis in splanchnic ischaemic shock. Crit Shock 18: 95–106
38. Ward PA, Till GO (1985) The autodestructive consequences of thermal injury. J Burn Care Rehabil 6: 251–255
39. Cheng CW, Fang ZY, Ge SD (1987) Observation of changes in mycardial contractility and regional blood flow after thermal injury in rabbits, Chin J Exp Surg 4: 160–164
40. Kadatz R, Kobinger W, Walland A (1976) RA 642 A pyrimidopurimidium derivative with vasodilating and hypertensive potency. Naunyn Schmiedebergs Arch Pharmacol 292: 97–103
41. Yin M, Liao XL, Tan SJ (1987) Effects of 2,2′-(4,8 bis(didiethylamino)-pyrimide-(5,4d)pyrimidine-2,6-diyl)di-(2-methoxyethyl)imino)diethanol (RA 642) on experimental scald shock. Acta Pharmacol Sin 8: 533–539
42. Xia ZF, Fang ZY, Ge SD (1988) Effect of FDP and DCA on mycardiac energy metabolism and intracellular pH of hearts of severely burned rats. Chin J Plast Surg Burn 4: 208–212
43. Xiao XG (1989) An on-line monitoring system of cardiovascular function by Sphygmogram. In: Proceedings of the 6th World congress on Medical Ingormatics (MEDINOF 89). Summary of Chinese papers, Beijing, 16–20 Oct 1989. p 60

4 Local Care in Severe Burn

Fang Zhi-yang

Following the initiation of fluid replacement therapy, the history of the burn is taken in detail and a physical examination is carried out. Local care of the burn wounds is started as soon as the general condition of the patient is stabilized with appropriate treatment, because severe infection of the burn wound can lead to life-threatening complications such as wound sepsis and septicemia.

All methods of cleaning, debriding, and treating the burn wound aim to control "burn wound sepsis", a concept proposed by Teplitz and characterized by bacterial infection of burn wound with the number of pathogens exceeding 10^5/g subeschar tissue and actively invading the underlying and surrounding tissue [1].

Colonization of the pathogen bacteria on the wound increases rapidly a few days after the burn. In superficial burns there is only partial damage of the dermis and the underlying blood vessels are partially obliterated, while in deep burns the whole dermis is burned and subcutaneous blood vessels thrombosed, which results in secondary ischemic changes. Hence, systematically administered antibiotics are unable to reach the area with bacterial colonization. Therefore, local care of the burn wound with topical antimicrobial agents seems to be of great importance.

Every effort is made to prevent secondary infection and ensure expeditious healing of the burn wound. Therefore, the following principles must be observed: (a) maintenance of the environment to suit the requirements for wound healing; (b) prevention of further contamination; (c) control of bacterial colonization and drainage of purulent exudation; and (d) removal of nonviable tissue.

4.1 Initial Burn Wound Management

Initial treatment and debridement of the local burn wound, especially in major burns, should be performed when the general condition of the patient has stablized. Prior to debridement, photographs may be taken and a swab culture obtained.

4.1.1 Analgesic and Sedative

Burn patients usually appear to be nervous and complain of local pain, particularly when the burn is superficial. Narcotics, such as merperidine 1–2 mg/kg i.v. or ketamine 1–3 mg/kg, may be given to the patient by the intravenous route.

4.1.2 Debridement

Debridement is initiated by cleaning and washing the surrounding skin with soap, detergent, or providone-iodine and the hair is shaved as necessary.. Then the wound is washed and cleansed with 0.1% benzalkonium chloride (geramine) or 0.05% chlorhexidine. The debriding technique is gently performed. It should be ensured that there is as little irritation as possible. On the other hand, the detached nonviable epithelium of ruptured blisters and soil should be removed as thoroughly as possible. As for superficial partial-thickness burns, large blisters can be drained and small blisters can be left intact. In deep dermal burns, particularly those caused by hot liquid, the loosely attached epithelium should be removed.

4.1.3 Circumferential Burns

4.1.3.1 Circumferential Deep Burns of the Extremities

In the case of circumferential deep burns of the extremities, constriction of the burn eschar, which can interfere with the blood supply of the distal part of the limb, is often seen at or above wrist level in upper extremity burns or ankle level in lower extremity burns. In brief, circumferential burn eschar can exert a tourniquet effect. Accumulation of edematous fluid undereath the eschar, especially rapid elevation of intracompartmental pressure interfering with lymphatic and venous drainage, compromises the arterial blood supply, leading to ischemic necrosis of muscles and nerves.

Signs of inadequate blood circulation include pallor or cyanosis of the distal end of the extremity with lowering of local skin temperature, loss of motor function, and absence of capillary refill and arterial pulsation, detected either by digital palpation or using an Ultrasonic Doppler flowmeter. Signs of the muscular compartment syndrome may be demonstrated in some cases.

Patients sustaining severe circumferential burns of the trunk, particularly the thorax, may show restriction of respiratory movement in the lower thoracic cage by the compression effect of the armor-like, while the movement of accessory respiratory muscles increases. Nevertheless, the overall ventilation is reduced. Furthermore, severe burn of the abdomen can compromise the ventilation due to restriction of the abdominal wall. The intraabdominal pressure is increased and the diaphragm is pushed upward, resulting in a decrease of vital capacity. The patient shows respiratory distress with tachypnea.

4.1.3.2 Operative Procedure of Decompression

The common sites of circumferential eschar formation requiring escharotomy, i.e., incisional decompression are the arm, hand, leg, thorax, and penis. The clinical indications for performing an escharotomy include [2]:

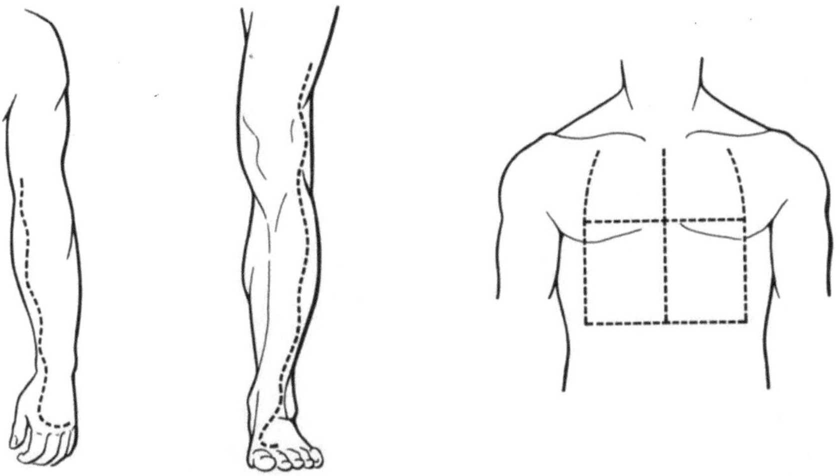

Fig. 4.1. Recommended sites of escharotomy incisions of upper and lower extremities and chest wall

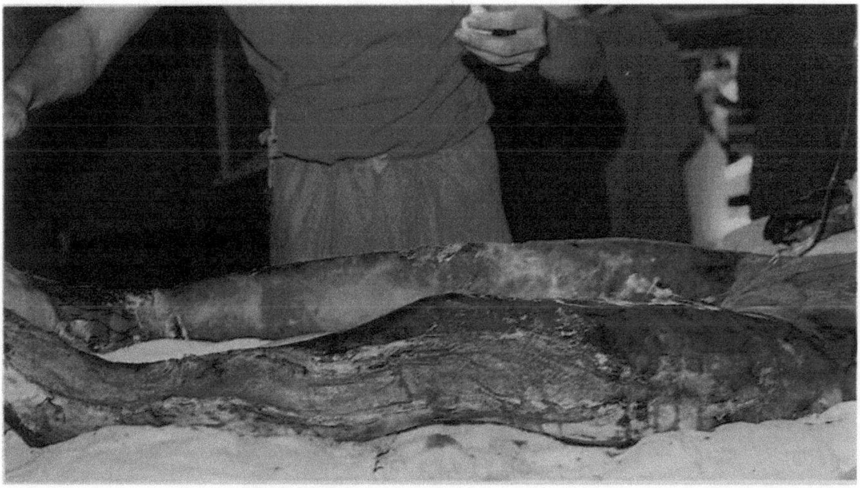

Fig. 4.2. Escharotomy of the lower extremity down to the deep fascia for relief of tissue tension

Absolute: (a) absent pulse, (b) cold extremity, (c) numbness
Relative: (a) decreased capillary filling, (b) cyanosis, (c) decreased sensation to light touch, (d) marked increase in edema in spite of continuous elevation of the injured extremity

1. Escharotomy and fasciotomy for circumferential burns of the extremities: The incisions are made along the medial and lateral aspects of the limbs. The

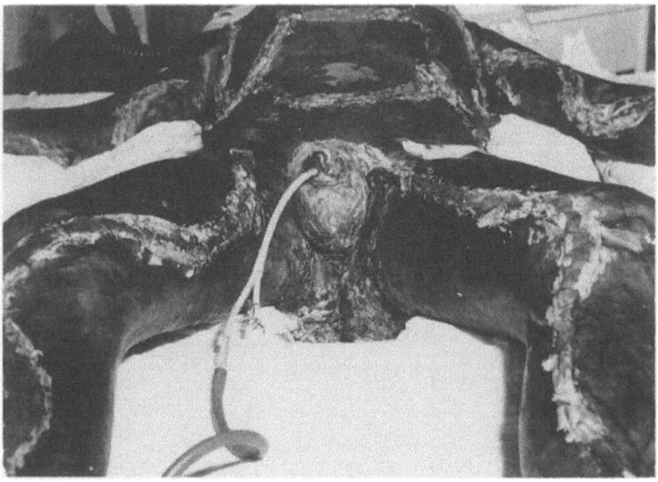

Fig. 4.3. Multiple incision escharotomy of upper and lower extremities and chest wall in a very severely burned patient

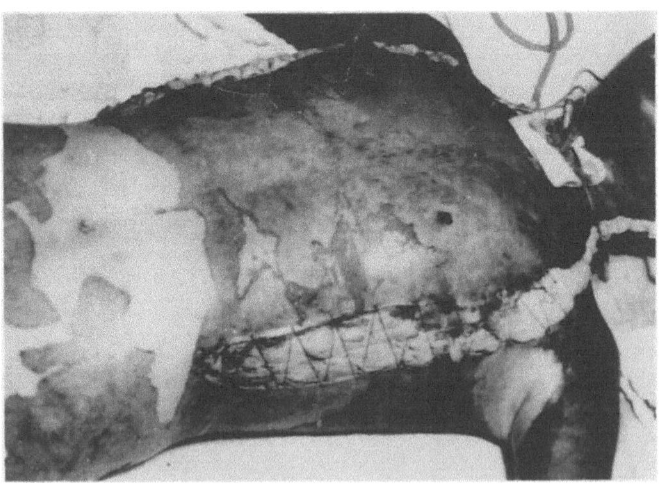

Fig. 4.4. Bilateral chest wall escharotomy with the incision extended through the circumferential eschar of the neck

proximal end of the incision should extend beyond the upper boundary of the burn wound. The distal incision should extend across the ankle or wrist joint. Escharotomy is performed simply by incising the burn eschar down to the deep fascia to relieve the tissue tension (Figs. 4.1–4.2). Deep burns, especially high-power electric burns, usually involve the underlying muscles to a certain extent; therefore, fasciotomy may be necessary to relieve the elevated pressure in the muscle compartment, which could not be relieved by simple escharotomy.

2. Escharotomy of the chest wall: Symmetrical incisions should be made bilaterally along the anterior axillary line down to the costal margin. For more severe transverse incisions should be made across the vertical incisions at the level of the nipple and the costal margin for adequate relief of tissue tension (Figs. 4.3–4.4).

The escharotomy and fasciotomy incisions should be widened by blunt dissection for thorough release of tissue tension. The surgical wounds should be covered with iodoform or povidone-iodine gauze.

These operations should be performed with the patient under general anesthasia with aseptic technique and electric cautery. They are better carried out in the operating room immediately after early debridement. Alternatively, they can be performed in the burn intensive care unit or the critical burn ward.

4.2 Definitive Local Care

Following early debridement the burn wound should be treated with definitive local care using either the exposure or the occlusive method. The semiexposure method can be applied as an independent measure itself, but also as an interchangeable measure or as a procedure following either of the methods mentioned above. Although each of the methods serves as a kind of definitive care of the local burn wound, they are usually used in combination for an individual patient, particularly in extensive burns, because the indication for each method varies with anatomical region. Moreover, the method which is used after debridement can be changed for another method when indicated.

4.2.1 Exposure Method

The exposure method is a simple measure for definitive local care. It simply involves exposing the wound to the open air. Although it might seem to be an open method, in essence it is a closed method, as a protective wound covering, i.e., a crust or eschar, will be formed through desiccation of the wound surface. This protective covering prevents the wound becoming bacterially contaminated. However, it is more predisposed to infection before the protective layer is formed. Therefore, an ideal ambient environment is mandatory, if this treatment method is adapted, in order to minimize wound contamination. Laminar flow, for which some burn centers are equipped, is the best choice. Nevertheless, contamination by direct contact, which is the main route of bacterial contamination, should not be overlooked, and aseptic techniques must be strictly followed by the medical staff.

The exposure method for local burn care is suitable for facial and perineal burns where frequent care is required. In China most extensive deep burn patients are treated with this method with the help of a Stryker turning frame, which offers most effective exposure of the wound.

A hot air blower is often used to promote drying of the wound. It is especially necessary underneath the Stryker turning frame when the patient is lying on the porous spongy mattress in the supine position without turning, as required in the early shock phase. In this way maceration of burn wounds on the back, the buttocks, and the dorsal aspects of the extremities is prevented.

An air-fluidized bed has been employed by some burn centers in China. It allows the patient to lie in the supine position for a long period without deepening of the wound over the pressure spots on the dorsal aspect of the body, and thus avoids formation of decubitus ulcers. The ambient temperature can be kept at 38°C, which is hostile to bacterial growth. As a result, the air-fluidized bed not only benefits the patient by preventing pressure injury to both skin and wound, and maintenance of environmental temperature, but also reduces the risk of infection. Meanwhile it also benefits the medical staff by simplifying and facilitating nursing care.

Room temperature should be kept constant to maintain warmth. Patients usually complain of cold, some of them even shivering due to heat loss from drying of the wound surface. Hence, the room temperature is kept in the range of 32°–36°C, not only to keep the patient warm but also to minimize caloric loss. At the same time relative humidity should be regulated to around 45%. Unfortunately an environment with such a room temperature and relative humidity is intolerable for the attending medical staff. Therefore, an electric heater, a single electric bulb, severl bulbs in a group with reflectors or shields, or infrared radiators can be used to keep the patient warm without raising the room temperature too much.

Although a high ambient temperature benefits the patient, an increase in insensible water loss, which affects the patient's homeostasis, is inevitable. The insensible water loss is more obvious when either a hot blower or an air-fluidized bed is used. An extra quantity of water should be administered in the early burn shock treatment. For the estimation of the amount of water to be supplied the following formula was proposed by Dong [3].

$$\text{Amount of water} = 2000\,\text{ml} + 49.93 + 4.43\,\text{ml}/\%\ \text{TBSA}$$

It is obvious that the amount of water to be replaced is actually the sum of daily requirement and extra insensible loss from the burn wound.

There are some disadvantages of the exposure method. Patients with superficial burns receiving this kind of local care usually complain of local pain, the wound being irritated even by a light breeze. There is inevitable damage to wound tissue, which leads to deepening of the partial-thickness burns to full-thickness burns. When the exposed burn wound is macerated or infected, the local care can be changed for the occlusive or semi-exposure method.

4.2.2 Occlusive Method

The purpose of the occlusive method is to protect the wound immediately after debridement from further contamination, thereby preventing infection, in order to obtain smooth healing. Hence aseptic technique should be strictly followed.

The conventional occlusive method used in China is as follows. The inner layer of dressing usually consists of one or two sheets of sterilized fine-mesh gauze impregnated with petrolatum, a topical ointment, or a medicinal herb paste. The outer layer is composed of multilayered, sponge-like, soft, loose, absorbent gauze or cotton pad, smoothly arranged and wrapped with a pressure bandage. Ordinarily, the dressings may be kept in place until epithelialization of the superficial burn is complete.

As for extensive deep burns, the occlusive dressing should be removed for reinspection at 4–5 days after the injury so that the depth of wound can be reassessed. At that time surgical intervention such as escharotomy or tangential excision can be decided upon. Since deep burns are more susceptible to infection, the surgeon must look out for early signs of infection. A decision can be made as to whether to continue with occlusive dressings, to change the dressings regular at intervals, or to change to the exposure and semi-exposure method.

In treating extensive burns, occlusive dressings are often applied to burned extremities to maintain better functional postures.

This method has some disadvantages. A large quantity of sterilized dressings are used, especially when there are mass casualities. A dressing change brings about unbearable local pain. Patients often ask for narcotics, which are seldom used in China in order to avoid adverse side effects and addiction.

4.2.3 Semi-exposure Method

The semi-exposure method is an intermediate method of local burn care. It may be used on a burn wound immediately after its debridement, or for a macerated burn wound. Sometimes it is a continuation of treatment with the occlusive method, i.e., simply removing the outer layers of the dressing, leaving the inner layer in situ.

A successful semi-exposure treatment is characterized by a dry and clean single layer of fine-mesh gauze. If the gauze is not clean, and a crust of exudation is formed, it is difficult to inspect the wound, and there may be an accumulation of purulent exudation underneath the dry crust.

4.3 Exposure Method with Topical Antibacterial Agents

The exposure method with topical antibacterial agents is the most popular treatment of burn wounds, for the following reasons:

1. Close daily examination of the wound is possible and infection may be detected at an early stage.
2. If infection of the wound occurs, a wound biopsy may be easily obtained.
3. The patient's temperature is more easily controlled, and hypothermia is prevented by keeping the ambient temperature at 34°–36°C.
4. A full range of motions can be performed in the burned areas.
5. Antibacterial drugs can be applied at an early stage.
6. Burned wound care is much easier for the house staff and nursing staff.

The common topical antibacterial agents in use today are described as follows.

4.3.1 Silver Sulfadiazine and N'-Sulfadiazine Compounds

One percent micronized sodium sulfadiazine in a water-soluble cream base is commonly used. When this compound is exposed to tissue, it gradually releases silver ion and sulfadiazine. Approximately 10% sulfa drug is absorbed. With absorption of silver sulfadiazine, the sulfa drug level is as high as 1.5%–4 mg%. This agent is able to interact with cellular DNA and thereby induces genetic change [4].

It has been reported that in 5% of patients treated with silver sulfadiazine over a large area, a transient leukopenia occurs after the first days of application. Drug rashes or urinary sulfur crystals are rare.

The 1% silver sulfadiazine cream may be applied to burn wound twice daily. When the cream is applied again, the previous drug should be wiped off. The penetration of silver sulfadiazine through the burn eschar is less than for mafenide (Sulfamylon). Painlessness is a advantage of silver sulfadiazine.

At present we are using 1% silver sulfadiazine mixed with 10% povidone-iodine (Betadine) powder for local treatment of deep second-degree or third-degree burns with good results.

To prevent and treat early infection of deep burn wound, it is desirable to apply 10% mafenide cream in the morning and 1% silver sulfadiazine cream at night. The penetrating power of mafenide is better than that of silver sulfadiazine.

More recently there have been may modifications of silver sulfadiazine, such as zinc sulfadiazine and cerium sulfadiazine. The water solubilities of the three drugs (SD_3-Ce, SD_2-Zn, SD_2-Ag) are 83, 56 and 0.19 mg/dl, respectively. Some investigators have reported increased effectiveness of SD_2-Zn, but we have found that individually it is no more effective than silver sulfadiazine.

4.3.2 Mafenide

Mafenide (Sulfamylon) has a large spectrum of antibacterial activity against both gram-positive and gram-negative pathogens in vitro, including *Pseudomonas aeruginosa* and *Clostridium tetani*. Mafenide causes pain on application, probably because of its high osmolarity [5], and mafenide acetate is a strong carbonic anhydrase inhibitor and may lead to metabolic acidosis. When mafenide is applied to over 40% of the total body surface area (TBSA), the acid-base balance is compensated by hyperventilation, until the drug is discontinued. Mafenide also induces polyuria as a result of either hyperventilation or increased urinary osmolarity.

Ten percent mafenide cream is liberally applied to the surface of burn wound to a thickness of 1–2 mm with a sterile gloved hand twice daily. The cream from the first application should be removed before the second application. The total amount applied should not exceed 450 g.

When this drug is applied to the burn wound within 30 min after injury, it is able to penetrate rapidly through the eschar. Five hours after its application, about 80%–90% of this drug is dissociated from its carrier and penetrates into the deeper tissue. The rapid absorption of the drug produces electrolyte disturbance. Eight to 10 h after application mafenide loses its bacteriostatic activity, which is why it must be applied twice daily.

4.3.3 Gentamicin

The use of aminoglycoside antibiotics as topical agents has become popular. They are used in a 0.1% concentration in a hydrophilic base and applied as a topical cream, or a 0.2%–0.5% gentamicin solution to the surface of burn wound. If gentamicin is applied to burns of over 75% TBSA for a relatively long duration, about 0.4% mg/kg of the drug is rapidly absorbed from the burn wound. So renal and auditory nerve toxicity may appear.

In our clinic it has been found that many pathogens are not sensitive to gentamicin. Since aminoglycoside antibiotics are often used systemically, their topical use should be limited.

4.3.4 Mixed Compounds for External Usage

1. SSC compound: 10% mafenide, 1% silver sulfadiazine, and 1:1000 chlorohexidine
2. SC compound: silver sulfadiazine powder 10 g in 0.5% chlorhexidine 100 ml in suspension, indicated for deep second-degree wound
3. SSD cream: 1% silver sulfadiazine, 0.5% $AgNO_3$ and 0.2% chlorohexidine diglucinide. It may be useful in gram-negative bacillus infection.

4.3.5 Povidone-Iodine

Povidone-iodine (Betadine) is commercially available for topical use on burn wounds as a 1% compound in a water-miscible cream or 10% ointment. Lee Tienzin et al. (1988, personal communication) reported 150 cases of burns of various sizes and depths treated with 10% povidone-iodine ointment. In superficial burns, exudation was remarkably reduced and a soft yellowish crust formed 24 h after 10% povidone-iodine ointment application. In deep burns the eschar was kept intact and separation of the eschar was delayed for about 4 weeks.

Blood thyroxine (T_4) and triiodothyronine (T_3) levels are decreased in the first 2 weeks with povidone-iodine treatment on the burn wound [6]. Occasionally some cases develop dermatitis, necessitating discontinuation of the drug.

4.3.6 Hydron Bandage

The bandage is applied directly by spraying liquid polyethylene glycol 400/H_2O and Hydron powder [poly(2-hydroxyethyl methacrylate)] alternatively onto the wound. Silver sulfadiazine (1% of dressing weight) is added to this mixture. Both components are nontoxic and compatible with body tissue and will not support the growth of bacteria. The intact dressing may remain in place for 3–5 days. When significant fluid accumulation occurs beneath the dressing, a small window may be made in the dressing and Hydron may then be reapplied on this open area. We have reported 50 cases where Hydron was used on second-degree wounds with good results.

4.4 Hydrotherapy

Hydrotherapy is one of the therapeutic measures in the management of burn wound, in addition to the measures mentioned above. It needs the necessary equipment and medical staff, particularly in the case of major burns, and has not yet been popularized as a regular measure in debridement.

Hydrotherapy is a regular program in some burn centers, where patients with extensive burns may be subjected to hydrotherapy every day, every other day, or twice a week. The burn center of the second Central Hospital of the Second Tienjin Medical College is quite experienced in treating extensive burns with hydrotherapy. It is suggested that only low-risk patients be subjected to hydrotherapy. This treatment is contraindicated in the case of extensive burns complicated by septicemia or disturbance of homeostasis, etc.

In most Chinese hospitals, hydrotherapy is only used in treating residual wounds of extensive burns. Residual wounds often result from deepening of deep partial-thickness burns, failure of skin grafting, or maceration of the newly epithelialized wounds by pressure or abrasion.

4.4.1 Procedure

Hydrotherapy brings about thorough cleansing of the wound, continuous debridement of deviatilized tissue, cleaning of the wound surroundings, reduction

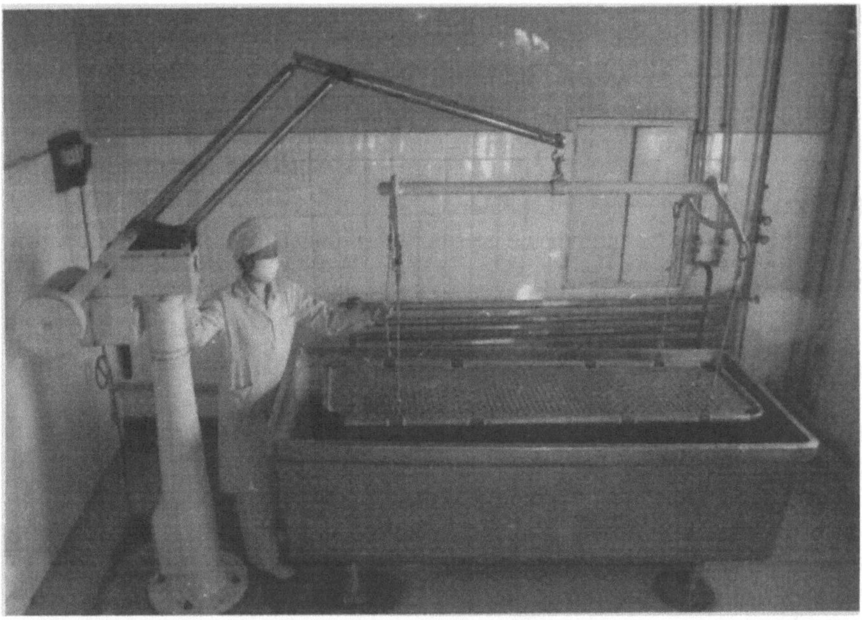

Fig. 4.5. Bath tank with hoist in the hydrotherapy room

in bacterial number, and preparation of the healthy wound for epithelialization or skin grafting.

In the hydrotherapy room, a bath tub or bath tank, usually fitted with a whirlpool, is the basic equipment. The patient is sent to the hydrotherapy room with the outer layer of the dressing removed and the inner layer left undisturbed. The patient is then lowered into the bath by means of a hoist (Fig. 4.5). When the inner gauzes are thoroughly soaked, they are gently removed by the whirlpool, or with the help of forceps. The purulent exudate is cleansed, and devitalized tissues are removed using forceps and scissors.

The attending medical personnel must closely observe the patient's general condition. During the bath, the patient's head is carefully rested on the head rest with the mouth, nose, and ears above the water surface. Attention must be paid to the tracheostomy tube if present, and intravenenous lines should be carefully protected. The nurses should keep a close watch on the pátient's vital signs. If there is any sign of collapse, the patient should immediately be lifted out of the bath by the hoist and appropriate treatment should be instituted. Ordinarily, the bath may last 30 min but should not exceed 45 min.

When the patient is lifted out of the bath, the body surface is immediately dried. The wound is promptly treated with an aseptic technique using various methods which are indicated.

4.4.2 Sterilization

Before starting hydrotherapy, the nurses in charge of the room must ensure that the bathtub and equipment is well sterilized and the room is neat and clean. This area should be kept warm with drafts at a minimum.

Various drugs can be added to the bath water suitable quantities, e.g., 1:20000 Bromogeramine, 1% povidone-iodine, or sodium hypochloride. The water should be warm enough and is usually maintained in the temperature range of 37°–39°C.

4.4.3 Cross-Infection

Hydrotherapy can be a source of cross-infection. Every effort should be made to prevent cross-infection. The bathtub should be disinfected with 3%–5% cresol or 3%–5% supernatant of bleaching powder, and the floor and wall should be washed with 2% peracetic acid as a routine. For the sake of the patient's safety, a special group of persons who have been strictly trained should be assigned to the work. Swab cultures are taken before and after the sterilization procedures.

4.4.4 Shower Bath

This procedure is performed simply by placing the patient in a special stainless steel frame covered with a network to allow leakage of water, or a stainless steel bed covered with a sterilized sheet. A movable nozzle is used for the shower. The patient may be more uncomfortable than if he or she were immersed in warm water. During the shower bath, cleansing of the wound and debriding of the devitalized tissue are performed, simultaneously. If the burn wounds are covered by a cream containing a topical agent, the area can be wiped clean during the shower.

Before finishing the bath the patient is thoroughly sprayed. Then the body surface is dried and the wounds are treated as appropriate.

A shower bath is not only simple, but also lessens the chance of cross-contamination compared with hydrotherapy carried out in a bathtub.

4.5 Cold Water Treatment

Cold water treatment is an old and effective method of treating thermal injury. It can be applied in a very simple way, as a first aid measure. Small or moderate-sized burns, such as a burned extremity, can be immersed in cold water. For major burns the burned area can be covered with large towels soaked with ice water as early as possible after the injury.

This measure benefits the patient not only in relieving the pain but also in reducing tissue damage and local burn edema by decreasing plasma, lymph, and intercellular fluid extravasation. It also reduces serum histamine and lactate levels within 8 and 24 h, respectively, after burn. Cardiovascular function, e.g., cardiac output, mean arterial blood pressure, total peripheral resistance, and hematocrit is improved particularly in severe burns [7]. Although early local treatment with cold water can benefit the patient, delayed cooling can result in more severe edema and delayed reabsorption of the extravasated fluid [8].

In experiments with rabbits, when there is a delay of as long as 3 h before the scalded hind limb is immersed in cold water at 10°–15°C, there is still a significant reduction in the amount of edema [9]. In mice with second-degree scalds of 7% TBSA, and a delayed cooling in water at 15°C 3 1/2 h after the injury, there was no significant increase in water content of scald wound, muscle beneath the wound, and lung compared with the control group. The mortality rate was reduced from 85.19% to 15.14% at 15 days after thermal injury [10].

It was suggested that cold water at a temperature of 8°–15°C is effective and safe in early local burn care, since cooling at 0°C is without the potential hazard of hypothermia. The duration of cooling should be relatively long—at least 30 min and as much as 1 h or more—for optimal pain relief and substantial abatement of pathophysiological alteration.

References

1. Teplitz C, Davio D, Mason HD Jr et al. (1964) *Pseudomonas* burn wound sepsis. I. Pathogenesis of experimental *Pseudomonas* burn wound sepsis. J Surg Res 4: 200–206
2. Mendelowitz D, Horton CE, Carraway JH (1975) Decompressional escharotomies in circumferential burns. Chir Plast 3: 85–90
3. Dong YL, Guo ZR (1987) The effect of an air fluidized bed on early fluid therapy in burned patients. Chin J Plast Surg Burns 3: 202–205
4. Rosenbranz HS (1979) Impermeability of human cells to silver sulfadiazine: a biological experiment. Burns 5: 312–314
5. Harrison HN, Shuck JM, Caldwell E (1975) Studies of pain produced by mafenide acetate preparations in burns. Arch Surg 110: 1446–1449
6. Prerssler P (1983) Änderungen der Schilddrüsenhormonspiegel nach schweren Verbrennungen bei Oberflächenbehandlung mit Poviden-Jod. Langenbecks Arch Chir 360: 9–15
7. Boyken JV, Cruts S (1982) Mechanisms of burn shock protection after severe scald injury by cold water treatment. J Trauma 22: 859–866
8. Demling RH, Majess RB, Woberg W (1979) The effect of immediate and delayed cold immersion in burn edema formation and resorption J Trauma 19: 56–60
9. Davis JWL (1982) Prompt cooling of burned area: a review of benefit and effector mechanisms. Burns 9: 1–5
10. Cheng YL (1985) Effects of cool water therapy in burned wound of mice. Chin J Exp Surg 2: 71–74

5 Management of Full-Thickness Burns

Ge Sheng-de

The most difficult and painstaking task in burn treatment is local burn management. Especially the management of deep burn wound, i.e., deep partial-thickness or dermal burns and full-thickness burns, is of crucial importance. It is obvious that the devitalized tissue is a culture medium for growth and proliferation of microorganisms. In other words, the damaged tissue offers a basis for bacterial colonization which allows bacteria to cause local burn infection. When bacteria invade the unburned tissue surrounding the burned area, burn wound sepsis will be the result, and when they invade the circulation septicemia ensues. Invasive and systemic infection may lead to a fatal outcome. Clinical analysis of the causes of death in some burn centers and burn units in China showed that death from infection accounts for 40%–60% of the total number of deaths. Hence, it is clear that infection is the most significant cause of fatality in burns [1]. It is obvious that local burn management, particularly in deep burns, is of extreme importance.

Although early debridement and definitive local care by either the occlusive or the open method offer better conditions for wound repair, application of topical agents is generally needed. In most of burn centers and burn units in China, topical antimicrobial agents such as silver sulfadiazine and mafenide (Sulfamylon) in cream are usually used. However, in the community hospitals some physicians prefer to use Chinese herbal medicines, such as decoction, extract, or tincture of *Ilex chinensis*, *Shangui sorba*, and *Polygonum*, and paste of *Coptis*, *Scutellaria*, and *Phellodendronum*. Most are astringents with a greater or lesser antibacterial effects. Despite various measures in local burn treatment, infection is inevitable in extensive full-thickness burns. Therefore surgery is indicated in the treatment of deep burns. The purpose of surgical intervention is to remove the devitalized tissue of deep burn wounds to eliminate the culture medium and colonizing ground for microorganisms. The surgical wound is then closed by skin graft or a substitute which prevents the open wound from subsequent contamination and infection. Development of surgical treatment in burns has been a milestone in the course of progress in burn treatment. One group of surgeons reported mortality of 31.5% in 76 patients with burns of over 30% total body surface area (TBSA). The main cause of death was wound sepsis, which was considered to be related to failure to carry out timely surgical treatment [2].

5.1 Surgical Treatment

Escharectomy and tangential excision are effective surgical procedures in removing devitalized tissue in full-thickness burns. The operating technique of escharectomy was first advocated in China by Fang Zhi-Yang and his colleagues in our burn center in 1959 [3]. The first patient who underwent escharectomy was a steel worker sustaining extensive flame burns covering 100% TBSA with 88% full-thickness and the rest deep partial-thickness burns associated with inhalation injury. There was no previous experience which could be followed in the treatment of such extensive deep burns. Excision of the eschar on the anterior trunk and both lower and upper extremities was performed on this patient. The surgical wound was covered by fresh skin allograft. Escharectomy was performed thereafter for the distal part of the extremities for extremely deep destruction, and the resultant wounds were treated in a similar manner. Because of shortage of skin donor site, allograft was applied and changed at certain intervals until fresh allograft was available. The patient finally died after aggressive treatment, but we began to learn the technique of escharectomy and skin transplantation using a large sheet of allograft in the management of extensive full-thickness burns.

Thereafter, escharectomy for full-thickness burn was gradually popularized. The area of deep burn to be excised may be large or small. At first, the extent of escharectomy was restricted to an area 15%–20% TBSA. It was gradually enlarged to 30%–45% TBSA. Recently, the extent of escharectomy was enlarged to 45%–65% TBSA in one setting. But such an extensive operative procedure has only been undertaken by some surgeons in a limited number of burn centers. Many problems will be encountered when too large an area of eschar is excised.

Tangential excision introduced by Janzekovic [4] was applied later in deep dermal mixed type and superficial full-thickness burns for better results in functional areas.

5.1.1 Timing of Surgical Treatment

In small-sized full-thickness burn, particularly when a functional area is involved, escharectomy may be performed as soon as possible. It is better carried out before local infection occurs, since the general condition is relatively good in this group of patients. In moderate full-thickness burns, escharectomy may be performed on the third or fourth postburn day after adequate fluid resuscitation in early burn shock. However, in extensive full-thickness burns, the first escharectomy is usually performed on the fifth to seventh postburn day, because a sufficient period is needed for stabilization of the patient's general condition after the early shock stage, i.e., to regain the state of homeostasis. It is important to allow the patient's general condition to improve so that he or she can better tolerate general anesthesia and a surgical procedure involving such an extensive area.

5.1.2 Perioperative Management

In order to perform a successful operation, correct perioperative management is of major importance. Attention should be paid to the general and local condition of the patient. Adequate treatment for existing problems should be instituted.

Systemic treatment should be focused mainly on fluid resuscitation in early burn shock, management of inhalation injury, and prevention and treatment of complications of the organ system such as stress ulcer, stress pseudodiabetes, renal insufficiency, toxic hepatitis, pneumonia, and urinary tract infection. In the meantime, maintenance of water, electrolyte, and acid-base balance and enhancement of nutritional support are of equal importance. The contraindications for major burns to receive surgical treatment are to be guarded against [5].

Local management includes maintenance on occlusive or exposure method treatment for the burn wounds, application of topical antimicrobial agents in solution, suspension, or cream, and use of antiseptics such as tincture of iodine, which is quite effective in promoting the formation of dry eschar.

Systemic antibiotics are usually prescribed and a combination of antibiotics are needed to obtain wide coverage of pathogenic bacteria. The drug sensitivity test of the bacteria isolated from swab culture of the burn wound may be used as a reliable guide in prescribing the antibiotics used in combination. If such information is not available, a combination of third-generation cephalosporins, e.g., ceftazidime or ceftriaxone with cephradine or amikacin, is considered to be the best choice for obtaining wide coverage of possible pathogenic bacteria, either gram-positive or gram-negative.

The most effective method of prophylactic use of antibiotics is to start intravenous administration of the drugs simultaneously with induction of general anesthesia. Administration of antibiotics in such a way will produce a sufficient level in serum higher than the minimal inhibitory concentration of the antibiotics given, so that pathogenic bacteria that enter the blood circulation or invade the surrounding healthy tissue due to surgical manipulation will be quickly eliminated. An additional dose of antibiotics is indicated in prolonged operations.

Antibiotics should be prescribed postoperatively at regular intervals. The duration of treatment course should be determined by the patient's specific condition.

Another important treatment is blood transfusion. Excision of burn eschar causes blood and fluid loss. The problem will be prominent when a large area of third-degree burn eschar is to be removed. Therefore adequate blood and fluid transfusion is important to guarantee a safe operation. Blood loss may be assessed preoperatively by following the rule of thumb that excision of burn eschar of an area of 1% TBSA may result in a blood loss of approximately 100 ml. It is advisable to have a sufficient quantity of blood prepared to meet the possible specific needs of the patient during or after the operation. Blood transfusion is better started early in the operation because not only should blood loss be replenished, it is also necessary to combat the deleterious anesthetic effect. For the sake of reducing the amount of blood to be transfused, plasma expander may be recommended before blood transfusion. There is no obvious harm if blood hematocrit is kept above 30%. Blood loss may be underestimated when the operation is performed on the trunk or when the operation is delayed 1 week or longer after the burn, when the inflammatory reaction has developed.

Tangential excision tends to cause more blood loss than escharectomy particularly when the procedure is performed on a functional area such as hands and face, which are richly vascularized.

It is important to minimize blood loss during the operation. Application of tourniquets to burned extremities and the use of electric cautery, carbon dioxide laser [6], and plasma scalpel are measures to this end.

5.1.3 Surgical Procedure for Escharectomy and Tangential Excision

5.1.3.1 Escharectomy

The incision is better made on the adjacent normal skin or second-degree burn wound. Be sure that areas of mixed-type deep burn, superficial third-degree burn, and relatively deep dermal burn wounds are included in the excision. This will help avoid granulation formation from the unexcised wound, which may become infected and cause graft failure. However, in extensive circumferential burns of the trunk and extremity, the incision is made right in the deep burn wound.

The classical way of performing escharectomy is to excise the burn wound down to the deep fascia with removal of subcutaneous adipose tissue and superficial blood vessels and nerves. In order to maintain venous return, veins are sometimes carefully preserved, such as the veins of the dorsum of the hand and the great saphenous vein.

In the case of deep burns involving muscles underneath deep fascia, the level of excision should be carried down to healthy tissue where active bleeding and contraction of muscle under stimulation is grossly found. When there are suspected deeper burns or when the fascial compartment is under high tension, fasciotomy is performed and the muscle underneath the deep fascia is inspected for its viability.

When the area of excision is limited in extent, the resultant wound is closed by skin grafting. Skin autograft is of course the first choice. A large sheet of split-thickness skin autograft is strongly indicated in the functional area, if it is available and the general condition of the patient permits. It is used in the treatment of deep burns of the dorsum of the hand with a beneficial effect [7].

In relatively extensive burns, meshed skin autograft may be used when a limited amount of graft is available. Meshed graft usually yields a fairly good functional result but with widespread speckles.

In the case of extensive deep burn, where there is a shortage of skin donor sites, total coverage of the resultant wound with autograft is impossible. Jackson developed a technique of combined transplantation of skin autograft and

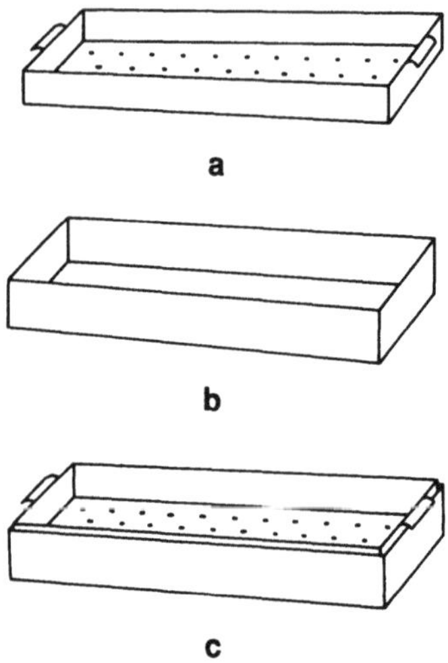

Fig. 5.1 a–c. Simplified equipment for micrograft skin transplantation. **a** An inner tray with holes punched in it. **b** An outer tray. **c** The two trays are put together for floating the micrograft

allograft [8]. The surgeons of the Burn Center of Ruijin hospital in Shanghai modified the experience and developed a new technique of intermingled transplantation of skin autograft and allograft [9]. The technique is composed of transplantation of a large sheet of punched skin allograft followed by insertion of small bits of skin autograft into the punched holes of the skin allograft. Epithelialization of epidermal cells takes place simultaneously with rejection of the epidermis of the allograft, which is often invisible under gross inspection. The ideal result may be obtained if the punched holes in the skin allograft are kept 1–1.5 cm apart and the skin autografts are 3×3 to $5 \times 5\,mm^2$ in size. Such a technique has offered an effective method of treating extensive deep burns, thereby greatly improving the results of treatment of extensive deep burns in China. It has been further developed for combined use of autograft and xenograft for skin transplantation [10].

The surgical technique has been further modified recently by Dr. Zhang Ming-Ling of Ji-Shui-Tan hospital in Beijing, and has been named "micrograft skin transplantation". The technique is designed on the basis of the different specific gravities of epithelium and dermis of the skin in normal saline. Epidermis is found to have a lipid content and its specific gravity is lower than that of dermis. Furthermore, the epidermal surface is more hydrophobic than the dermal surface. Due to these characteristics, when the minute pieces of skin float in normal saline, the epidermal side of all the micrografts will face upwards while the dermal surface faces downwards, thus facilitating the fishing out of the micrograft with dermal side up. The procedure begins with mincing skin autograft into micrograft or by cutting autologous split-thickness skin with a pair of scissors, knife, or the recently developed electric cutting machine into minute pieces not larger than $2 \times 2\,mm^2$. A double-bottomed tray with the inner bottom punched like a sieve is prepared (Fig. 5.1). At the bottom of the tray a layer of silk

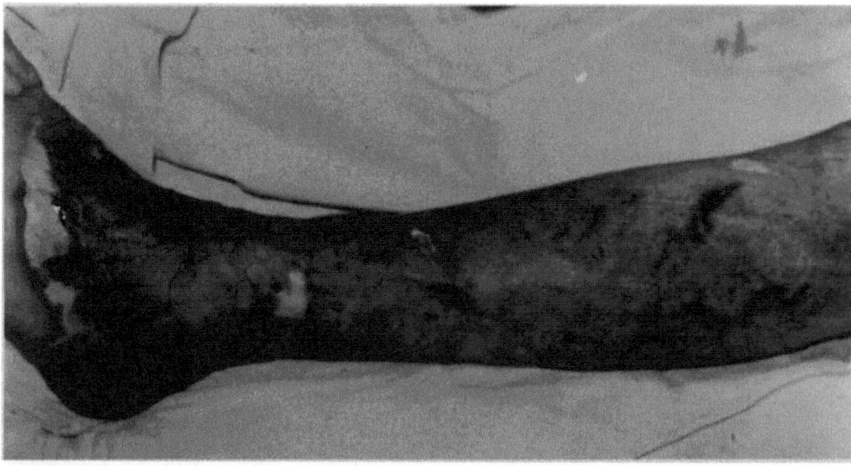

Fig. 5.2. Preoperative appearance of third-degree petrol burn

fabric is laid. The tray is then filled with normal saline and the micrografts are transferred into the tray. The micrografts float on the surface of normal saline with their epidermal side upwards. The screen is lifted up and moved back and forth, in order to obtain even spread of the micrografts. When the inner bottom of the tray is lifted out, the micrografts spread evenly on the silk fabric. The silk fabric is pulled out and kept taut, and then applied to the dermal side of a large sheet of fresh or cryopreserved skin allograft or fresh or lyophilized glutaraldehyde-treated porcine skin. Then apply the large sheet of skin allograft or xenograft together with the micrografts toward the surgical wound surface created by escharectomy. The operated area is then wrapped with sterilized dressing and the operating procedure is completed. New techniques have been developed such as using skin allograft with epithelium and dermis split with a part undetached followed by spreading of autogenic micrograft homogenate on the allograft dermis after fixation on the excised wound of third-degree burns (Figs. 5.2–5.6).

Recently another new technique for intermingled skin transplantation has been developed. Crisscross grooves 1–2 cm apart were made on the dermis of an allogeneic skin graft by using a scalpel. Epithelial cells harvested from the patient were seeded into the dermal grooves. The allograft thus prepared was used to cover excised wound of full-thickness burns [11]. A follow-up study showed that the new skin was soft and elastic with no contraction 1 year later. Cultured epithelial cells [12, 13] and skin pulp epithelial cells [14] have been tried clinically for the same purpose. All these developments and modifications were aimed at saving the amount of skin autograft needed, since the extreme shortage of skin donor sites in extensive deep burn patients was the most difficult problem encountered. However, they are still under clinical trial. More experience should be gained before they can be popularized. Scalp is an ideal skin donor site,

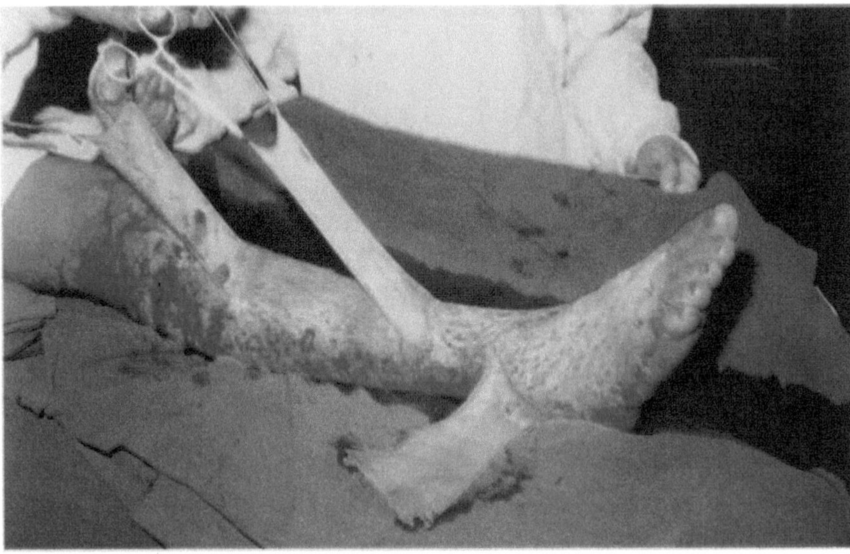

Fig. 5.3. Punctured allograft dermis is fixed on an excised wound of third-degree burn. Note that three undetached superficial split-thickness allografts have been lifted from their dermal base

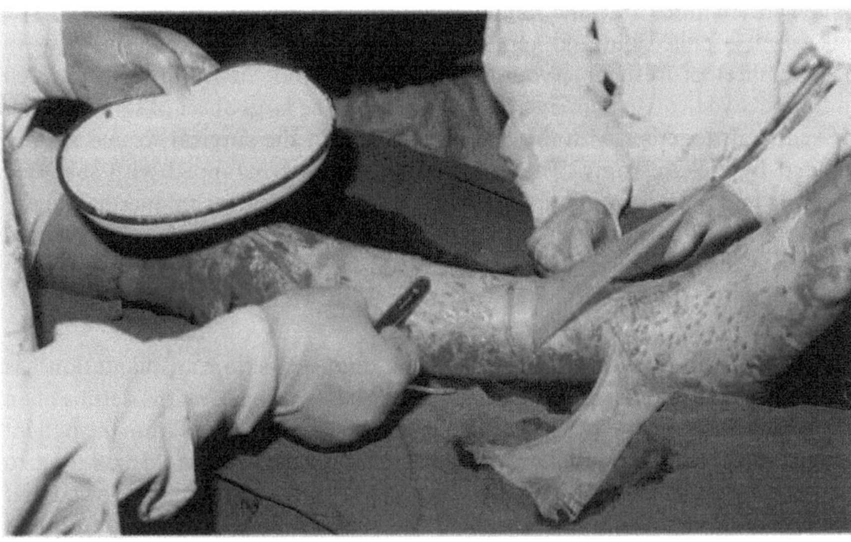

Fig. 5.4. Homogenate of an autogenous micrograft is then evenly spread on the fixed dermis of the skin allograft. A superficial split-thickness allograft is finally covered and fixed on the homogenate spread dermis of the skin allograft, and the operated wound is wrapped with sterile dressings

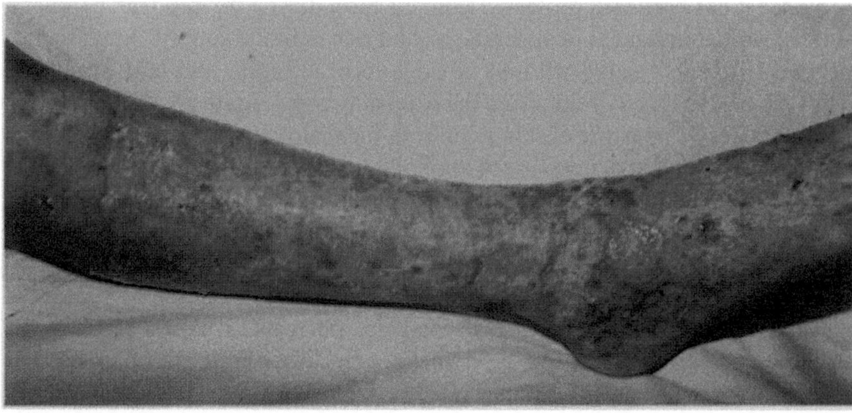

Fig. 5.5. Healing of the wound 3 weeks postoperatively

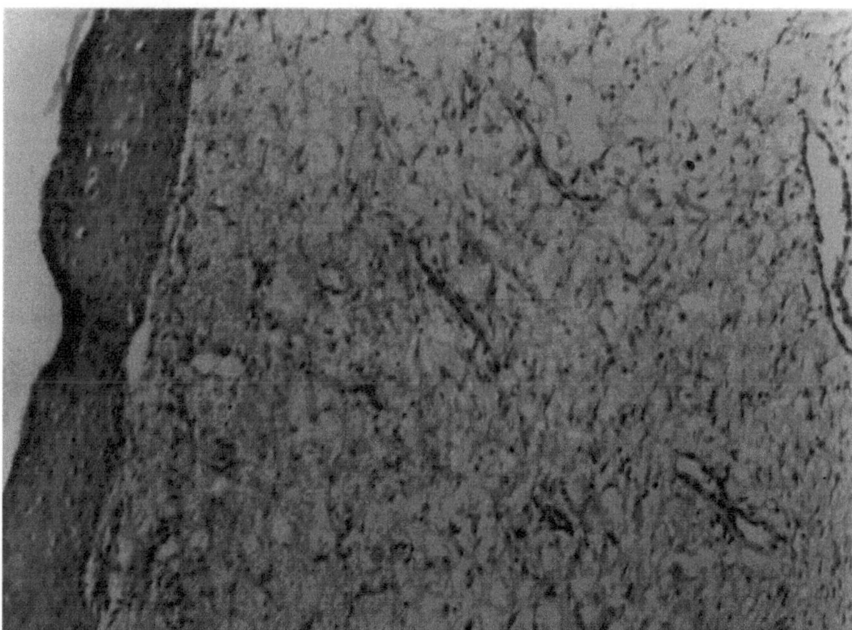

Fig. 5.6. Microscopic examination of a biopsy sample showed newly generated epithelium generally resembling the basic configuration of normal skin with the exception of a thinner layer of epithelial cells and lack of skin appendages

provided it has been well protected from the burn during the accident, because it is thick with abundant skin appendages, and rich in blood supply. When treated properly, it heals readily without obvious local infection and scar formation. Thus repeated harvest of skin from the scalp may compensate greatly for the lack of donor sites. Harvesting of skin graft from the scalp causes more bleeding than other donor sites. Local injection of normal saline or local anesthetic with a small amount of epinephrine is beneficial in reducing blood loss. A tourniquet may be applied for the same purpose.

A technique has been introduced to double the amount of skin harvested from a limited area of donor site. A piece of skin graft is first obtained by means of a Padgett dermatome, and the graft is again split while it is still stuck to the surface of the drum. Thus two layers of split-thickness graft are obtained. The superficial or outer layer is transplanted in the usual way, while the deeper or inner layer can be transplanted with either side facing the wound surface. This type of skin autograft is not suitable for micrograft transplantation, as the split layer is too thin to meet the technical requirement.

5.1.3.2 Tangential Excision

A tangential excision is used to excise devitalized tissue in the deep dermal mixed type, or superficial third-degree burns [15]. It is often used in the treatment of deep dermal burns of the hand [16]. It can offer a better functional and cosmetic result. Some surgeons recommend tangential excision in the treatment of facial burns in order to obtain a better functional and cosmetic effect. However, there may be profuse bleeding due to rich blood supply in this specific area.

The technical difficulty of a tangential excision is in deciding the right plane of excision. It is better to perform the excision in one single shaving, i.e., the excision should be deep enough to remove the divitalized tissue as expected. If the first shaving is inadequate, a second excision can be done. However, the second excision will be more difficult to perform, because of the reduced tissue tension and slippery dermal base, so that the excision is often too deep, resulting in undue tissue loss and damage to deep anatomical structures which are expected to be preserved.

A shiny porcelain-white dermal base with evenly scattered spotty active bleeding of fresh blood indicates an adequate tangential excision. If the wound base is not porcelain white and the spotty bleeding is dark red in color and not active, the excision is inadequate, and another shaving should be performed. In some burn centers and burn units, methylene blue is applied preoperatively as an aid in judging the adequacy of tangential excision [17].

An ideal operating instrument ensures a successful excision. The Humby knife, a freehand knife with an adjustable protective roller, is easy to manipulate even in inexperienced hands. An electric dermatome will be of help in performing an extensive excision. A newly developed instrument, the miniature electric dermatome, is available for operating with a high degree of proficiency. Such an instrument is suitable for tangential excision in some special areas such as the webs between the fingers in hand burns. It also facilitates harvesting of skin graft in special donor areas such as scalp and foot, particularly the toes and sole.

A tourniquet is not necessarily recommended for performing tangential excision, since gross inspection of bleeding is often a criterion of adequate excision. However, in excision of extensive deep burn wound or when there is inflammation in the operating area, a tourniquet may be applied in order to prevent massive blood loss.

Occasionally, when there are some areas showing necrosis or hemorrhagic necrosis. Care should be taken in choosing the best type of operation. Local necrosis or hemorrhagic necrosis of deep dermal burns may be caused by hemorrhage, trauma, fungal infection, invasive infection, or wound sepsis. The necrotic lesion is usually deeper than the surrounding burn wound. Hence, tangential excision may be inadequate for total removal of the devitalized tissue. Since the above-mentioned possible lesions are not readily differentiated by gross inspection, biopsy for bacterial count has been used. At present some burn centers prefer to make a diagnosis by tissue section. Some individual units are starting to use frozen section for rapid diagnosis. For fear of inadequate removal of devitalized tissue by tangential excision, and because of the possibility of spread of infection by the operating procedure, excision down to the fascia should be performed to ensure complete removal of the possible infected focus.

5.1.3.3 Wound Closure

5.1.3.3.1 Free Skin Grafting

Skin grafting is the most important means in securing wound closure. Skin autograft is the first choice. It may be grafted in the form of a large sheet, as a mesh graft, or as micrograft in intermingled transplantation with fresh or liquid-nitrogen-preserved allograft, lyophilized glutaraldehyde-treated xenograft, or xenograft preserved by other means such as alcohol.

5.1.3.3.2 Local Skin Flap

When a localized deep third-degree burn of limited area, such as an electric contact burn or a hot metal contact burn, is excised, repair of the defect with a local skin flap is strongly indicated. In the case of deep burns in specific areas where deep anatomical structures, such as large blood vessels and nerves, are exposed, a local pedicle flap is used because it has adequate blood supply to protect the exposed tissues, and healing is promoted. Sometimes an island flap is used to meet special purpose needs. Occasionally, a regional flap such as a forearm radial artery flap is used to repair localized deep burn of the hand. A number of local skin flaps have been designed by plastic surgeons. Some have been applied in the treatment of burns. So far, a specially designed 83 × 43 cm lumbosacral-gluteal-hip composite flap is the largest local flap that has been used in treating burns in China [18].

5.1.3.3.3 Free Skin Flap

Since the development of microsurgical technique, tissue and organ transplantation has been widely used in surgical treatment. Free skin flap, musculocutaneous flap, and composite tissue flap have been popularized in plastic surgery, and they have also been adopted in the treatment of severe burn for the preservation of deep anatomical structures, where free skin grafting is usually unsuccessful, or local skin flap is not available.

Free skin flap is designed so that the blood vessels can be anastomosed to the blood vessels of the recipient site. Free composite tissue flap transplantation is better used in the early postoperative days. The end results of the operation are different in various postburn stages. The therapeutic effects in a group of patients are shown in Table 5.1 [19].

Blood vessels should be manipulated with care and anastomosed with meticulous surgical technique to ensure patency at the site of anastomosis. Although the result with a free skin flap is better in the treatment of deep burns, it should be used with care. Blood vessels of the recipient site available for anastomosis are usually damaged. Gross examination is important, and the vessels are carefully dissected and cut a distance away from the damaged segment, because in thermal burns it has been found that the intima of the blood vessel is usually damaged up-to 3 cm from the damaged segment. More attention should be paid to electric contact burns, since a longer segment of blood vessel damage is often encountered. Anastomosis of damaged blood vessels will certainly lead to thrombus formation, resulting in failure of the flap transplantation.

The operative indication is more strict for the use of free skin flap than for other operative procedures, because the patient will sustain more stress in undergoing the free skin flap transplantation, both anesthesia and operating procedure being more prolonged.

Table 5.1. Result of vascular anastomosis of composite tissue flap transplantation at different postburn stages

Group	Cases (number)	Survival rate of tissue flap (%)	Rate of excellent wound healing (%)
Emergency	9	100	100
Acute stage	16	80	66.3
Infection stage	18	73	50
Late stage	11	82	64

5.1.4 Anesthesia

General anesthesia is usually used. Inhalation anesthesia is infrequently employed, whereas intravenous anesthesia is often used in most hospitals. Nowadays intravenous ketamine is the drug of choice. The anesthetic course of ketamine is relatively smooth.

Although inhalation anesthesia is not frequently used, intratracheal intubation is usually performed in patients with severe burns of the face, neck, and thorax for better control of respiration and to ensure a patient airway and adequate oxygen supply.

Local and regional anesthesia are seldom used, although they are simpler and safer, because of their inadequate anesthetic effect and because multiple areas, including skin donor sites, are often to be operated on. However, they are sometimes indicated individually or in combination with another anesthetic modality in burn patients with special problems and complications that render general anesthesia contraindicated. Local and regional anesthesia are occasionally used in patients with small full-thickness burns or in separate areas of skin donor sites.

Acupuncture anesthesia is not indicated in burns. Only a limited number of surgeons prefer to use it for harvesting small areas of split-thickness skin graft.

5.2 Autolysis and Associated Treatment

5.2.1 The Process of Autolysis

Autolysis is a natural process in local burn wound which is not excised in the early postburn period. It occurs in the zone of circulatory stasis. Inflammatory reaction produces demarcation between viable and nonviable tissues and granulation. The course of autolysis is accelerated by local infection. Devitalized tissue is separated from the healthy tissue by the process of autolysis, and is then removed en masse or piecemeal during subsequent dressing changes.

5.2.2 Topical Treatment

Topical agents suitable for burn treatment are usually astringents and antimicrobial agents. Herbal medicine used topically usually has the same effects as these agents. Topical agents of these types delay autolysis of deep burns by either crust formation or control of local infection.

Drugs with enzymatic properties are indicated in promoting autolysis of deep burns. Petrolatum (Vaseline) also serves the same purpose with less effect. Some pastes of herbal medicines are found to be effective in promoting autolysis of burn tissue and formation of granulation wound. Drugs, for these purposes either enzymes or herbs, are mentioned elsewhere in this volume.

5.2.3 Closure of Granulation Wound

5.2.3.1 Healing by Natural Process

Granulation wound of full-thickness burns of a limited area may heal spontaneously by proliferation and coverage of epithelial cells from the edge of surrounding skin or healed area of partial-thickness burn. In the case of patients with a large area of granulation wound which is difficult to close, the natural healing process will be protracted if the patient refuses operative treatment. The prolonged natural healing process is painful for the patient and time-consuming work for the medical staff and results in abundant scar tissue formation and contracture with functional loss and disfigurement.

5.2.3.2 Skin Grafting

5.2.3.2.1 Split-Thickness Skin Graft

Split-thickness autograft is used to cover granulation wound of a large area. In most circumstances small pieces of autograft about 1 × 1 cm in size are used. Stamp graft is seldom used in current clinical practice. However, it may be used, even in larger pieces, for specific functional and cosmetic requirements such as for burns of the face, neck, and hands. Attention must be paid to the preparation of the recipient granulation wound to prevent infection and grafting failure. Mesh graft can be used to cover granulation wound of a relatively large area with a fairly good functional result.

As for extensive granulation wound, skin allograft, either fresh or preserved, may be used intermingled with skin autograft in a mosaic pattern to circumvent the shortage of skin donor sites. If allograft is not available, fresh xenograft may be adopted for the same purpose. Meshed autograft may used with onlaid meshed or large-size allograft, xenograft, or even artificial skin in order to promote healing and control infection.

5.2.3.3 Management of Residual Granulation Wound

Residual granulation wounds in burns are those which have lasted a protracted period without signs of healing or have resulted from failure of skin grafting due to infection, trauma, etc. Some of them are small wounds left unhealed. The granulation tissue is not fresh enough to support epithelialization or to receive skin grafting. The granulation tissue is usually edematous and fibrotic with formation of fibrous plate underneath which interferes with the blood supply. Local resistance of this type of wound is reduced; hence there is obvious local infection with copious amounts of purulent exudation at the time of dressing changes.

The wound is not ready to heal although topical antimicrobial agents have been used and skin grafting has been performed. The course of treatment is protracted by a stay in hospital, with all its consequences for both patients and staff.

Many therapeutic measures have been tried in the management of residual granulation wound, and some are considered promising. Among these, hydrotherapy is relatively effective. Some of the wounds are healed by hydrotherapy accompanied by dressing changes. Some topical agents are also thought to be effective, and trimming of the overgrown granulation tissue may be beneficial. However, these measures are not useful in the treatment of protracted granulation wound of a large area. In such a case skin grafting is to be considered. However, the area be should be well prepared by removing all the edematous and fibrotic granulation tissue. Occasionally a fibrous plate underneath the granulation tissue should be removed concomitantly.

5.2.3.3.1 Hydrotherapy

A specially designed tank is used for hydrotherapy. An overhead trolley is used to help the patient lowering into and getting out of the bath. The hydrotherapy room should be kept warm, and the temperature of the bathing water is best maintained in the range of 40°–41°C. Bromogeramine and salt are usually added to the bath water in our hydrotherapy room.

Patients subjected to hydrotherapy should have a relatively stable general condition and should be advised not to become overexcited, particularly on first treatment. While in the bath the patient should be carefully observed. Hydrotherapy is terminated should there be any disorder. It has been reported in the medical literature that some patients may collapse while in the bath. However, no such problems have been encountered in our Burn Center, probably due to hydrotherapy being used at a late stage, when the general condition of the patient is usually much improved.

Before the patient is lowered into the bath, the outer dressings are removed. The inner layer of gauze may be left intact if it sticks fast to the wound surface. While in the bath, the inner layer gauze is soaked and will be easily removed by the whirling motion of the bath water or solution. The wound is then thoroughly cleaned and treated as indicated. The patient is rinsed when getting out of the bath. The body surface is immediately dried, and the wounds are quickly dressed.

After the hydrotherapy tank is used, it should be thoroughly washed, cleaned, and sterilized to prevent cross-infection between burn patients.

5.2.3.3.2 Topical Agents

Topical agents are prescribed by some surgeons to promote healing of the residual wound.

5.2.3.3.3 Treatment During Convalescence

Treatment is required during convalescence in some patients, particularly in most patients with deep burns. Deep burns usually result in scar formation, hypertrophic cicatrization, and even keloid. Contraction of scar tissue may result in disfigurement with functional loss and cosmetic problems.

Splinting of the burned extremities especially right after the surgical treatment mentioned above seems to be important. It is advisable to continue these during the course of convalescence. Passive and active exercises are mandatory in promoting functional recovery. A pressure garment may be of help in controlling formation of hypertrophic scar.

Detailed discussions on this subject can be found in Chap. 18.

Other physical therapy measures such as microwave treatment, iontophoresis, and acupuncture may bring about beneficial effects with at least relief of symptoms.

Treatment of contracture of scar tissue and consmetic problems resulting from healing of the burn wound may be further continued or followed by plastic surgery, when nonoperative treatment cannot lead to further improvement. Surgical repair and reconstruction is very often necessary. However, detailed discussion of plastic surgery is beyond the scope of this book.

References

1. Tian FQ, Liu JC, Fu YM et al. (1987) Major causes of death in burn patients. Chin J Crit Care Med 7(3): 6–10
2. Zhu CT, Xu XF, Zhang YF (1985) Clinical analysis of 76 extensive burn cases. Jiangsu Med 9(4): 33
3. Fang ZY (1959) Experience of treatment of critical major burn patients. 2nd Milit Med Coll (restricted publication, p 1)
4. Janzekovic EA (1970) New concept in the early excision and immediate grafting of skin. J Trauma 10(12): 1103–1108
5. Sheng ZY, Liu SH (1983) Contra-indications to early escharectomy in major burns. In: Yang ZJ, Sheng ZY, Shi JX (eds) Treatment and research in burns. Science Press, Beijing/Wiley, New York, pp 9–20
6. Xiao YR, Yang ZJ, Zhuo RP et al. (1983) Excision of burn eschar with CO_2 laser. In: Yang ZJ, Sheng ZY, Shi JX (eds) Treatment and research in burns. Science Press, Beijing/Wiley, New York, pp 40–45
7. Wang XZ (1985) Treatment of dorsum of deeply burned hand using whole sheet split-thickness autograft. Chin J Surg 23(8): 501–503
8. Jackson DA (1954) Clinical study of use of skin homografts for burns. Br J Plast Surg 7: 501
9. Shi JX, Yang ZJ, Xu WS (1982) Burn treatment. Chin J Surg 20(5): 259–261
10. Yang ZJ, Xu WS, Liao ZJ et al. (1983) Intermingled transplantation of fresh porcine and human skin in treating extensive third degree burns. In: Yang ZJ, Sheng ZY, Shi JX (eds) Treatment and research in burns. Science Press, Beijing/Wiley, New York, pp 46–53
11. Feng GD, Zhao CA, Zhang ST (1987) Seeding of autologous epithelial cells into allograft dermis as coverage for full-thickness burns. Proceedings of the 2nd Sino-American conference on burn injury and trauma, Beijing, p 118

12. Zhao XF, Lu SZ, Ju JN et al. (1987) Preliminary experience of wound coverage using cultured human epithelial cells. Chin J Surg 23(5): 297
13. Hu JN, Li N, Huan WH et al. (1986) Preliminary clinical observation of application of epithelial cultured membrane of skin allograft on burn wound. Chin J Plast Surg Burns 2(1) 52
14. Sun YH, Li S (1989) Skin pulp autoepithelium and homo-derma in the treatment of extensive full-thickness burns. A new method of skin grafting. Proceedings of the 2nd Sino-American conference on burn injury and trauma, Beijing, p 115
15. Sun YH, Chang ZD, Zhang ZM et al. (1987) Problems encountered during tangential excision for the treatment of deep burns. In: Yang ZJ, Sheng ZY, Shi JX (eds) Treatment and research in burns. Science Press, Beijing/Wiley, New York, pp 93–98
16. Sun YH, Wang XW (1980) Treatment of deep hand burn using tangential excision. Chin J Med 60(6): 358–361
17. Davies MRO, Adendorff D, Rode H et al. (1980) Colouring the damaged tissue on the burn wound surface. Burns 6: 156–159
18. Sun YH, Zhang ZM, Cao DX et al. (1984) Successful treatment of an extensive deep burn patient complicated by sequela of severe carbon monoxide intoxication. Beijing Med 6(1): 58
19. Shen ZY, Chang ZD, Wang NZ et al. (1988) Repair of super-deep burns. Beijing Med 10(4): 252

6 Burns of Special Areas

Wang Shi-liang and Li Ngao

Burns in certain regions of the body present several special problems and need specific treatment.

6.1 Burns of the Head and Neck

6.1.1 Burns of the Scalp and Skull

Except in electrical and chemical injury, full-thickness burn of the scalp is rarely seen. Partial-thickness burns of the scalp are usually treated conservatively by clipping the hair every week, cleansing the wound every 1–3 days, and daily application 5%–10% mafenide (Sulfamylon) cream or 1%–2% silver sulfadiazine cream. Every now and then, tangential excision is needed in the case of a deep partial-thickness burn in order to eliminate the necrotic tissue and drain the infection existing in hair follicles and sweat glands. After excision, the wound is simply dressed or covered with homograft. Full-thickness burn of the scalp with intact pericranium is suitable for early excision and grafting. Because of the potential profuse bleeding during excision, it is better to use an electric knife or laser. If the viability of the pericranium is in doubt, it is safer to cover the pericranium with a local skin flap after early removal (within 1 week) of dead soft tissue. If a local flap is not available, a distant free skin flap is indicated, using microsurgical anastomosis of the blood vessels. Treatment is often handicapped in the case of extensive necrosis of the scalp and skull. One of the difficulties is estimating the depth and area of the bone injury. In the early postburn period, X-rays or even computed tomography (CT) scans of the skull have proved to be of little value. Pegg [1] advocated the use of technetium scanning in the diagnosis of full-thickness bone loss. The conventional tactic of dealing with necrotic skull is to wait for its sequestration, then to drill holes down to the dipolë, or chisel off the outer table, and postpone the skin grafting until firm granulation tissue forms [2]. This method is not only time consuming, it induces intracranial infections such as brain abscess and meningitis. The alternative method, adopted currently, by many surgeons, is to excise the burned scalp together with the damaged outer table of the skull and to cover the inner table, which is left in situ regardless of its viability, with a local skin flap or remote skin flap with its blood vessels anastomosed with regional vessels, or with a composite greater omentum and skin grafting, i.e., a large sheet of free skin graft is placed on a piece of free autogenous greater omentum which has been laid on the inner table of the skull and anastomosed with the regional vessels [3,4]. The advantages of using omentum are: (a) it is big enough to cover the extensive skull wound and (b) its blood vessels are large and anastomosis is relatively easy. Its shortcomings are also twofold trauma of laparotomy and risk of infection of the abdominal cavity. Yang and Zhai [5] reported an 8-month-old baby with an extensive skull burn in whom sequential excision of the necrotic scalp and outer and inner tables of the skull except the area of the sagittal suture were performed, and the wound was covered with autografts on the dura mater immediately after excision.

6.1.2 Burns of Face and Neck

Our data [6] reveal that the face is involved in nearly 50% of all burns victims (788 of 1505 patients). In burns of face and neck it is of immediate importance to determine whether inhalation injury is present. Because the facial skin is flaccid and rich in blood supply, edema of burned face is usually marked, especially in the regions of the eyelids and lips. The eyelids may completely everted or even closed, and the lips thickened and protruded, often preventing the mouth from opening. In deep burns of face and neck, the inelastic dense eschar often confines edema fluid to the deep tissue, resulting in swelling of the laryngeal area and sometimes obstruction of the respiratory tract. Severe pharyngeal swelling can also disturb normal swallowing and clearing of vomitus from the mouth and pharynx, and thus aspiration may ensue.

Secretions from eyes, nose, and mouth will prevent eschar formation on the facial burn wound or often already formed eschar, and infection of the wound ensues. In addition, infection of facial wound sometimes complicates or exacerbates infection of ear and eyes. However, the healing of facial wound is facilitated by the rich hair follicles, sweat glands, and blood supply of the facial skin.

Superficial partial-thickness burns of the face and neck are usually treated with the exposure method. It is imperative to cleanse the burn wound, remove the debris and detached epidermis, and frequently remove secretions with sterile cotton swabs to keep the burn wound dry. Intact blisters are protected or evacuated at their dependent parts. If the blister epithelium is removed, the remaining burn wound surface should be protected with petrolatum gauze, biological materials (amnion, etc.), or artificial skin in order to protect the dermis from desiccation and necrosis. A topical antimicrobial agent such as 5%–10% mafenide and 3%–5% clotrimazole cream can be used.

In the case of moderate or minor burns affecting less than 30% of total body surface area (TBSA) cold therapy is indicated. Cold water (5–15°C) is used to rinse the burn wound, or the wound is covered with a cold compress for about 1 h or until pain abates after stopping the therapy. Cold therapy should be initiated as early as possible, and it is best done immediately after the burn injury.

The conventional treatment for deep partial-thickness burns is the same as that for superficial partial-thickness burns mentioned above. By virtue of the

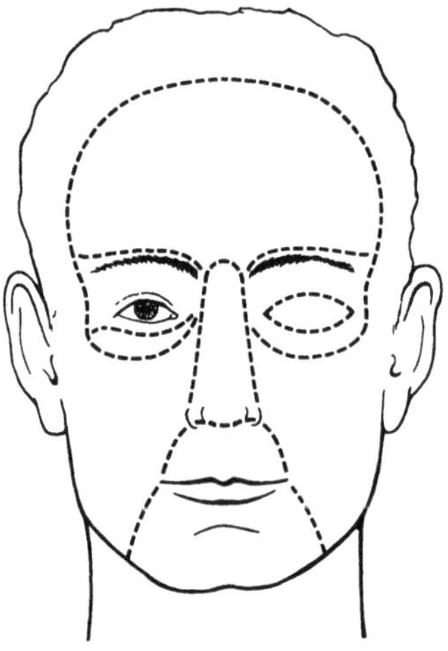

Fig. 6.1. The face is divided into eight regions, which are usually covered individually using one sheet of skin graft for each region

abundant supply of dermal appendages and capillary circulation, most of these wounds will heal spontaneously, but may leave hypertrophic scars with severe contractures. However, our institute [7] and others [8, 9] have now adopted early tangential excision with immediate skin autografting, and better cosmetic and functional results have been achieved. Krob et al. [10] also reported the use of serial debridement and allografting of facial burns to promote spontaneous healing with encouraging results. Nevertheless, the crucial problem with tangential excision is the judgment of the depth of the facial burns. Warden et al. [8] recommend excision therapy when the burn wounds are not expected to heal by 14 days, while Engrav et al. [9] assert that primary excision and grafting of face burns should be performed if the burns are judged not to be healed at 10 days. However, further clinical studies are needed to confirm their experience. Profuse bleeding is also a knotty problem during facial excision. Infiltration of isotonic saline or 0.25% procaine hydrochloride (Novocain) containing epinephrine (1:200000, or 1 drop/10 ml) into subcutaneous tissue beneath the area to be excised seems to be a simple and preferable way of controlling bleeding. The choice of the thickness of skin autograft depends on the depth of skin layer excised. The deeper the wound, the thicker the graft should be. It is not suitable to cover the superficial wound with a thick split graft, for this may impede the secretions of the sweat and sebaceous glands, resulting in the development of cyst and infection. On the contrary, it is also not advisable to cover the deep wound with thin graft, because it may end up forming more serious scar and deformity. Moreover, it is better to use a large sheet than mesh or small-piece grafts to achieve better cosmetic and functional results. The face and neck are divided into several esthetic regions for split-thickness grafting [2, 6, 10]. Usually there are eight regions of the face: the frontal region above the arcus superciliaris, two orbital regions, two faciobuccal regions, the nose, the upper lip (labionasal), and the lower lip(labiomental). The neck may be divided by the wrinkle between the

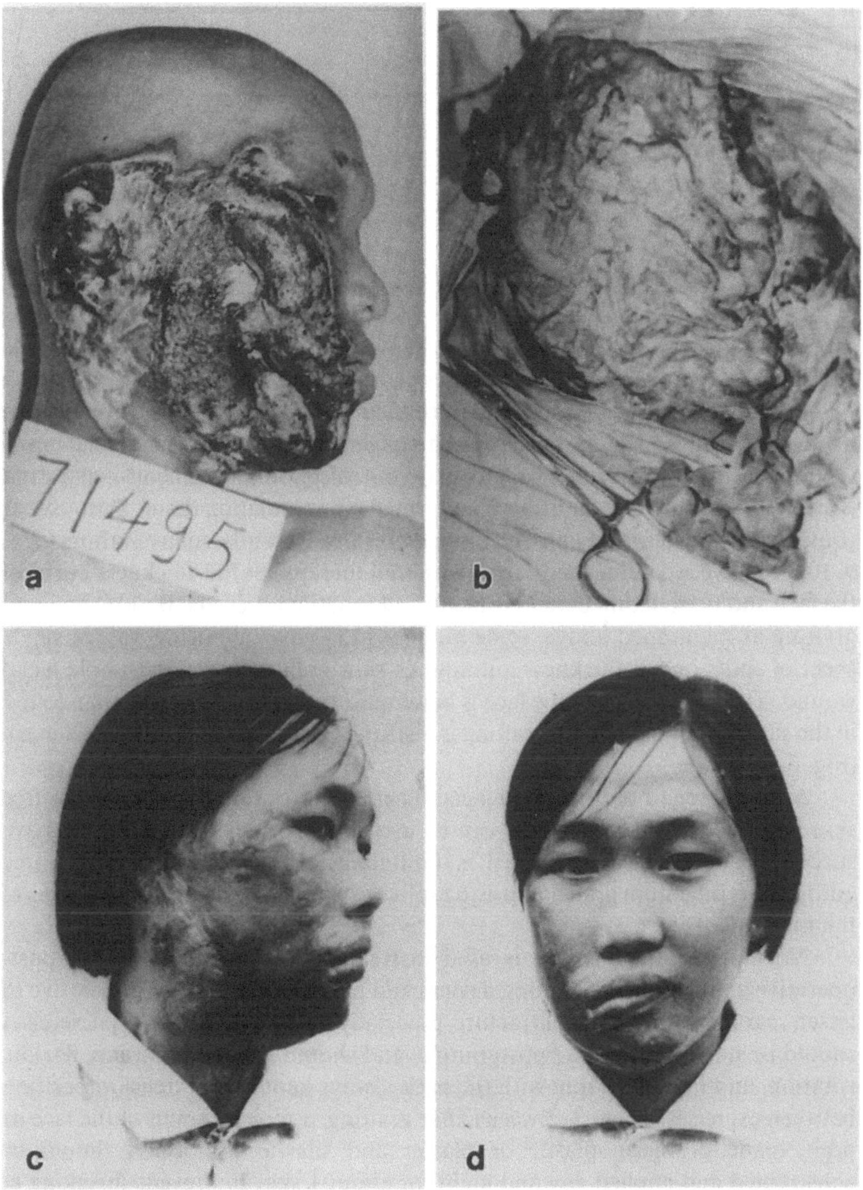

Fig. 6.2 a–d. Repair of a perforated electrical burn of the face using free omentum graft. **a** Perforated electrical burn of face, preoperation. **b** Free omentum graft covering the perforated region and anastomosed to regional verssels; split-thickness skin graft used as liner. **c** 15 months after operation (*lateral view*). **d** 15 months after operation (*front view*)

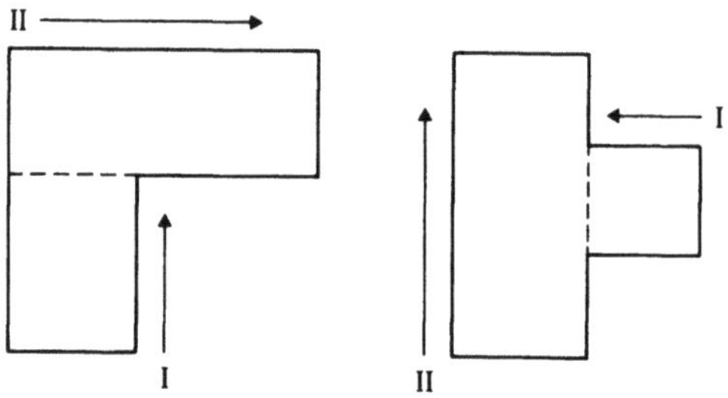

Fig. 6.3. Method for cutting a single sheet of graft of "T" or "L" shape

submandibular triangle and neck into lower jaw and neck regions. Generally, it is advisable to use one sheet of graft to cover one region (Fig. 6.1).

Because of profuse bleeding and the difficulty in identifying the depth of burn wound, the traditional approach to the management of full-thickness facial burns is nonoperative: the wound is kept dry to avoid infection, spontaneous separation is awaited, and then skin grafting is performed on granulation tissue. Serious scar contracture and deformity are the ultimate results. Recently, many authors [7, 8, 9, 10, 11] have recommended early excisional therapy for full-thickness burns of the face and neck, citing better cosmetic and functional results. Besides regional grafting as mentioned above, some authors [12] advocate using a large single sheet of split- or full-thickness autologous skin graft to cover the whole facial wound. The appearance of the face is better and there is less scarring than found in the suture lines of regional grafting is lost, and the appearance is that of a mask (Fig. 6.2).

As to the repair of perforated facial burns, two free skin flaps or a single free skin flap folded to form a linear can be used [13]. In our clinic [14], we have successfully repaired a perforated mandibulofacial electrical burn with a free autogenous omentum graft comprising split skin grafts placed on both surfaces of the omentum (Fig. 6.3).

No matter what method is used in treating face and neck burns, postoperative application of splinting devices and pressure garments is imperative to lessen scar formation and contracture, especially in the neck area [15]. Exercises should be started 1–2 weeks postgrafting, and should include extension, flexion, rotation, and lateral flexion, with the neck always kept in its extension position between exercises. Then, 2–3 weeks after grafting, a molded splint of the face or neck, made of thermoplastic or plaster and silastic conformer, should be constructed and applied day and night for about 1 year to prevent shrinking of the graft.

6.1.3 Burns of the Eyes

There have been 195 cases of eye burns among the 1505 burns patients in our institute, giving an incidence of 12.9%. In most instances, because of the blink reflex of the eyes, usually only the eyelids are injured. The cornea, conjunctiva, and sclera are rarely involved except in cases of explosion, splashes of hot liquids or chemicals, and flash injury due to short circuiting of an electric current.

The management of superficial eyelid burn resembles that for superficial facial burns. In deep burns of the eyelids, the problems are the rapid ectropion formation during the early swelling stage and the subsequent contracture of eyelids first by eschar and later by scar. Incomplete closure of the lids causes exposure and dryness of the cornea, often resulting in ulcer formation, and sometimes severe infection, cornea perforation, and panophthalmitis may supervene. Tarsorrhaphy is one of the methods of choice to protect the cornea from damage. However, suturing of the lids or tarsal plates together may lead to distortion of the lid margins with subsequent trichiasis and may hamper the inspection of the cornea and the inner portion of the eye, especially for early detection of infection. Tarsorrhaphy if needed at all, is mostly a temporary measure. Use of the moisture chamber [16] seems to be a simple expedient to protect the exposed cornea from drying. It is constructed by placing a supporting ring around the eye, covering it with a plastic wrap, and sealing around the rim with ophthalmic lubricating ointment. A preferable method, however, is to correct the contracture and ectropion of the eyelid by early escharescomy of the eyelid with free skin autografting. The incision should be close to the lid margin (usually, because of the blink reflex, the lid margin is not burned), and the excision should include the devitalized skin inside the orbital margin. Any contracture of scar tissue should be released to overcorrect the affected eyelid. Properly selected and color-matched full-thickness skin grafts, usually obtained from the medial aspect of the upper arm or the superaclavicular area, are applied.

Chemical Burn of the Eyes. The crucial point is to wash the eyes promptly and thoroughly with large amounts of water or isotonic saline. Attention should be paid to irrigating the conjunctival sac. This procedure should be continued for at least 20–30 min at the scene of the accident or during first aid. The same procedure should be repeated at the clinic when the patient is first seen. In explosive burns, all particles and foreign bodies in the conjunctival sac need to be carefully removed. Early ophthalmological consultation is indicated if the cornea is injured. All eye treatment is directed toward preventing exposure, infection, ulceration, and perforation of the cornea.

Antibiotic drops and/or ointments (0.5% chloramphenicol, 1% polymyxin B, 1% gentamycin, etc.) and subconjunctival injections of antibiotics should be used every 2–6 h to prevent or control infection. Atropine drops for mydriasis, Dionin (ethylmorphine hydrochloride) or tolazoline drops for dialating vessels, and 0.5%–1% dicain for analgesia are needed. Because of the possibility of promoting bacterial invasion and ulcer formation, steroid-containing ophthalmic drops and ointment should be administered only after the healing of corneal ulcer for the purpose of lessening inflammatory reaction and scar formation.

In addition, the damaged cornea can be protected with amniotic grafts or local conjunctival flaps. During the treatment of eye burns, especially with corneal ulcer, attention should be paid to aseptic technique and avoidance of the prone position and pressing the eyeball. Adhesions of the conjunctival sac should be separated once or twice a day with sterile glass rod to prevent symblepharon.

6.1.4 Burns of the Ears

Of the 1505 burns patients admitted to out institute, 359 (20.3%) have had burns of the auricle. Burn of the external auditory meatus is exceedingly rare; occasionally it occurs when hot liquids or chemicals are splashed into the meatus. The management of superficial partial-thickness burns of the auricle is the same as facial burns. Care must be taken to prevent infection which might invade the deeper layer to produce chondritis. Of our 359 patients with auricle burns, 29(8.1%) developed chondritis [2]. Chondritis occurs infrequently in superficial partial-thickness burns, whereas it occurs much more frequently in deep burn superimposed by infection during the 3rd–5th week postburn. In a group of 76 patients with auricle burns, chondritis developed in only 1 of 40(2.5%) superficial partial-thickness burns, but in 19 of 36(52.8%) deep burns [17]. The subcutaneous tissue of the auricle and the poor blood circulation make the ear cartilage vulnerable to infection. Therefore, it is important to note that pressure on the auricle should be avoided, because it will not only make the burn wound become macerated and liable to infection but also further impair the local circulation, hastening the development of chondritis. A ring-shaped pad or pillow should be provided to protect the ear from bending or pressure when the patient is lying on that side. Topical chemotherapy is beneficial in reducing the incidence of chondritis following auricle burns. In one report, it is claimed that only one in seven of the patients treated with 1% silver sulfadiazine cream developed chondritis [17], and the rate of chondritis was significantly reduced from 24.9% to 9.4% by the topical use of silver sulfadiazine suspension [18]. Frequent removal of the secretions accumulated in the areas of the triangular fossa, external auditory meatus, and around its entrance should not be neglected, especially during the early postburn stage, so as to keep the wounded ear dry. However, whenever the infection becomes inevitable, an antibiotic wet compress can be applied to facilitate drainage of exudate and control superficial infection. Some authors recommend laser therapy to prevent chondritis, and good results were found in an experimental study [19].

The conventional treatment for chondritis of the burned ear is thorough drainage of the infected soft tissue with excision of the involved cartilage under general anesthesia as soon as the diagnosis is made. All the involved cartilage should be thoroughly removed, otherwise the infection will not subside and repeated surgical excision is needed. As a result of partial or total loss of the ear cartilage, disfigurement of the auricle may ensue. In order to avoid or minimize the deformity surgery should be performed early, and a policy of waiting for localization of infection is undesirable. In our institution, early incision and drainage followed by alternating frequent irrigation and wet compress with a sensitive antibiotic solution resulted in cure without apparent disfigurement in six cases of chondritis.

6.1.5 Burns of the Nose

Singeing of the nasal hairs indicates the presence of nostril burns. After cleansing of the nostrils with 3% H_2O_2, they should be examined with a sterile speculum to determine the severity of the burns. Application of antibiotic ointment every 4–6 h is beneficial. Moreover, attention should be paid to burns of the deeper respiratory tract. Burns of the nose are usually handled together with facial burns. Early excision and grafting of deep burns, for example, are performed concurently. To prevent stenosis or atresia of the nostrils after deep burn of the nasal alae, soft plastic tubes may be inserted into the nostrils, especially during the healing stage. Care must be taken not to use hard rubber tubing and to avoid continuous pressure against the vestibular wall so as to prevent ischemic necrosis. Care should also be taken to remove the crusts from the nostrils to facilitate nasal breathing, especially in the early stage.

6.1.6 Burns of the Mouth

Burns of the mucosa of the oral cavity, not infrequently complicated by inhalation injury, are sometimes seen after swallowing of erosive chemicals or hot food. These burns are usually superficial and healing can be expected within several days, sometimes helped by frequent gargling and cleansing of the mouth cavity. Deep burns of the mucosa of the oral cavity do occasionally occur and are usually followed by severe infection with sloughing of mucosa. Not only is healing often delayed, but there will also be severe pain during eating. Therefore, tube feeding is helpful. Burns of the lips are usually associated with facial burns. Solitary severe lip burns are seen in the case of electrical injuries, almost exclusively in children. Treatment for lip burns is similar to that for facial burns. In deep lip burns, however, the prevention of microstomia, which may tend to result from scar contracture, is important. Silverglade and Ruberg [20] introduced several differnt splinting appliances for burns involving the lips and commissures. Each provided physical resistance to contracture of the scar and was utilized until the scar had lost its contractile potential. Delaplaza et al. [21] considered that, in mild cases, a good result could be achieved with conservative treatment. In severe cases, with extensive destruction of the lips or the tongue, their experience favored surgery, to be performed as early as possible.

Besides the common occurrence of scar contracture, restriction of mouth opening may also suggest septic arthritis involving the temporomandibular joint [22], though this is rare.

6.2 Burns of the Hand

Because the hands are important in living and working and are nearly always exposed, the incidence of hand burns is very high. There were 644 cases of hand burns in our group of 1505 burns patients, giving an incidence of 44.1%. Although the surface area of both hands accounts for only about 5% of TBSA, deep burns of the hand often lead to serious deformity and disability. Therefore, they are classified as severe burns. Because the skin of the dorsum of the hand is thinner and more likely to be exposed, especially when the hands are clenched, burns, of the dorsum is more common and serious than of the palm. The palm is usually burned by electricity, by chemicals, or by grasping hot metals or other materials. Because of its thicker epidermal layer, burn of the palm is usually not deep. Severe deeper injury may occur in electrical burns, hot metal burns, or burn injury due to heat and pressure.

6.2.1 Principles of Management

Besides promotion of early wound healing, prevention of hand deformity to achieve a good functional result is of great importance.

6.2.1.1 Early Wound Coverage

Waiting for spontaneous separation of dead tissue in the deep burn wound would provide a favorable medium for the proliferation and invasion of bacteria, and this would inevitably lead to further deepening of the wound. In the case of wound healing by natural epithelialization of the granulating surface, hypertrophic scar, scar contracture, and deformity are inevitable. Moreover, early active and passive exercises of burned hands are often restricted due to local pain, inelastic eschar, tendon contracture, muscle rigidity, and stiff joints, and the result will be severe functional loss. Therefore, early burn would excision with immediate autologous skin grafting to achieve early wound coverage and better function is of primary importance, unless the patient's general condition contraindicates. Needless to say, in the extensively burned patient, life-saving is the first priority, and early operation of burned hands is often delayed due to the performance of life-saving procedures. If early excision cannot be performed, the next choice is delayed excision and autografting within 3 weeks after injury, removing all the dead tissues and overgrown granulations and covering the wound with a large sheet or stamp-sized pieces of autograft. Postoperative active and passive exercises of the hands are permitted. Stiffness of the joints can be prevented, and a better functional result may be obtained.

6.2.1.2 Reduction of Acute Edema

Edema from fluid exudation due to increased capillary permeability usually reaches its peak at 2–3 days postburn. Depositions of the protein-rich exudate along tendons, muscle layers, joint capsules, and periarticular tissue become organized. Elastic fibers, tendon sheaths, fasciae, small muscles, and joint capsules, especially in small joints, become bound by fibrous tissue, resulting in ankylosis and loss of function of the hand. Therefore, it is important to reduce the extent and duration of edema. The simple and proper procedure is to elevate the hand and to encourage active motion as early as possible. A pillow covered with a sterile envelope is used to keep the hand 15–20 cm above the bed. In the case of circumferential deep burns, immediate escharotomy is indicated when there is inadequate blood flow. Escharotomy should be performed along both sides of the forearm, extending both beyond the elbow and down to the fasciae so as to release the constriction completely. Sometimes, fasciotomy should also be performed to relieve the pressure on muscular compartments and interosseous muscle bundles. It appears that no obvious improvement in reducing acute burn edema will be obtained by using compressive dressings, and sometimes this may even produce more compression which will retard or block circulation in the burned extremity and thus worsen the edema. In the case of deep circumferential finger burns, escharotomy along both sides of the burned finger should also be performed as early as possible.

6.2.1.3 Encouragement of Early Movements and Splinting

Edema, eschar, dressings, and pain are factors limiting the movement of burned limb. After resorption and subsidence of edema, it is better to encourage the patient to move the burned extremity actively, and try to take care of her- or himself in daily life as much as possible. When active movement is not allowed due to the presence of open wounds, fractures, or peripheral nerve injuries, and also during rest, the burned limb should be splinted to prevent deformity, no matter whether the occlusive dressing or the exposure method is used. The deformity caused by a dorsal hand burn is usually in the form of a claw, with flexion of the wrist, adduction of the thumb, full extension of the metacarpophalangeal joints, and full flexion of the interphalangeal joints. The splints should be applied with slight extension of the wrist (20–30°), abduction and opposition of the thumb, flexion of the metacarpophalangeal joints (90–120°), and mild flexion of the interphalangeal joints (20–30°). Thermoplastic splint is recommended, because it is economical and convenient to use.

6.2.1.4 Control of Infection

Following initial debridement, topical antibacterial agents such as cream or paste of 1%–2% silver sulfadiazine or 5%–10% mafenide and an antifungal agent

(4%–5% clotrimazole) should be applied. Moreover, any one of the following concentrated herbal decoctions can be used topically (usually 1 ml decoction is equivalent to 1 g herb): *Coptis chinensis*, *Scutellaria baicalensis*, *Phellodendron amurense*, *Allium sativum*, *Lonicera japonica*, *Ilex chinensis*, and *Eucalyptus robusta*. All of these decoctions kill most of the microorganisms that commonly colonize the early burn wound surface, and some are claimed to be able to stimulate the reticuloendothelial system, improve phagocytosis, and augment the lymphocyte transformation rate [23]. Some burn physicians in China prefer combined use of a topical chemotherapeutic agent and a concentrated herbal decoction and claim better clinical results.

6.2.2 Treatment of Superficial Burns of the Dorsum of the Hand

No special care is necessary for first-degree burns of the dorsum of the hand except good analgesia and protection from further trauma. In superficial partial-thickness burns, blisters should be well protected from rupture. A large blister is only drained by aspiration or incision at its dependent border. It has been found that the burn wound will heal better if the blister is kept intact. However, if the blisters have already been broken or badly contaminated, all detached epidermis should be removed and after a thorough cleansing the burn wound is covered with an artificial or biological membrane. We have compared the therapeutic effect on healing of superficial wounds under four materials after removal of blisters: herb decoction (*Eucalyptus fobusta*), 1% silver sulfadiazine cream, semi-open with a single layer of oil-impregnated fine-mesh gauze, and type T-41 artificial skin. The best result is seen with artificial skin [24]. Aminotic membrane can also be used with good results. Proper drainage and prevention of infection are still the points to which attention should be paid in using these membranes.

6.2.3 Treatment of Deep Partial-Thickness Burns of the Dorsum of the Hand

To date, tangential excision with transplantation of a single large sheet or pieces of autologous skin graft is the best way to treat deep partial-thickness burns of the dorsum of the hand, provided there is no coexisting life-threatening injury or condition. For instance, in the case of patients with quite extensive burns, which may be life threatening, it is wise to treat the burned hand conservatively with topical chemotherapy and/or a herbal decoction until the patient's general condition has stabilized; then a delayed excision may be performed, or skin grafting may be instituted after separation of dead tissue. It should be pointed out that the web areas are usually only superficially burned, because the hand is often clenched when a burn occurs, and can therefore be left unexcised during the tangential excision and allowed to heal spontaneously. Better cosmetic and functional results can be obtained in this way [25].

6.2.4 Treatment of Third-Degree Burns of the Dorsum of the Hand

If a third-degree burn of the dorsum of the hand involves only loss of full-thickness skin, the total burn area is not too extensive, and the patient's general condition permits surgery, early excision of eschar with split-thickness skin autograft is advisable, and is best performed within 2 weeks after the injury. Skin grafting is usually carried out immediately after excision. Some surgeons prefer to delay skin grafting for 2 days in order to avoid hematoma underneath the graft and to remove any nonviable tissue left during the previous operation. However, the incidence of infection seems to be higher in delayed skin grafting. In our experience, cosmetic and functional results are better if the dorsal venous system and superficial fascia of the hand are conserved during excision. For the same reason, as stated in the description of deep partial-thickness burns of the dorsum of the hand, we also conserve the triangular areas of the finger webs. The tip of each triangular web area reaches the level of the metacarpophalangeal joints. In order to lessen scar formation, sometimes a T- or L-shaped single skin sheet about 300 cm^2 area, obtained with a Padgett dermatome, may be used to cover the whole dorsum of the hand [2]. A split sheet of autograft about 10 × 8–10 cm in size is harvested but the end is not cut. The drum is removed from the loose skin, rotated 90°, and another sheet of 10 × 20 cm is harvested which is in continuation with the perpendicular flap. The harvested skin can thus be in a T form or an L form (Fig. 6.3). The T- or L-shaped skin flap is often used in cases where the wrist region is included in the excision of the dorsum of the hand. If more than one piece of skin graft is used to cover the dorsal area, the suture lines between the grafts should not be located over the joints in order to avoid any interference in joint function after healing. Use of mesh graft should be restricted unless there is a shortage of donor sites. When a deep burn is excised from the dorsal part of the finger, the excision is better extended beyond the distal interphalangeal joint, and the lateral incisions should be planned slightly ventral to the midlines and in a zigzag fashion so as to prevent linear scar contracture after healing. If the burns on the dorsal aspect of the digit involve extensors, tendons, bone, and joints, the cortex of the digital bone can be removed by rongeur and an immediate skin graft applied directly to the raw bone surface [26]. In the case of circumferential loss of soft tissue around the digital bone, the bare phalangeal bone can be first wrapped with a free autologous omental graft, to be covered by skin autograft. The length of the digits can thus be preserved and a certain amount of function restored [27]. Burns, of the dorsum of hand can be so deep that the extensor tendons or bones are exposed after escharectomy. As free skin grafting usually would not be successful in such a case, a radial or ulnar forearm islet flap can be transplanted to cover the excised dorsal surface, provided the radial and ulnar arteries together with the palmar arch are intact. Otherwise, a free skin flap from another part of the body or a lower abdominal pedicle skin flap should be considered.

6.2.5 Treatment of Deep Burns of the Palm

Because palmar skin is thick and tough, deep burns of the palm are less frequent. Deep partial-thickness burns are better treated with tangential excision followed by split-thickness skin grafting. In the case of full-thickness burns with the palmar aponeurosis still intact, escharectomy and skin autografting can be used, although controversy exists over the choice of full-thickness or split-thickness skin graft to cover the defect [28, 29]. If the aponeurosis is burned and tendons and vessels are exposed, either islet skin flap from forearm on the ipsilateral side or free skin flap from any part of the body can be used after thorough debridement of the devitalized tissue. One to two weeks after grafting, when the graft has firmly adhered to the bed, physical therapy should be initiated. Either active or passive motion to ensure joint flexibility is encouraged. Splinting is also important to maintain the injured hand in extension in the intervals between active or passive movements and thus prevent flexion contracture of palms and digits. Hypertrophic scar formation can be lessened by pressure dressings if started early.

6.3 Burns of the Axilla

Usually, no special care is necessary in the case of superficial burns of the axilla except the use of pads or gauze to prevent adhesion. For deep burns, early excision and skin grafting is indicated. Either local myocutaneous or fascio-cutaneous flap can be selected according to local needs after excision. The axilla should be splinted in abduction and physical therapy should be started early after grafting.

6.4 Burns of the Perineum

Some 298 (19.8%) of the 1505 burn cases hospitalized in the Burn Research Institute of the Third Military Medical College, had burns involving the perineal region. Because the perineal region is constantly soiled and moist, the exposure method is usually adopted. The patient lies the supine with legs kept apart, and a mattress is put under the patient's back so as to elevate the buttocks and keep the perineum away from the bed. It is advisable to place children in the prone position so that better exposure can be achieved. A topical agent can be applied. The perianal region should be thoroughly irrigated with 0.05% chlorhexidine or 2%–3% hydrogen peroxide after each bowel movement. Usually an enema is given before skin grafting tincture of opium is then used after operation in order to constipate the patient for 4–5 days. Some authors [30] prefer to use temporary colostomy to divert the fecal flow. However, in the majority of cases this does not seem necessary, and it is especially inadvisable in the case of burns involving the abdominal wall. There exists a risk of intraperitoneal contamination in performing a colostomy. In the case of deep burns, in order to eliminate the possibility of anaerobic or fungal infection, oral administration of metronidazole (Flagyl 0.2–0.4 g tid), nystatin (1 000 000 units tid), or other anti-anaerobic or antifungal drugs can be used especially during the pre- and postgrafting periods.

An indwelling catheter is usually needed in females, and also in males if the penis is deeply burned. Owing to the high incidence of urethritis or even ascending urinary infection after prolonged indwelling catheterization [31], some authors advocate suprapubic cystostomy or an indwelling catheter introduced through a suprapubic puncture by means of a trocar. Good results have been obtained even in the presence of suprapubic burns. In our experience, if bladder irrigation can be carried out carefully two to three times a day together with systemic use of effective antibiotics which are excreted via the renal route, the danger of ascending infection from the indwelling catheter is minimal, especially when the catheter is removed within 2–3 weeks.

Early surgical excision of deep partial-thickness burns and even mixed deep second- and third-degree burns of the perineal region is usually not adopted. However, thorough debridement and skin grafting should be performed as early as possible [30, 32, 33] if third-degree burn is proved. In light of the relatively low survival rate of free skin graft in this region, some authors [32, 33] advocate the use of skin flaps, either local or islet, for early repair of third-degree burns. It must be pointed out that viable tissues should be conserved as much as possible during the excision, especially in the area of the penis, scrotum, testis, labium, and anal sphincter. The seam of a skin graft applied to the penile shaft should not be placed on the ventral aspect, to prevent subsequent chordee. After operation, oral stilbestrol can be administered to prevent erection of the penis and thus help assure that the skin graft takes. The foreskin can be split and spread to cover the penile shaft and its surrounding area [31]. The urethal meatus should be carefully everted with sutures to prevent stenosis. If the area of necrosis of the skin of the scrotum is no more than one-third of its total area, the defect left by the excision can be closed with sutures by virtue of the extensibility of the scrotal skin. Any linear or circular suture should be avoided; instead, multiple Z-plasties are used to minimize linear or annular scar contracture or constriction. Stent dressings are usually applied to hold the skin graft in place.

References

1. Pegg SP, Jenkins AM (1987) Deep electrical burns to the scalp. Burns 13(1): 62–65
2. Burn Research Institute of the Third Military Medical College (ed) (1977) The treatment of burns. People's Health Publisher, Beijing. pp 254–278
3. Sun YH, Tsao DS, Ma RL et al. (1985) Use of autogenous omentum for grafting electrical injury affecting the scalp and skull. Burns 11(4): 289–292
4. Liu HS, Xu BD, Huang FR et al. (1986) Treatment of necrotic skull burns using autogenous free omentum graft—report of two cases. Abstract of the 11th burn and plastic surgery conference of the PLA, 5–9 Dec, Beijing, pp 136–137
5. Yang SW, Zhai JH (1987) Severe skull burn in an infant—report of a case. Chin J Plast Surg Burns 3(1): 23–25

6. Artz CP, Moncrief JA, Pruitt BA (1979) Burns. A team approach. Saunders, Philadelphia, pp 309–329
7. Ai SH, Li A, Kang SY et al. (1986) Repair of deep facial burn using large sheet of split-thickness skin graft. Abstract of the 11th burn and plastic surgery conference of the PLA, 5–9 Dec, Beijing, p 146
8. Warden GD, Saffle JR, Schnebly A et al. (1986) Excisional therapy of facial burns. J Burn Care Rehabil 7(1): 24–28
9. Engrav LH, Heimbach DM, Walkinshaw MD et al. (1986) Excision of burns of the face. Plast Reconstr Surg 77(5): 744–751
10. Li CL, Yang KF, Pan DH et al. (1987) Early escharectomy and grafting in the treatment of deep facial-cervical burns. Chin J Plast Surg Burns 3(3): 200–201
11. Krob MJ, Jordan MH (1987) Serial debridement and allografting of facial burns: a method of controlling spontaneous healing. J Trauma 27(2): 190–194
12. Wang JD (1985) Repair of facial burns using a single sheet of full-thickness skin. Proceedings of the 1st Sino-American conference on burn injury, Chongqing, p 143
13. Shi HR, Yang ZN, Cao L et al. (1987) The repair of severe perforated facial burns — report of 4 cases. Chin J Plast Surg Burns 3(1): 1–2
14. Zeng XZ, Ou BP, Ma SZ et al. (1984) Free omental transplantation for treatment of severe electric burn of the face. Med J Chin PLA 9(1): 59–60
15. Yang ZJ, Xu WS, Shi JX et al. (1985) Burn treatment, 2nd edn. Shanghai Science and Technology Publisher, Shanghai, pp 155–204
16. Hupp SL, Galanos AN, Luterman A (1987) A simple moisture chamber for the early treatment of corneal exposure in patients with facial burns. J Burn Care Rehabil 8(2): 115–116
17. Zhu WL, Li JY (1988) Treatment of burns of ear. Chin J Plast Surg Burns 4(2): 114–115
18. Zhang QZ, Wang XW, Josephine I et al. (1985) Prophylaxis and treatment of auricle burns complicated with perichondritis of ear cartilage. Proceeding of the 1st Sino-American conference on burn injuries, Chongqing, p 165
19. Chen SZ (1982) The effect of laser on the chondritis of the burn ear and scattering wound. Abstract of the 9th burn and plastic surgery conference of PLA, Shanghai, pp 72–73
20. Silverglade D, Ruberg RL (1986) Nonsurgical management of burns to the lips and commissures. Clin Plast Surg 13(1): 87–94
21. Delaplaza R, Quetglas A, Rodriguez E (1983) Treatment of electrical burns of the mouth. Burns 10(1): 49–60
22. Hilbert L, Peters WJ, Tepperman PS (1984) Temporomandibular joint destruction after a burn. Burns 10(3): 214–216
23. Chen XQ (1982) Pharmacology, 11th edn. People's Medical Publishing House, Beijing, pp 103–127
24. Wang JH, Chen GX, Li A (1989) The comparison of the effect of wound healing of superficial thickness burn among four different materials. Acta 3rd Milit Med Coll
25. Hu JN, Ling SZ (1985) Treatment of 102 cases with deep second degree burns of the hand. Proceedings of the first Sino-American conference on burn injuries, Chongqing, p 149
26. Zhong DC, Lin LY (1985) Prevention of deformities by early grafting in special areas of burns. Chin J Plast Surg Burns 1(4): 253–254
27. Sun YH, Yin DQ, Zhao XG et al. (1985) Repair of burnt metacarpals and phalanges with free greater omentum grafting. Chin J Plast Surg Burns 1(1): 43–44
28. Pensler JM, Steward R, Lewis SR et al. (1988) Reconstruction of the burned palm: full-thickness versus split-thickness skin grafts—long-term follow-up. Plast Reconstr Surg 8(1): 46–49
29. Merrell SW, Saffle JR, Schnebly WA et al. (1986) Full-thickness skin grafting for contact burns of the palm in children. JBCR 7(6): 501–507

30. Kim KH, Tsuneda K (1987) A case of perianal burn. Burns 13(5): 396–397
31. McDougal WS, Peterson HD, Pruitt BA et al. (1979) The thermally injured perineum. J Urol 121: 320–323
32. Zhu ZX, Yang H, and Wang TJ et al. (1988) Early repair of deep burns in male perineal region. Chin J Plast Surg Burns 4(2): 101–102
33. Yu SH, Zhou YP, Fei TX (1986) Early escharectomy of third degree burns in perineal region—report of two cases. Chin J Plast Surg Burns 2(2): 142

7 Burns of Special Causes

Ge Sheng-de

Burns induced by causes other than thermal injuries such as chemical, electric, and irradiation burns, are defined as burns of special causes. Generally, burns of special causes only account for a small proportion of burns – usually about 15% of the cases treated at a burn center. With the development and popularization of modern technology in industrial plant and in research as well as in the home, the incidence of burns of special causes is likely to increase.

Although the basic principles for treatment of thermal burns also apply to burns of special causes, it is important to emphasize that principles specific to the mechanism of various burn causes should be followed.

7.1 Electric Burns

The progress and technical innovation in industry and agriculture, the improvement of military equipment, and the upgrading of domestic facilities have all made for more widespread use of electricity. This in turn has led to an increase in the incidence of electric burns. Special treatment appears to be important owing to the severity of the damage that can be caused by such burns. Therefore, further study of the mechanism of electric burns, continuous improvement of diagnostic techniques, and constant development of therapeutic measures are mandatory.

According to the mechanism and clinical features of the injury, electric burns are usually classified into two categories, i.e., contact burns and flash burns. Sometimes electric burns are associated with thermal burns due to ignition of clothing. The associated flame burn injury enlarges the area of electric burn, and it should be managed according to the principles for thermal burns.

The systemic effect of acute electric injury is electric shock, which may lead to a fatal outcome. It may occur without skin damage and is, therefore, an internal medicine problem. Hence, it will not be discussed in this chapter.

7.1.1 Mechanism of Electric Burns

7.1.1.1 Factors Influencing Electric Burns

The electrical conductivity of the skin predisposes it to electric injury and allows the electric current to pass through it. On the other hand, the skin also offers resistance to electric current. Consequently, skin damage due to contact burns is produced not only by the electric current itself, but also by the heat generated when the current meets a resistance. There are many influencing factors that should be taken into consideration. These factors are circuit type and voltage, pathway of the current through body tissues, current amperage, body resistance, and duration of contact.

7.1.1.2 Joule's Law

Electric burn is produced by the electric thermal effect, which follows Joule's law: $P = 0.24\, I^2\, Rt$, where P = heat produced, I = amperage, R = resistance, and t = time(s). The amount of heat produced when the electric current passes through the body tissue is in direct proportion to the square of amperage, tissue resistance, and duration of contact. At a fixed amperage and a given duration of contact, the greater the tissue resistance against the current, the greater the heat produced and the more severe the burn injury will be.

7.1.1.3 Electrical Conductivity of Various Tissues

All other factors being equal, the greater the skin resistance, the greater the local damage and the less severe the systemic injury. Clinical experience shows that some patients sustain electric shock without showing any local damage of the skin, while others have local burn of the skin but no systemic disturbances. If the skin resistance happens to be low at the time of the electrical contact, the electric current passes readily through the body tissue, leading to severe systemic disturbances. If the skin resistance is normal, the current may cause local damage while the systemic influence may be small or absent.

The electric current after penetrating the skin passes through various tissues in order of resistance. Nerve offers the least resistance, followed by blood, muscle, skin, tendon, and fat, while bone exhibits the greatest resistance. Therefore, nerves and blood vessels are readily involved during the burn. The result is damage to endothelium and formation of thrombi, producing secondary damage to the extremity involved.

7.1.1.4 Types of Electric Current and Voltage

Contact electric burn is defined as the injury produced by direct contact of the body surface with electric current of voltage varying from 110 to 250 000 V. Burns produced by an electric current with a voltage above 380 V are referred to as high-tension electric burns. Direct current with a low voltage is not as dangerous as the corresponding alternating current, though direct current with high voltage is dangerous. Body tissue is more prone to damage by alternating current than by direct current; practically only circuits of 24 mA or less may be safe.

7.1.1.5 Amperage

Electric current with low amperage of 1 or 2 mA will produce a tingling sensation. When a current of 8–12 mA enters the body, muscle contraction occurs, enabling the victim to withdraw from the circuit. When the current is above 20 mA severe burns will result. A current of 100 mA passing through the body from hands to feet is sufficient to cause ventricular fibrillation. An electric current of low frequency (15–150 Hz) can cause electric injury, and alternating current of 50–60 Hz is especially dangerous. An electric current with a very high frequency is harmless as it only produces a heating effect, such as in diathermy.

7.1.2 Mechanism of Contact Burn

7.1.2.1 Dynamics of Thermal Response [1]

The magnitude of heat produced during an electric burn is a function of current density, tissue conductivity, and spatial arrangement of the tissues. Energy will be dissipated at different rates in various tissues because of differences in electrical conductivity. The heat produced is inversely proportional to tissue conductivity.

The maximum power density is dissipated in the skin, since dry skin has a conductivity much lower than that of the other tissues. Hence, skin burn is readily produced. Severe damage is produced in the tissues with good conductivity, such as nerve, muscle, and blood vessels.

The tissue temperature response to electric current changes along the current path. The temperature rise near a joint can be much greater, since the cross-sectional area of soft tissue and the ratio of soft tissue to bone are lower.

Other factors may influence the temperature in the burned area. Heat is transferred from warmer to cooler areas by conduction and surface convection, and blood removes heat from the local tissue. After current ceases to flow, the temperature change is determined by blood perfusion rate, heat conduction, and convection on the skin surface.

During the flow of electric current, heating is an adiabatic process. The rise in local temperature is equal to the energy dissipated at that point divided by the specific heat.

Muscle sustains the greatest temperature rise during the current flow. The bone which is surrounded and heated by the muscle equilibrates with the latter in temperature in about 10 min. The skin temperature frequently does not rise to a lethal value because the heat is lost by surface convection. This will mask the extent of damage to the muscle underneath. However, local swelling often serves as a guide in clinical diagnosis.

Blood flow is critical for cooling of the deep tissues damaged by heat. Restoration of tissue perfusion may be crucial in improving survival of tissues.

Although tissue injury is produced by heat during electric current flow, tissue injury may also occur in the absence of obvious thermal effects, which implies that cellular damage can be produced by electric current through nonthermal mechanisms.

7.1.2.2 Electrical Breakdown of Cell Membranes [2]

Perforations in plasma membrane large enough to change the electrochemical balance between intracellular and extracellular compartments may result in cellular metabolic disorder and finally lead to cell damage or even cell death. This mechanism may be partially responsible for late neurological sequelae to electric injury and progressive muscle necrosis. Membrane rupture inflicting injuries on muscle or nerve cells remains to be proven.

Thermal injury is probably irreversible, since denatured proteins do not spontaneously resume their original configuration. If electric breakdown of cell membrane is mainly responsible for the injury of muscle and nerve, it may be possible to save these tissues, since cultured cells do survive transient membrane rupture sustained in the process of electrocution.

It is possible to rupture the plasma membrane of muscle cells within an electric field which is too weak to produce lethal thermal injury. It is concluded that electrical energy may play an important role in the pathogenesis of electric injury.

7.1.3 Clinical Diagnosis

Typical history and typical local wound will lead to correct diagnosis of an electric contact burn. The general conditions, particularly the vital signs such as consciousness, pulse, and respiration, are important for the diagnosis of electric shock. Electrocardiography may be necessary to detect cardiac arrhythmia. Physical examination should be regularly performed. Attention should be paid to the signs of thoracic and abdominal problems requiring surgery. Neurological examination is helpful in assessing mental status, hemiplegia, paralysis, seizures, etc. Ophthalmological examination for cataract is important. For the evaluation of muscle damage, [^{99}Te]pyrophosphate muscle scan and ^{133}Xe muscular blood flow determination may be performed [3]. Electric injury can cause serious vascular damage which will be evident 15 min postburn and will progress for 48 h. Although therapeutic measures such as anticoagulation and sympathectomy may delay the appearance of vascular injury, they do not affect the ultimate degree of damage [4]. Arteriography using meglumine diatrizoate may be carried out to evaluate the arterial blood supply. In addition, biochemical determination of 5-ornithine carbamyl transferase and creatine phosphokinase are important in supplementary diagnosis.

7.1.4 Types of Electric Burns

7.1.4.1 Contact Burns

7.1.4.1.1 Pathological and Clinical Features

Electric contact burn is characterized by multiple wounds produced by the entrance and exit of the current. The injury at the entrance point is usually more severe than that at the exit site. The wounds are commonly small in size and circular or oval in shape. The lesion is usually dry and ischemic, whitish yellow or whitish gray in color, with a concave coagulated center which may appear to be charred. Its edge is clear-cut with a narrow, circular reddish band of congestion.

The wound is also characterized by extensive necrosis. The necrosis originally produced by electric injury, is followed by secondary necrosis due to damage of the cellular membrane or local ischemia caused by vascular thrombosis. The area of ischemic necrosis may be large; for instance, a whole extremity may be involved. Severe tetanic contraction of the muscles may cause open fractures and dislocations of the extremities, particularly the hands.

Contraction of flexor muscles induced by electric injury causes flexion of the extremities. Burns may be demonstrated in the antecubital fossa or the armpit. The wounds are usually oval in shape due to direct contact of the opposing skin during flexion of the extremity. Progressive damage of the muscles may occur due to direct electric injury or secondary ischemic necrosis as a result of either vascular thrombosis or an increase in tissue tension in the muscular compartment. The degree of damage of muscle bundles or fibers is uneven, i.e., some areas are viable and some are not. The viable and nonviable tissues may have a sandwich-like configuration.

Electric burns of the face can cause severe damage of the sensory organs, which may lead to destruction of facial features and result in severe cosmetic problems. Burns of the cranial area usually cause deep damage of the scalp, aponeurosis, and the flat bones underneath. In some cases the loss of soft tissue will bring about exposure of the flat bones. The conventional method of treatment focuses on the surrounding burn wound. The devitalized tissue or eschar is removed by surgical debridement or autolysis. The course of the latter will be hastened by local application of a paste of the Chinese herbal medicine Huafu Shengji Gao, which promotes autolysis and enhances proliferation of tissue cells. Split-thickness skin grafting is performed on either the open surgical wound or the granulation wound. Healing of the surrounding wound facilitates surgical treatment of the devitalized bone under relatively clean conditions. The conventional surgical operation consists in drilling of the outer table to a depth where active bleeding is seen. Granulation tissue then forms in the drilled holes. The rest of the outer table is gradually covered by the granulation tissue during its growth. The wound is closed by performing split-thickness skin grafting. The drawback of this method is that sequestra may be expelled through the grafted area accompanied by local infection, the treatment of which may take a long time. An alternative method is to chisel off the devitalized outer table of the skull and then carry out split-thickness skin grafting on the granulation wound when it has formed. Sometimes early surgical debridement with removal of devitalized soft and bony tissue is performed. The bony defect, usually involving only the outer table, is covered by a local skin flap, with split-thickness skin grafting to close the wound of the donor area. Occasionally, when the supplying blood vessels are available in an extensive electric burn of the skull, free greater omentum obtained by laparotomy is grafted on the debrided wound with anastomosis of the arteries and veins by microsurgical technique, and the exposed greater omentum is covered with split-thickness skin graft [5]. For more severe burns where the inner table of the skull is involved, the cranial bone can be removed at the time when the sequestrum is separated and the wound then closed by the method mentioned above. The bony defect can be closed later with a prosthesis, or the patient can wear a helmet or a special cap to protect the brain tissue from further trauma.

Electric burns of the thorax and abdomen may cause severe damage, even defects of the thoracic or abdominal wall with exposure and injury of the viscera. These defects, which may be seen in high-tension electric burns, are closed with local skin flaps. Greater omentum can be used for closing the defect, and the wound is finally closed with split-thickness skin graft.

Hemorrhagic necrosis and rupture of intestine, colon, urinary bladder, and gallbladder are occasionally seen in high-tension electric burns of the abdomen. Close observation and careful assessment of signs and symptoms of acute abdomen is very important in the early postburn stage, especially on the second day.

Renal damage may occur following electric injury. There are many factors which influence the occurrence of acute renal failure, e.g., injury by electric current with ischemic damage of renal tissue caused by vascular occlusion due to thrombosis, damage resulting from initial shock, and damage of the nephron from sedimentation of hemoglobin and/or myoglobin in the renal tubules due to the breakdown of red blood corpuscles and muscular tissues particularly the latter, which usually occurs in severe electric burns. Clinical observation for hemoglobinuria and myoglobinuria or anuria is of great importance. More fluid should be given during fluid resuscitation the amount being adjusted according to the increase in hourly urine output, provided no contraindication such as pulmonary or brain edema is observed. Alkalinization of urine using sodium bicarbonate and diuresis using either mannitol or furosemide may be helpful in preventing renal tubular damage. Attention must be paid to the clinical picture of respiratory alkalosis. Alkalinization of urine can bring about iatrogenic metabolic alkalosis, resulting in mixed metabolic and respiratory alkalosis, a serious condition which can have a fatal outcome. In the case of acute renal failure, gastrointestinal dialysis, intraperitioneal dialysis, or hemodialysis may be instituted. Respiratory paralysis and ventricular fibrillation and even respiratory and cardiac arrest may occur in some patients, which can result in early fatal outcome. Hemiplegia may appear due to injury to the spinal cord.

A delayed complication or sequela of major electric injury is the development of cataract, which may be uni- or bilateral. The incidence is about 6%. Cataract is usually first suspected when visual acuity decreases at 1–12 months, on average about 4 months, after the injury. Most patients require eye surgery for vision loss at 3 months to 2 years postinjury, or even later. An operation can restore vision excellently [6].

7.1.4.1.2 Treatment

Although the general principles of thermal burn management are to be followed, specific treatment is required for electric burns.

First Aid. The victim should first be removed from the electric current. Immediate care should be given. If cardiac and respiratory arrest has been observed, mouth-to-mouth artificial respiration and cardiac massage should instituted without delay. The victim should be sent to a nearby hospital for ECG monitoring. If there is ventricular fibrillation, prompt defibrillation should be performed.

Fluid Resuscitation. Fluid formulae used for thermal injury are not appropriate for electric injury. No formula can be used as a reliable guide for fluid replacement therapy in electric burns, because a certain amount of body fluid has been sequestrated within the interstitial space, especially in the fascial and muscular compartments, where devitalized muscle is located. Hence, the amount of fluid required cannot be estimated only by the body surface area burned.

Urinary output is taken as a clinical guide for fluid replacement therapy. A higher hourly urinary output is desirable, provided there are no contra-indications to massive fluid infusion. Adequate fluid infusion not only increases renal perfusion but also promotes excretion of hemoglobin and myoglobin in the presence of hemoglobinuria and myoglobinuria. Solute diuresis using mannitol is indicated. Emergency surgical debridement of devitalized tissue or amputation of a severely damaged extremity is beneficial not only in recovery from burn shock but also in protecting renal function.

Management of Local Burn Wound. The basic principle of early management of the local burn wound is to follow a wait-and-see policy, followed by cautious periodical and sequential debridement, if there is obvious progressive muscle damage, a potential risk of irreversibility of burn shock, renal damage due to hemoglobin and myoglobin precipitating in the renal tubules, or anaerobic infection, especially clostridial infection. It is better to perform any surgical operation immediately or soon after early debridement. If the general condition of the patient permits, vigorous fluid therapy is given, and local burn eschar is excised first. The incision may be sufficiently prolonged by cutting through the skin of the edematous area of over the swelling muscle compartment for decompression and exploration of the muscle compartment. Devitalized muscle bundles are removed. Blue tetrazoline can be locally applied for further gross differentiation of dead muscle. Gentian violet and methylene blue have also been used for this purpose. Damaged large blood vessels should of course be securely ligated, or else secondary hemorrhage will occur in the later course of treatment. The open wound can be dressed or covered with either biological dressing or artificial skin. Secondary transplantation of skin autograft is later performed if the underlying wound proves healthy after removal of the covering substance. Instantaneous transplantation using skin autograft is strongly indicated. The graft may not take in the case of inadequate removal of the devitalized muscle. When parabiotic tissues cannot be adequately removed because of the danger of exposing important anatomical structures, e.g., local blood vessels and nerves, the open wound can be closed by either a local skin flap or a free composite cutaneous, fasciocutaneous, or musculocutaneous flap. In order to save a damaged extremity, the technique of replanting a severed limb has been introduced in the treatment of major electric burns by surgeons from Ji-Shui-Tan Hospital, Beijing. Devitalized tissues are adequately excised, the devitalized segment of bone shaft is resected, and the bony ends are approximated by internal fixation. The exposed bony structure with or without periosteum is wrapped and covered with viable muscle bundles. The damaged blood vessels and nerves are resected and reapproximated using microsurgical technique. The open wound is then closed by instantaneous transplantation of skin autograft or is first closed temporarily using biological or artificial skin, followed several days later by secondary transplantation of skin autograft for permanent closure.

Case Report. A 28-year-old male electrician was admitted to our Burn Center, Changhai Hospital, Second Military Medical College of the PLA, Shanghai, with a history of contact burn produced by a high-power electric current of 6600 V half an hour previously. The accident occurred when the cut-off power suddenly returned to a machine while he was working on it. He sustained third-degree burns of 45% of his body surface area. The wounds on his head and neck were very deep, resulting in mask-like eschar covering the face. There were defects due to charred soft tissue with exposure of the nasal cavity, the oral cavity, and the right orbital fossa, which was partially occupied by the charred eyeball. The left eye was also severely damaged, resulting in electric cataract. The frontal bone was partially denuded, exposing brain tissue of the frontal lobe with leakage of cerebro-spinal fluid through a perforation. The maxillae and most of the hard palate with all but the last two molar teeth were destroyed (Fig. 7.1 a, b). The abdomen was also seriously burned. There was a total defect of the abdominal wall 18 cm in diameter located at the lower center of the abdominal eschar. The small intestine, colon, and urinary bladder were exposed and perforated, and the external genitalia were totally burned off (Fig. 7.2). Both lower extremities were seriously damaged. A large defect at the femoral triangle of the left thigh was seen in the center of an extensively charred eschar. Extensive devitalized muscles were exposed, and the left femoral artery, vein, and nerve were also exposed. Most of

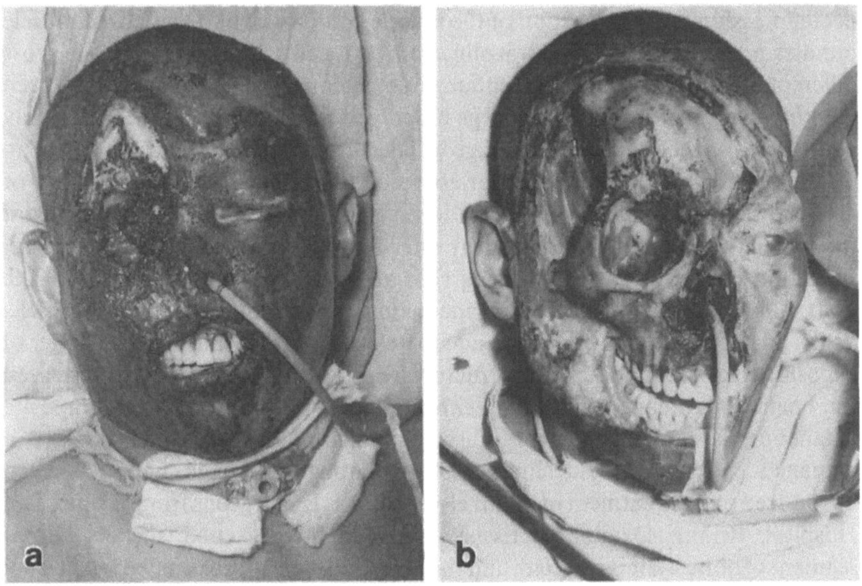

Fig. 7.1 a, b. Severe burns of head and neck produced by high-power electric current (6600 V). **a** Facial burn with a mask-like eschar. **b** Facial burn after partial debridement with exposure of devitalized bony structure

the right leg was burned with severe damage of the knee joint, i.e., destruction of the periarticular tissue and synovial capsule, with only a part of the soft tissue located in the popliteal fossa remaining intact (Fig. 7.3). There were small areas of third-degree burns in the upper extremities.

After fluid resuscitation, amputation of the left lower extremity was performed with the beneficial outcome of elimination of hemoglobinuria and myoglobinuria, and thus acute renal failure was prevented. The right knee joint was fixed with a stainless steel pin, and the right leg was not amputated (Fig. 7.3). The perforated intestinal segment was resected through the abdominal wall defect, which was later successfully closed using greater omentum, followed by subsequent autologous skin grafting. The perforations of the colon and the urinary bladder were successfully treated by conservative methods the latter being drained with an indwelling catheter. After removal of the devitalized bony structures of the face, skin autograft was applied on the granulation wound and the exposed dura with a successful result. During the treatment course many difficult complications, such as hemolysis associated with the inability to identify the subgroup in conventional blood typing, were surmounted. The patient survived after a long and complicated period of treatment.

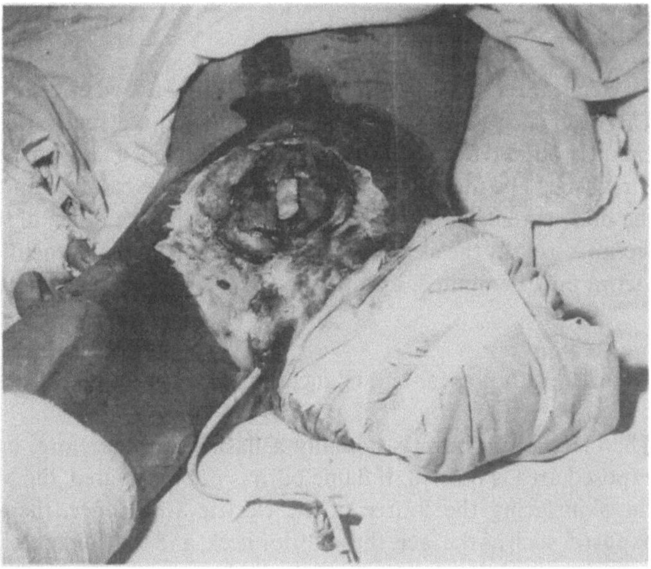

Fig. 7.2. Severe burns of the abdomen with a total defect of the abdominal wall and injury and perforation of the small intestine, colon, and urinary bladder. The external genitalia were burned off

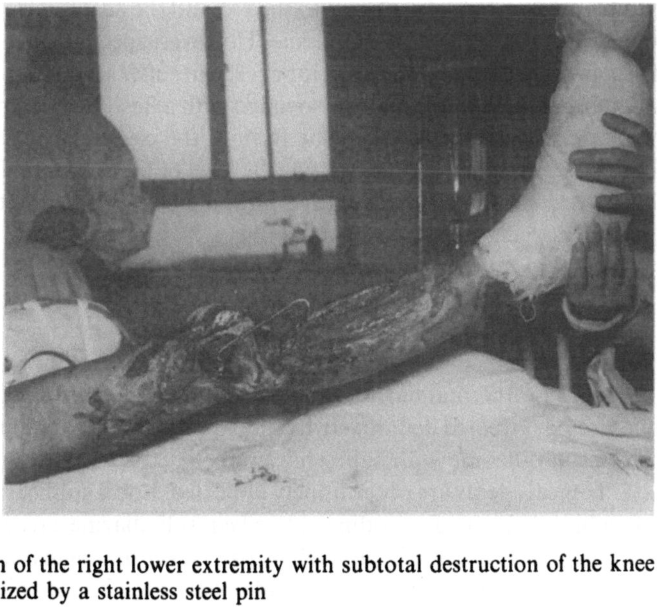

Fig. 7.3. Severe burn of the right lower extremity with subtotal destruction of the knee joint, which is stabilized by a stainless steel pin

7.1.4.2 Arc Burns

An electric arc burn is produced by an electric arc when a short circuit is formed. The burn is caused by the heat released from the spark. In the case of a short circuit produced from high-tension electric current a temperature of 2500°–3000°C is reached. The instantaneous high temperature can certainly produce burns of the body surface if the victim is located within the range of the electric arc. The victim is usually the user of some form of electrical equipment. The clothing of the victim may be ignited, and the arc burn area can be enlarged by flame burns.

7.1.4.2.1 Pathological and Clinical Features

The electric arc burn is actually a flash burn; therefore, only the skin of the exposed area is burned. If flame burn is not associated, the burn wounds are on the skin facing the source of the electric arc. Hence, the areas most usually exposed, such as the face, the anterior neck, and the dorsum of the hand, are likely to be involved. If other parts of the body are exposed, more extensive burns are produced. The patient may suffer pain during the accident, or may feel no pain at first due to fright, with dull pain following later.

An arc burn often gives the local appearance of a deep burn wound, and even exhibits the characteristics of a third-degree burn because of the high temperature. In fact, in most arc burns the deep dermis is not involved due to the very short duration of exposure to the arc, and the heat is not transferred down to the dermis and subcutaneous tissue. However, specific areas with thinner skin, such as the eyelids and the anterior neck, can suffer severe third-degree burns. An arc burn of the face is usually associated with a flash burn of the cornea, since the winking reflex is slower than the flash of the electric arc. Diagnosis is usually based on a transverse cloudiness at the level of the palpebral fissure. If diagnosis by gross inspection is not definitive, it should be confirmed by the fluorescein test.

7.1.4.2.2 Management

Early debridement of electric arc burn wounds follows the principles and measures for thermal burns. The devitalized epithelium is usually removed, and the wound is treated definitively by the exposure method, which usually leads to a successful outcome with subeschar epithelialization.

Topical agents are not routinely indicated. Local application of 2.5% tincture of iodine, 1% povidoneiodine, 1% silver sulfadiazine cream, or decoction or tincture of a herbal medicine such as *Ilex chinensis*, *Sanguisorba*, or a mixture of *Coptis*, *Scutellaria*, and *Phellodendronum* may be beneficial in preventing bacterial and fungal infection.

The exposure method is often used in treating second-degree burns after early debridement, since the area prone to electric burns is usually exposed. The occlusive method may also be used as indicated, and the semiexposure method may be used as well. The dressing should be changed when there is local infection. Topical antimicrobial agents such as 0.1% chlorhexidine and the above-mentioned topical agents are locally applied. In the presence of drug-resistant bacterial strains, topical antimicrobial agents such as Dermazin, a micromolecular silver sulfadiazine cream prepared by the LEK Pharmaceutical and Chemical Works, and silver salts of quinolones are recommended. Burn wound sepsis will be controlled with effective local treatment. Obviously, however, systemic antibiotic therapy is also recommended.

Treatment of Deep Burns by Surgical Operation. The attitude toward excisional therapy should be conservative, since the burn is often more superficial than judged on gross inspection. Tangential excision is the operative measure of choice, because most of the wounds are deep second-degree burns or at most superficial third-degree burns. After removal of the devitalized tissues, skin grafting is performed. Large-sheet skin autografting is recommended for permanent coverage in areas where either cosmetic or functional requirements have to be met. Occasionally other skin grafting procedures may be used under certain conditions.

Treatment of Cornea Burn. Treatment of corneal damage caused by an electric arc burn is of great importance. Cornea burn is usually superficial. Timely appropriate treatment will bring about recovery. Ignorance of the importance of corneal burn and neglect of its management, particularly in the case of severe damage, can result in disturbance of vision due to sequelae from the damage per se or from its complications, such as corneal nebula and leucoma.

When the diagnosis of electric arc cornea burn is made by gross inspection or confirmed by the fluorescein test, ophthalmic treatment is instituted; it consists of application of eye drops and ointment containing antimicrobial agents. Mydriatic eye drops, e.g., 1% atropine, 2% homatropine, or 0.1%–0.25% scopolamine, are indicated when congestion of the bulbar conjunctiva is present. The above-mentioned therapeutic measures proved effective when used properly in treating certain complications such as keratitis, corneal ulcer, keratoconjunctivitis, keratoiritis, and keratoiridocyclitis.

7.1.4.3 Lightning Injury

Lightning injury is a special type of electric burn. It manifests itself as an arborizing or serpiginous pattern of cutaneous injury. It usually occurs during thunderstorms and is caused by electric currents of 12000–200000 A. It takes 1/1000–1/100 s for lightning to travel from its usual height to the ground. The accident usually happens in the open. Victims of lightning injury may sustain not only skin burns but also deeper injury, or may even be killed instantaneously. Lightning injury may be associated with complications such as shock, premature ventricular contraction, subendocardial infarction, bilateral rupture of tympanic membranes, and neuropathy.

7.2 Chemical Burn

Chemical burns constitute the most commonly seen group of burns of specific causes. It usually occurs in industrial accidents, particularly in chemical works, and can also occur in laboratory and domestic accidents. Chemical burn is defined as acute skin damage caused by direct irritation, corrosion, and/or heat produced from reactions of chemical agents. It may be associated with thermal injury produced by chemicals at high temperature, eye burn, and/or inhalation injury [1].

A pooling of experience in the management of chemical burns at the First National Conference on Chemical Burns held in Shanghai in October 1988 showed that the most common cause of chemical burns was industrial accidents, brought about by breakage of equipment and containers, breaches of rules and regulations, etc. [7]. Other causes included laboratory mishaps such as breakage of glassware and spillage of chemicals, domestic accidents, and deliberate criminal assault. Chemical weapons may also be employed in wartime.

The mechanism of chemical burn is more complex than that of thermal burn. Jelenko (1974) asserted that oxidation and reduction, corrosion, protoplasmic toxic effect, dehydration, and bleb formation were involved [8]. Although chemical burns may present some of the characteristics of thermal burns, they nevertheless have some typical features. Therefore surgeons, especially burn specialists, must be familiar with the chemicals commonly involved. An understanding of their chemical and physical properties, the tissues or organs they tend to act upon, and their adverse and toxic effects is the key to successful treatment.

Since first aid is of the utmost importance in the acute management of chemical burns, its basic principles and simple methods of treatment should be widely taught to workers and management in chemical works, so that first aid can be instituted immediately at the scene of the accident. One of the modern trends in emergency medicine is prehospital treatment, which is very important in the treatment of chemical burns.

When skin comes into contact with a chemical agent that burns, local destruction is produced not only on the surface but also in deeper layers due to the agent's penetrating nature, which will cause continuous injury until the chemical reaction ceases. First aid at the scene of the accident comprises not only prehospital management but also measures to halt damage to the deep tissues. Rinsing with copious amounts of water is the most effective measure because water is often more readily available than specific antidotes. If specific antidotes are available at the scene of the accident in suitable concentrations, they should be used, if they are not available, one should not wait for antidotes, and rinsing with water should be instituted without delay.

Comparative studies have shown that prolonged rinsing is important in preventing continuous damage by chemicals. Therefore, it is advised that rinsing should be carried out for as long as 30 minutes or even longer.

An analysis of approximately 10 000 cases of chemical burns showed that 179 different chemical agents were involved. The most commonly seen types of chemical burn are discussed below.

7.2.1 Acid Burn

7.2.1.1 General Considerations

Acid burn is one of the most frequent types of chemical injury. It is often caused by spillage of an acid, producing minor burns which appear spotty or sometimes take on a rivulet form. This kind of incident frequently occurs in chemical laboratories.

Acid burns involving more of the body surface often occur as an industrial injury in chemical works. Sometimes a worker sustains extensive deep chemical burns by falling into acid slurry.

Obviously, burn area and depth depend on the area exposed, the concentration of the acid involved, the duration of contact, and the mode of immediate local care and first aid.

Clothing may protect against acid spillage. However, it can be harmful if it becomes soaked with acid, and the burn area can be enlarged by careless handling.

The mechanism of acid burns includes the actions of exothermic reaction, cellular dehydration, and protein precipitation.

Because of the continuous chemical reaction of an acid, the victim often feels long-lasting local pain. The superficial local wound is red and soft in texture, while deeper wounds have a leathery appearance and display various colors, e.g., gray-yellow, brown, or black, depending on the causative acid, the depth of the burn, and the duration of exposure. Although an acid burn wound often resembles a third-degree burn eschar, in most cases it is deep second-degree burn, because the leathery eschar hinders further acid penetration. Usually no significant systemic complications of acid burn are seen, except in extensive hydrofluoric acid burns, in which clotting mechanisms may be affected.

Breathing of the acid fumes may cause inhalation injury, which may result in respiratory dysfunction due to chemical tracheobronchitis and other respiratory complications.

It is well known that local treatment is very important in acid burns. A topically applied alkaline solution such as sodium bicarbonate will neutralize the acid, thereby stopping the burn. In most cases, appropriate alkaline solutions are not readily available in suitable concentrations and adequate amounts. Therefore, thorough rinsing with copious amounts of water is the measure of choice in both first aid and definitive local treatment. This measure has been proved to be simple and effective, since water is nearly always available. Local debridement by removal of loose and devitalized tissue follows. Continuous rinsing, particularly with running water, may still be needed and a specific neutralizer of an appropriate concentration may be used if available.

Most burn surgeons prefer the exposure method to the occlusive method in definitive local treatment. The exposure method is carried out without topical agents. Since the leathery eschar, which does not readily undergo autolysis, forms a natural protective cover, less local infection occurs in acid burns. Most of the wound will epithelialize under the eschar during exposure treatment. In deeper acid burns where demarcation and separation of the devitalized eschar eventually take place, granulation wound is formed. If the open granulation wound is too large to be epithelialized by proliferation of the surrounding epithelial cells, skin grafting is needed. Other measures in the local treatment of acid burns resemble those for thermal burns. The basic principles of systemic treatment are also similar to those for thermal burns. Nevertheless, the amount of fluid required for volume replacement in the early stage may be less than that for thermal burns. This may be due to less exudation and insensible water loss.

7.2.1.2 Specific Acid Burns

7.2.1.2.1 Phenol Burns

Phenol is obtained in fractional distillation of coal tar and is used as a raw material in the production or preparation of substances such as asbestos, coke, medicinal materials, explosives, paints, spices, synthetic resins, and plastics. It is often widely used in the petroleum, leather, papermaking, soap, and dye industries. Phenol is a plasma toxin which can damage various kinds of cells, i.e., skin on direct contact or respiratory tract on inhalation of its fumes [9].

A low concentration of phenol causes protein degeneration, while a high concentration induces protein precipitation. Phenol absorption via the skin, digestive tract, or respiratory tract can cause acute systemic intoxication, characterized by effects on the central nervous system, with trembling and spasm, circulatory and respiratory collapse with slow and weak pulse, and accompanying cyanosis, changes in pupil reflex, and fluctuation of body temperature. Systemic intoxication can result in impairment of renal function [10, 11]. Acute phenol intoxication may be fatal.

Most of the absorbed phenol may be oxidized or combined with glucuronic acid and then excreted through the excretory system. A small part of the absorbed phenol is excreted in its original form.

Clinically phenol is recognized as a corrosive agent. Most of the phenol burns are second degree with local pain and numbness. The local wound is primarily light gray or grayish white in color, and light brown later. Little swelling is observed.

First aid for phenol burns consists of removal of the causative agent as soon as possible. This may be achieved by rinsing with water or taking a shower. Since phenol is insoluble in water, it is better treated by wiping with 10% ethyl alcohol or polyethylene glycol 300. Cleansing of the wound be repeated during early debridement until the characteristic smell of phenol disappears. The subsequent rinsing with water or shower bath is followed by application of 5% sodium bicarbonate for neutralization. Definitive local care is instituted using conventional methods.

Although there is less fluid loss with phenol burn, a large quantity of lactated Ringer's solution is infused to effect solute diuresis; thereby hourly urinary output is increased to enhance rapid excretion of phenol in order to prevent renal damage. If there is no contraindication, the hourly urine output should be as high as 200 ml. In the case of extensive phenol burn complicated by acute renal failure, peritoneal dialysis or hemodialysis may be instituted.

During emergency treatment blood gas analysis should be performed. If necessary, an appropriate amount of sodium bicarbonate is prescribed.

Inspiration of phenol fumes may cause inhalation injury, which can result in chemical pneumonitis. It is suggested that methylprenisolone be prescribed. Respiratory support, by ventilator, may be given. Diazepam and pentobarbital may be used for sedation. For inspection of the damaged tracheobronchial tree, fiberoptic bronchoscopy is indicated.

During the course of treatment, in addition to blood gas analysis, determinations of urinary phenol and reticulocyte count are indicated. Nutritional support is of great importance. Various vitamins may be helpful. Although local infection of phenol burn is rarely seen, as phenol itself is a disinfectant, antibiotic therapy should be prescribed in the case of extensive burns.

7.2.1.2.2 Hydrofluoric Acid Burns

Hydrofluoric acid, produced from the reaction of concentrated sulfuric acid and calcium fluoride, is irritating, corrosive, and highly toxic. It is used in preparing inorganic fluorides and carbofluoro compounds, in metal refining, and as a catalytic agent in organic chemical reactions. It is also applied as a corrosive agent in glasswork and pottery.

Hydrofluoric acid skin burns are often seen in the semiconductor industry. Most patients only sustain minor burns with involvement of one or more fingers. Burns involving a larger body surface area are rarely seen. The mechanism of hydrofluoric acid burn resembles those of other acid burns, with liquefaction and decalcification as additional features. Furthermore, hydrofluoric acid penetrates more deeply than other acids. Destruction of the phalanges may occur if the fingers are involved. The wound is often painful, due to the continuing chemical reaction, and shows a leathery eschar with necrosis in the center and erythema at the periphery. The basic principles for local treatment resemble those for thermal burn. In addition, however, the neutralizing agent, calcium gluconate, which helps to halt the burn and relieve the pain, should be administered by local infiltration or arterial injection. Magnesium oxide or its glycerin paste may also be used for the same purpose. The wound may also be soaked with magnesium sulfate in local treatment particularly of minor burns. A new preparation containing calcium chloride, betamethasone, lidocaine, and dimethyl sulfoxide was recently used for local treatment of hydrofluoric acid burn, with obvious therapeutic effect [12].

7.2.1.2.3 Phosphorous Burns

Phosphorus burn is caused by inorganic phosphorus, known as white or yellow phosphorus. It is occasionally seen in chemical works, particularly in those producing agricultural chemicals. Inorganic phosphorus is a protoplasmic toxic agent that has a relatively low melting point and ignites at a temperature of 34°C. Hence, the mechanism of phosphorus burn is complex, the injury being a combination of chemical and thermal damage including cellular dehydration and oxygen deprivation caused by diphosphopentoxide. Phosphoric acid is formed from the latter in the presence of water and induces protein precipitation. Thermal injury is caused by the heat produced in the chemical reaction. Similar injuries may occur in the respiratory tract from phosphorus fumes, particularly when diphosphopentoxide is inhaled. Inorganic phosphorus can be absorbed via either burned skin or damaged mucosa. The serum phosphorus concentration rises 1 h after injury, gradually increases to a peak 10 h postburn, then returns to normal levels by 20 h. The urinary phosphorus level increases 11–22 h postburn, reaching its peak 25–30 h postburn. It then decreases slowly, the level still being higher than the average preburn level at 2–3 days postburn [13, 14]. Laboratory determination of the serum and urinary levels of inorganic phosphorus is of diagnostic importance in phosphorus intoxication. However, since less phosphorus enters the serum than the red blood corpuscles—the ratio of serum phosphorus to erythrocyte phosphorus is 1:6 [15, 16]—diagnosis of phosphorus intoxication cannot rely on serum phosphorus alone [17].

Absorption of phosphorus may cause systemic intoxication even in minor burns. Phosphorus intoxication is usually characterized by renal, hepatic, and cardiac damage. Pathological examination of the kidney shows cloudy swelling with loss of clear-cut demarcation between renal cortex and medulla and congestion of renal tubules with hemoglobin casts in their lumina. The liver shows loss of hepatic lobules, cloudy degeneration of hepatic cells, congestion and swelling of hepatic sinuses, and enlargement of Kupffer's cells. The heart shows exudation and focal hemorrhage of pericardium and degeneration and local hemorrhage of the myocardium.

The clinical features of phosphorus burns are local pain, leathery eschar of various colors, such as gray, bluish-green, blue-black, or, in severe burns, black. Subcutaneous fat, muscles, and bones are involved in more severe burns, which appear black in color on surgical operation. Glowing of phosphorus particles on the wound surface can be seen when the patient is examined in a dark room. Patients with systemic intoxication may show weakness, dizziness, headache, nausea, jaundice, and pain the right upper quadrant of the abdomen. Petechiae, bilirubinuria and proteinuria, oliguria or anuria, tachycardia, lowering of blood pressure, clonospasm, and hepatic coma can be seen in patients with more severe burns.

First aid in phosphorus burns consists of cleaning the wound immediately, removing as many of the phosphorus particles as possible. This can be done by means of rinsing with copious amounts of water, followed by draping the wound with a wet towel or immersing it in water to pervent ignition of the residual phosphorus particles. During emergency treatment in the operating theater, further removal of the phosphorus particles must be performed with patience and meticulous technique. Topical application of 1% copper sulfate can be helpful in removing phosphorus particles, for this substance reacts with phosphorus to form cupric phosphide, a black, insoluble compound. Formation of cupric phosphide on the surface of phosphorus particles not only stops the phosphorus igniting but also facilitates detection and removal of the particles. Since absorption of copper sulfate during topical application might result in copper intoxication, characterized by hemolysis and renal dysfunction, it is clear that copper sulfate should only be applied during early debridement of the local wound, and not used as a topical agent for soaking. An alternative measure, topical application of 3% silver nitrate, has been introduced [18]. A black compound, silver phosphide, is formed on the surface of the phosphorus particle when silver nitrate is applied topically to the local wound. For neutralization of phosphoric acid and nitric acid, which are formed in chemical reaction , 5% sodium bicarbonate is applied locally. Experience has shown that silver nitrate is as effective as copper sulfate. This method is recommended and should be popularized.

The subsequent definitive local treatment of the burn wound is usually the occlusive method, with gauze soaked with 3%–5% sodium bicarbonate often used as the inner layer of the occlusive dressing. In this way phosphoric acid, which is usually formed, can be neutralized. Since phosphorus is readily soluble in petrolatum and grease, the conventional occlusive method of using petrolatum gauze as the inner layer, with various kinds of ointments and herbal medicine pastes, should be prohibited, for the reason that it may hasten the absorption of inorganic phosphorus to produce systemic intoxication.

So far, there is no efficacious antidote for inorganic phosphorus, and effective local treatment of phosphorus burns is also lacking. Surgical operation is, therefore, mandatory. Emergency escharectomy for deep dermal and full-thickness burns is of great importance. Amputation of severely burned extremities with extensive damage of muscles and bones should be performed as quickly as possible.

In addition to the conventional principles and measures of systemic treatment in burns, more attention should be paid to the special requirement in the treatment of phosphorus burns. It is recommended that more fluid be given in early fluid replacement therapy in order to obtain a higher urine output, i.e., to maintain urine volume over 50 ml/h. Mannitol and furosemide can be used for diuresis. Sodium bicarbonate can be prescribed for alkalinization of urine to prevent precipitation of hemoglobin in the renal tubules when there is severe hemolysis. The above-mentioned measures are helpful in promoting phosphorus excretion and preventing severe renal damage. Nutritional support by hyperalimentation using a high-caloric diet supplemented with an elementary diet and parenteral amino acids and human albumin is valuable. Transfusion of blood and plasma is important. Glucurolactone, corticosteroids, vitamin B_1, vitamin B_{12}, and glucose with potassium and insulin are recommended for protection of hepatic function.

7.2.2 Alkali Burns

7.2.2.1 General Considerations

Alkali burn is another frequently seen chemical injury. Although the circumstances of alkali burns are similar to those of acid burns, the mechanism of injury is different. It mainly consists of hygroscopic cellular dehydration, saponification of fatty tissue, and precipitation of protein.

The most commonly seen alkalis which cause burns are caustics such as sodium hydroxide and potassium hydroxide. Alkali burn is painful and appears erythematous with bullae in superficial burns, or a slick eschar giving a soapy sensation in deeper wounds.

Alkali readily penetrates through the wound, so that continuous deepening of the local wound is often seen. Therefore prolonged rinsing with copious amounts of running water is recommended in first aid. During debridement of the wound in emergency treatment 0.5%–5% acetic acid or 5% ammonium chloride can be used for neutralization. Meanwhile, loose devitalized epidermis should be removed. The alkali burn eschar is soft in texture, in contrast to that of acid burn, and thus tends to undergo autolysis. It is wise to perform escharectomy and skin grafting instead of the conventional conservative measure of skin grafting on the granulation wound after autolysis.

7.2.2.2 Ammonia Burns

Ammonia is widely used in the production of fertilizers such as ammonium sulfate, ammonium nitrate, and urea. It is also used in refrigeration to produce artificial ice. Aqueous ammonia is employed for medical and agricultural purposes. Ammonia burn accidents usually occur in refrigeration plants, in electroplating, heat treatment, printing and dyeing, etc., and in chemical works and laboratories.

Ammonia dissolves in water to form ammonium hydroxide, a weak alkali that is able to cause skin burn. Respiratory irritation will be found when the density of ammonia in inspired air exceeds $10\,mg/m^3$. A higher density can damage the central nervous system, leading to convulsions.

Immediate local washing with copious amounts of water is important. During early debridement, the local wound can be treated with 5% acetic acid in addition to washing with water. For inhalation injury, a steam aerosol with a little acetic acid may be helpful. For relief of dyspnea, oxygen therapy is instituted.

7.2.2.3 Lime Burns

Calcium oxide and calcium hydroxide are referred to as lime. Lime is used in producing refractory materials, in tanning hides, in the manufacture of bleach, and in the paper industry. It is also used in steel plants and is employed as a building material. In China, lime burn is frequently due to the victim falling into a line pit near a construction site.

Calcium oxide is irritating and corrosive, and releases large amounts of heat when mixed with water. Calcium hydroxide is a weak alkali. Lime may damage the skin by its alkalinity and the heat produced.

Initial cleansing of the local burn wound should be performed using mineral or vegetable oil or alternatively by gentle brushing followed by washing with large amounts of water. Washing with water can also be employed without any previous local treatment, as the heat produced during washing is rapidly dissipated by the running cold water. The principles of local management for thermal burns can of course be applied routinely.

7.2.2.4 Cement Burns

Cement alkali burns can cause skin damage, inhalation injury, and eye damage. Cement burns usually occur at cement factories or on construction sites. Severe cement burns are rarely seen.

Three patients with severe cement burns were admitted to the burn center of Changhai Hospital, Shanghai. The victims were workers at a cement factory. The accident happened in a cement kiln when there was a sudden downpour of a large amount of cement at a temperature of over 300°C. All the patients sustained extensive deep dermal and full-thickness burns with moderate to severe inhalation injury. After the early burn shock stage all the patients showed signs and symptoms of inhalation injury. One patient who was some distance away from the center of the cement downpour showed coughing, wheezing, and dyspnea for more than 2 days after the shock stage. This patient responded fairly well to a combination of therapeutic measures including salbutamol aerosol, intravenous administration of aminophylline, and intravenous dexamethasone drip. The pulmonary complications subsided within a few days. The other two patients—one fell with the hot cement from a height of 3 m and the other was near the center of the downpour—showed severe inhalation injury. Cement was found in their sputum in the emergency room. Tracheostomy was performed soon after their admission. On the 4th postburn day they showed dyspnea, wheezing, and decrease of normal breathing sounds in both lungs. They did not respond well to the therapeutic measures mentioned above. Debris and fragments of necrotic mucous membrane were sucked out during irrigation of the tracheobronchial tree. The clinical picture in combination with X-ray proved that the patients had necrotic purulent tracheitis and bronchitis as complications. The most critically ill of the three patients died a week postburn. The other two patients survived with successful treatment of deep burns and inhalation injury.

7.2.3 Chemical Burns in Warfare

7.2.3.1 Mustard Gas Burns

Mustard gas is a type of vesicant which is used in chemical warfare. When it comes into contact with the skin, its irritating effect produces local pain. Blisters or bullae are formed with progressive enlargement due to the vesicant effect. Mustard gas enters the blister fluid by penetrating through the epithelium. In liquid form, mustard gas is absorbed by the skin within 30 min. After an incubation period of about 2–6 h, the victim will feel a mild pricking and itching sensation followed by erythema. Blisters are formed 18–24 h after direct contact. Local pain is obvious in severe burns, which may progress to ulceration with local infection.

When skin is exposed to mustard gas vapor, absorption is slow with mild local damage. However, the vapor is apt to induce eye damage and inhalation injury.

Precautions must be taken during early debridement. Blisters should be left unbroken, and no rinsing of the wound with water is allowed lest more extensive burns be produced by direct contact of the surrounding skin with blister fluid containing mustard gas. The burns are usually superficial while deeper ones may be encountered due to more severe damage or subsequent infection. The principles and measures of local and systemic treatment are similar to those of thermal burns.

First aid for mustard gas burns usually consists of the application of bleaching powder followed by rinsing with water. An alternative, simpler method is to use soap and water.

Systemic treatment, for use particularly when there are symptoms of systemic intoxication, consists of intravenous injection of 25% sodium thiosulfate and intramuscular injection of British antilewisite. Systemic antibacterial therapy should be instituted as indicated. For eye injury, 2% sodium bicarbonate or 0.5% chloramine is used. These can be used together with antibiotics in inhalation injury, administered with the aid of an atomizer.

Medication for relief of various symptoms of systemic intoxication may be indicated. The agents often used are sedatives, inotropic drugs respiratory stimulants, oxygen, and fluids, as well as blood and plasma, amino acids, and vitamins for nutritional support.

7.2.3.2 Incendiary Bomb Burns

On explosion, incendiary bombs scatter their contents, which consist of an incendiary agent, napalm, and an igniting agent, usually inorganic phosphorus. The latter ignites the napalm when it is exposed to the air.

Combustion of a primary napalm bomb generates heat reaching 800°–1000°C. Inclusion of polystyrene, thermite (Thermit), or magnesium can raise the temperature to 2500°–3000°, and 4000°C, respectively. A magnesium-containing incendiary bomb not only causes deep burns during combustion but also results in ulcer formation, since magnesium is an ulcer-forming element.

The most important thing to do immediately is extinguish the fire, using, for example a wet sheet or raincoat. To attempt to put out the fire with the hands is inadvisable, because napalm is sticky and will thus cause severe hand burns and enlarge the burn area.

Definitive treatment is as for thermal burns in general. Escharectomy and skin grafting may promote wound healing. Surgical intervention appears to be effective in preventing ulcer formation.

7.3 Radiation Burns

Radiation burn is rare, but its incidence is gradually increasing in China. A number of patients are orthopedic surgeons who have burnt their hands due to frequent exposure to X-ray radiation under fluoroscopy during manipulative reduction of fractures and dislocations. Some patients are burned by receiving an overdose of irradiation during radiotherapy with X-ray, ^{60}Co, or linear accelerator devices. Occasionally, radiation burns are caused by careless handling of radiotherapeutic apparatus or radioactive sources, and the patient is unexpectedly exposed to radiation energy. It is also possible that radiation burns could be seen in thermonuclear warfare [19, 20].

Acute radiation burns due to an overdose of irradiation are divided into four stages. The early reaction stage features erythema and swelling, with itch and pain several hours or 2–3 days after radiation. The incubation stage features recovery from local symptoms and signs, and lasts 4–5 days or even longer, up to about 3 weeks. The reaction stage features erythema with loss of hair, desquamation, pigmentation, blistering, and ulceration. The convalescent stage features subsidence of pigmentation, skin atrophy, capillary congestion, and chronic ulceration which might lead to cancer.

Treatment of radiation burns should follow the basic principles of burn treatment, but should also consider and manage the problems specific to radiation injury per se. As a whole, burn injury and its associated trauma should be actively treated with the aim of achieving healing before the reaction stage sets in. To control and accelerate subsidence of inflammatory reaction, the appropriate topical agent should be applied to the local wound. Blisters should be drained using aseptic technique, and the open wounds and ulcers should be treated with antimicrobial agents for the prevention of infection. Appropriate treatment for acute radiation injury should, of course, be instituted. Deep radiation burn wounds, particularly ulcers, should be treated surgically, with timely excision and subsequently skin transplantation for permanent coverage [21].

It is inadvisable to operate during the acute reaction stage, but surgery may be undertaken when this stage is over. Ulceration usually develops secondarily to chronic radiation dermatitis or minor injury. The ulcer will be infected and becomes indolent if surgery is not performed. The lesion should be extensively excised but without exposing important deeper tissues. If the excision bed is superficial and well vascularized, the wound can be closed with a split-thickness skin autograft. A thinner skin graft is advisable for a better take. For closure of a surgical wound resulting from excision of chronic ulcer, a local rotating flap, pedicle flap, island skin flap, musculocutaneous flap, or free skin flap may be used. Usually the excision of the radiation burn is incomplete; therefore, long-term follow-up is necessary to detect the early signs of malignancy.

References

1. Lee RC, Kolodney MS (1987) Electrical injury mechanisms: dynamics of thermal response. Plast Reconstr Surg 80(5): 663–671
2. Lee RC, Kolodney MS (1987) Electrical injury mechanisms: electrical breakdown of cell membrane. Plast Reconstr Surg 80(50): 672–679
3. Clayton JM, Hayes AC, Hammel J et al. (1977) Xenon-133 determination of muscle blood flow in electrical injury. J Trauma 17: 293–298
4. Lazarus HM, Huttow W (1982) Electric burns and frostbite: patterns of vascular injury. J Trauma 22(7): 581–585
5. Sun YH, Wang SH, Cao DX et al. (1982) Early repair of extensive electric burns on the skull. J Chin Med Assoc 62(9): 513
6. Saffle JR, Crandall A, Warden GD (1985) Cataracts. A long term complication of electrical injury. J Trauma 25: 17–21
7. Shanghai Institute for Prevention and Treatment of Professional Diseases in the Chemical Industry (1991) Diagnostic criteria and principles for chemical skin burns. National Standard
8. Jelenko (1974) Chemicals that "burn". J Trauma 14(1): 65–72
9. Yang ZJ, Xu WS, Shi JX (eds) (1985) Chemical burns, 2nd edn. Shanghai Scientific Press, Shanghai p 238
10. Wu Sy (1984) Cresol burns associated with acute renal failure—a case report. Chin Prev Med J 18(3): 145
11. Zhang LX (1987) Acute renal failure caused by phenol burns with two case reports. Chin J Crit Care Med 7(2): 55–56
12. Zhang ML et al. (1989) A new preparation for treatment of hydrofluoric acid burn. Chin J Plast Surg Burns 5(1): 40–42
13. Wang W (1981) Pathological changes and inorganic phosphorus determination after phosphorus burns in rabbits. Med J Chin PLA 6(3): 136–138
14. Xia SF (1982) Experimental study of systemic effect of phosphorus burns in rats. Chin J Surg 20: 411–416
15. Ben-Hur N, Giladi A, Applebaum J et al. (1972) Phosphorus burns: the antidote, a new approach. Br J Plast Surg 25: 245–249

16. Ben-Hur N, Giladi A (1978) Phosphorus burns in primates. A conducive experimental study of a new specific therapy. Burns 4: 26
17. Gao DX, Ma RL, Zhang ML et al. (1979) Treatment of extensive phosphorus burns. Chin J Surg 17(5): 357–360
18. Zibo Occupational Disease Hospital (1979) Management of phosphorus burn wounds using silver nitrate and sodium bicarbonate. Collection of reference material from the 2nd national academic conference on labour hygiene and occupational disease, p 156
19. Pillsbury RD, Artz CP (1956) Necessary compromises in therapy of burns sustained in nuclear warfare. JAMA 162: 956
20. Langevin JL, Greenstone R, Elder CO (1958) Effectiveness of troops exposed to thermal radiation from nuclear weapons. Operations Res 6: 710
21. Guo ET, Ji ZL, Zhang ML (1986) Surgical management of radiation ulcer. Chin J Plast Surg Burns 2(2): 81–83

8 Inhalation Injury

Yang Zong-chen and Li Ngao

Inhalation injury is a common occurrence among burn victims and has been found in as many as 3%–33% of patients admitted to hospital for treatment of thermal trauma [1]. It can also occur in cases without cutaneous burns, in which it has proved equally fatal. In the period January 1959 to December 1985, 5258 patients with burn injuries were admitted to our burn institute and 395 (7.5%) of them were found to have inhalation injury. It is generally asserted that inhalation injury is one of the causes of death after major burns, and its mortality may reach 30%–89% [2–7].

Although the seriousness of inhalation injury was pointed out after the Coconut Grove fire in 1942, its significance was not widely realized until the 1970s. In recent years, early diagnosis of inhalation injury and evaluation of its severity have aroused the interest of burn physicians, but so far the pathophysiological events have not been clarified and no definite improvements have been made to the therapeutic measures. It is still one of the most difficult problems in the treatment of burns.

8.1 Pathogenesis

Inhalation injury is caused by the inhalation of heat or smoke or both generated in a fire. It is difficult to induce pulmonary burns by heat alone, particularly with hot air, for the airway has the ability to reduce the temperature of inspired hot air to a remarkable extent because of its low heat capacity. Studies in dogs have shown that air at a temperature of 350°C blown through the larynx via a thermally insulated endotracheal tube cools to 50°C at the level of the tracheal carina [8]. The injury caused by heat is usually limited in the upper respiratory tract, but dust particles may carry heat into the lower respiratory tract. However, increasing the humidity of hot air being inhaled will significantly aggravate the injury. Steam, by its nature, has a heat-carrying capacity approximately 4000 times that of dry air [6]. Hot air at 142°C transfers only 13 calories of heat to the respiratory tract in a single breath, while steam transfers about 200 calories to the airway with each breath. In our institute we have produced severe pulmonary burns in animals by delivery of steam through a cuffed endotracheal tube.

In fire accidents, hot air or steam is rarely the only cause of damage to the respiratory tract; more often damage is also caused by smoke. Smoke contains carbon particles and noxious gases. The increasing use of synthetic materials has caused greater production of smoke when these materials are burned and has therefore increased the potentially toxic effects of smoke. Almost all the noxious gases in smoke such as chloride, phosgene, hydrogen chloride, cyanide, acrolein, aldehydes, and nitrogen oxides are pulmonary irritants and can produce bronchospasm, and bronchiolar and pulmonary edema. Smoke may be undetectable. Toxic chemicals may travel all the way down to the alveoli during inhalation and cause inflammation thoroughout the respiratory tract, but the most significant damage occurs in the small airway and alveoli.

There are many factors that influence the nature of pathological alterations following inhalation injury, most important of which is the direct injury by heat or smoke or both. However, other modifying factors may also play significant roles in causing pathological changes. As is well known, cutaneous burn alone can result in significant lung damage [8]. In addition, many therapeutic methods may have a role in determining the course of events in patients with inhalation injury.

The body has many ways of reacting to injury. A variety of cellular, humoral, and neural mechanisms have been recently described as causing the events which comprise the body's reaction to injury. Humoral factors implicated include histamine, serotonin, kinin, prostaglandins, complement metabolism product, proteolytic enzyme, superoxides, fibrin degradation products, and fatty acid. A series of experimental studies on inhalation injury in our institute have indicated that many humoral factors which primarily affect the vascular tonicity, such as serotonin, catecholamine, angiotensin, $PGF_{1\alpha}$, and cGMP, change slightly. They may increase transiently within 1–2 h after the inhalation injury and then fall to baseline levels [9] (Figs. 8.1–8.3). In contrast, those mediators which affect the vascular permeability, such as histamine, fibrin degradation product, anaphylotoxin, free radicals, and thromboxane have markedly elevated levels after inhalation injury. Inhalation injury activates the complement system, as evidenced by the fact that T-CH50 and AP-CH50 contents decrease and the

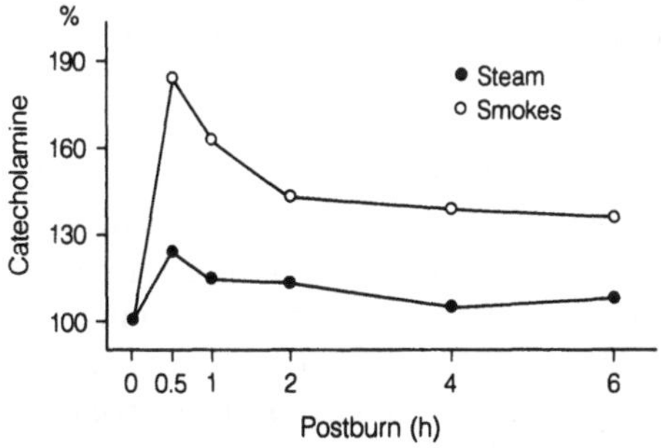

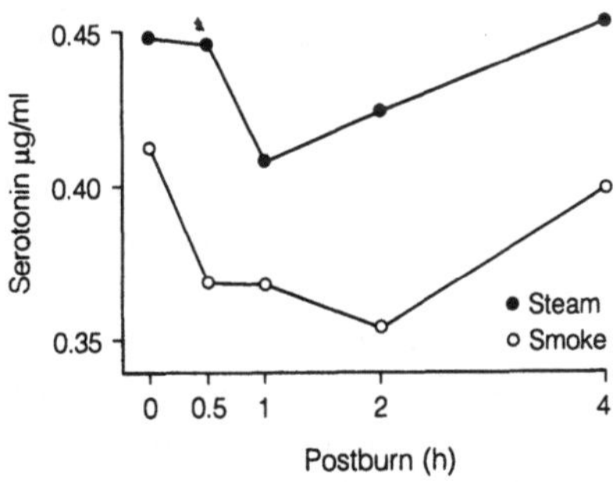

Fig. 8.1 (*left*). Changes in epinephrine and norepinephrine content in left ventricular blood in dogs after inhalation injuries. ●, dogs with steam inhalation; ○, dogs with smoke inhalation

Fig. 8.2 (*right*). 5-Hydroxytryptamine content in left ventricular blood. ●, dogs with steam inhalation; ○, dogs with smoke inhalation

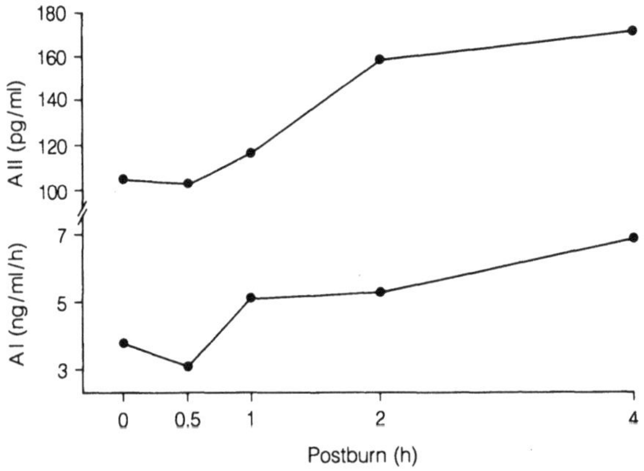

Fig. 8.3. Contents of AI and AII in left ventricular blood in dogs after inhalation injuries

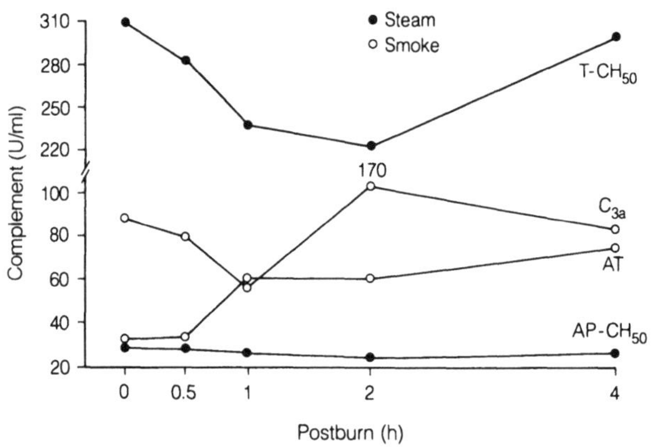

Fig. 8.4. Changes in complement product contents in left ventricular blood after inhalation injuries. ●, dogs with steam inhalation; ○, dogs with smoke inhalation

anaphylotoxin content increase (Fig. 8.4) [10, 11]. C3a and C5a can provoke constriction of smooth muscle and damage the endothelial cells, or activate mast cells to release histamine, granulocytes to release protease and oxygen radicals, and endothelial cells to release prostaglandins and leukotrienes. Histamine has been well known as a mediator which increases capillary permeability. It can provoke constriction of capillary endothelial cells, widening of the intercellular gap, and an increase of the lung lymph flow and lung water content. Our studies have shown that the histamine content in left ventricular blood increases significantly after inhalation injury [12] (Fig. 8.5). Arachidonate metabolites have also been postulated as possible mediators of lung injury. Arachidonic acid is normally bound to the phospholipids of cellular membranes, including neutrophils. These phospholipids may be released when cellular injury occurs

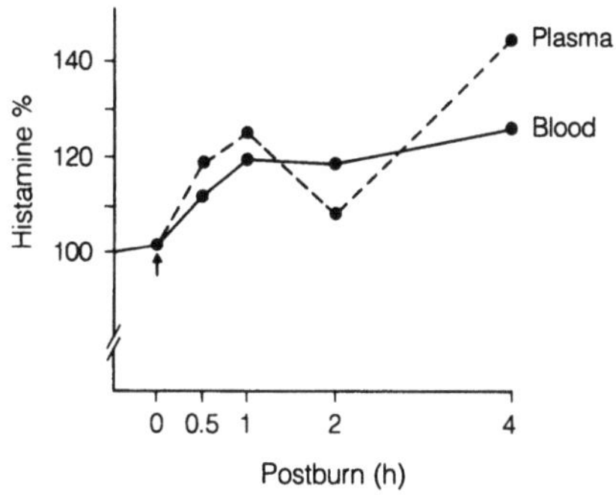

Fig. 8.5. Histamine contents in left ventricular blood in dogs after steam inhalation injury

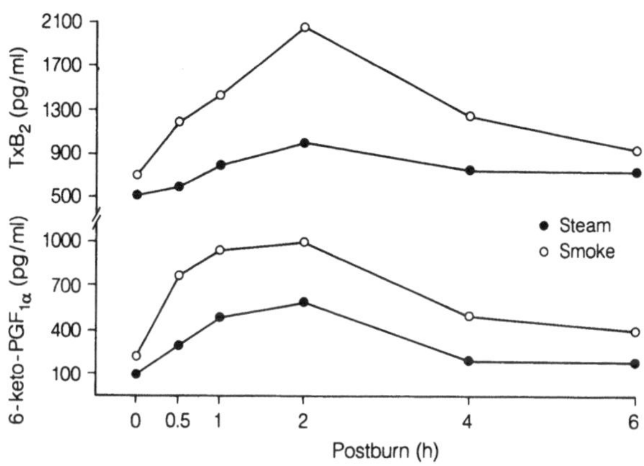

Fig. 8.6. Changes in TxB2 and 6-keto-$PGF_{1\alpha}$ in arterial blood, lung lymph fluid, and lung tissue in B goats after inhalation injuries. ●, steam inhalation; ○, smoke inhalation

and result in release of free arachidonic acid by interacting with phospholipase. This serves as the substrate for many vasoactive substances, such as prostacyclin, a powerful vasodilator, and thromboxane A_2, a vasoconstrictor. However, PGI_2/TxA_2 ratio is more important in influencing the vascular tonicity. Our studies have shown that the TxB_2 and 6-keto-$PGF_{1\alpha}$ contents in the left ventricular blood and lung lymph in goats after smoke inhalation injury significantly elevated. TxB_2 increased more markedly and rapidly. Therefore, the TxB_2/6-keto-PGF_{1a} ratio also increased [13] (Fig. 8.6). This may be one of the primary etiological factors leading to increasing pulmonary vascular resistance. Meanwhile, TxA_2 may damage the capillary directly. Recent studies have shown that leukotrienes may play an even more important role in participating in producing respiratory failure after inhalation injury than the vasoactive products of the cyclo-oxygenase pathway. In addition, attention has been paid to the effects of free radicals, including superoxide radicals, hydrogen peroxides, and hydroxyl radicals. Under normal circumstances, a quantity of free radicals may be released, but most are cleared by scavengers. However, under certain pathological

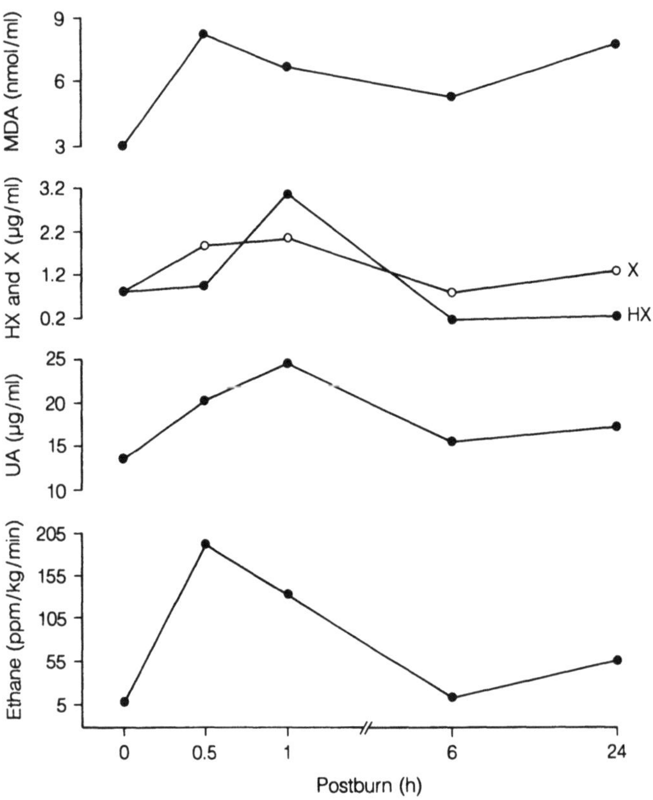

Fig. 8.7. Changes in plasma monodehydroascorbate (*MDA*), hypoxanthine (*HX*), xanthine (*X*) uric acid (*UA*), and ethane in expired air in dogs with smoke inhalation injuries

conditions, such as hypoxia, oxygen toxicity, leukocyte aggregation, and high arachinoid metabolism, the amount of free radicals produced increases. These oxygen by-products can cause lipid peroxidation and in turn destroy the cellular membrane. It has been proved that they can directly injury endothelial cells, pneumocytes, and fibroblasts. Oxygen intermediates are also capable of inactivating protective enzyme inhibitors, such as α-1 proteinase inhibitors. Moreover, after interacting with arachinoid products, they can destroy the cellular membranes, membranous protein, and pulmonary parenchyma. In our experimental studies of smoke inhalation injury, superoxide dismutase (SOD) activity and the contents of xanthine, hypoxanthine, uric acid, monodehydroascorbate (MDA) in animal blood, and ethane in expired gases were all increased [14] (Fig. 8.7), proving that free radicals play a major role in causing lung damage after inhalation injury. Oxygen-derived free radicals may be produced from three sources: (a) ischemic and hypoxic lung tissue, (b) complex arachidonic acid metabolic cascade, and (c) radical-activated neutrophils. The neutrophil is an important effector cell. In response to heat and/or smoke inhalation, the

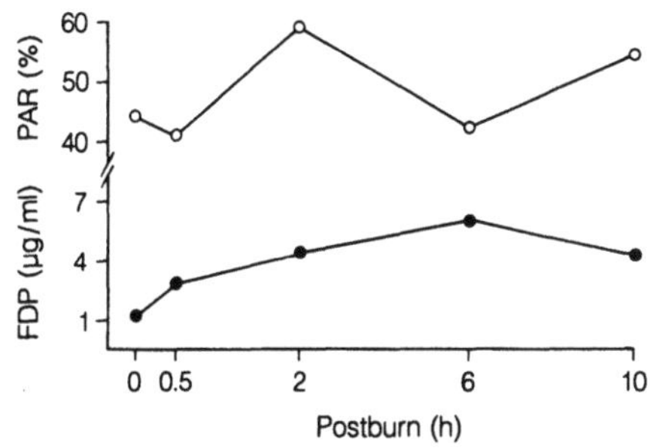

Fig. 8.8. Changes in platlet aggregation rate and fibrin degradation product (*FDP*) contents in rabbits after inhalation injuries. ○, smoke; ●, steam

polymorphonuclear neutrophils (PMNs) aggregate and form microemboli. The aggregations or microemboli are trapped in the microcirculation of lung tissue. The subsequent release of deleterious proteinases and oxygen intermediates produces cell toxicity and potential oxygen dysfunction. Another important effector cell is the platelet. Our studies have shown that the blood platelet count declines and the largest platelet aggregation rate increases [15] (Fig. 8.8). Platelet aggregation causes release of ATP, ADP, histamine, serotonin, and thromboxane. It has also been demonstrated that fibrin degradation products increase in rabbits after smoke inhalation (Fig. 8.8). Fibrin degradation products, particularly fragment D, can induce thrombocytopenia, neutropenia, endothelial cell damage, and respiratory failure.

8.2 Pathology

A study of the pathology of inhalation injury reveals a wide range of severity. Intensity of injury also varies from minor subclinical smoke poisoning to immediate death. Besides the direct damage to the respiratory tract, inhaled agents can be absorbed, causing systemic effects. The most commonly encountered irritant gases are chlorine, phosgene, ammonia, sulfur dioxide, nitrogen oxides, and ozone. Their effects are modified by the concentration and duration of exposure as well as by the solubility of the gases. All of these toxic agents can cause edema of the mucous membrane, inflammation, capillary damage, and bronchospasm. Some patients develop severe oropharyngeal edema with upper airway obstruction. Injury to the bronchial mucosa induces bronchospasm and exudative inflammatory bronchitis associated with plugging of the small bronchi and atelectasis. Damage to the alveolo capillary membrane will cause noncardiogenic pulmonary edema.

Early pathological changes result from the immediate injury. The primary early changes are limited to the respiratory tract epithelium and superficial tissues. There are areas of focal hemorrhage, necrosis, and carbon soots in the trachea and bronchi, the epithelial cells may be desquamated and the cilia lost, and the lung is heavier than normal soon after inhalation injury. Gross examination of the lung may reveal generalized congestion and scattered subpleural hemorrhages. Microscopic study shows congestion of the capillaries, mild interstitial edema, and red cell extravasation in the early postinjury period. Electron microscopic study of the animals sustaining inhalation injury 2 h postburn reveals that the endothelial cells are swollen, the cytoplasmic matrix of type I epithelial cells has become markedly edematous with vacuole formation, and the organelles are damaged to some extent; type II epithelial cells are essentially normal. Subsequently, alveolar edema, atelectasis, a further increase in lung weight with emphysematous blebs and hemorrhagic foci on the surface, and diffuse hemorrhage with fluid oozing from the cut surface may be found. In addition to the laryngeal damage, serious injuries to the trachea and bronchi with diffuse pseudomembranous tracheobronchitis are often found. Pseudomembranes, edema, fibrinous exudate, mucosal slough, and bloody fluid are all present. Microscopic study demonstrates epithelial desquamation and bronchiolitis. Debris composed of leukocytes, erythrocytes, epithelial cells, carbonaceous material, and proteinaceous fluids is found in all levels of the respiratory tract. Peribroncial as well as perivascular edemas are often seen. In some cases, peribronchial pneumonic infiltration, necrotizing areas, and pseudomembranous inflammation are found. Widespread interstitial and alveolar edemas are frequently seen. As time passes, hyaline membranes may be formed as a result of the deposition of protein. Red cell extravasation and cellular debris are common findings in some alveoli. The ultrastructural changes are often remarkable. Our experimental animal studies [16] showed that the cilia of epithelial cells are reduced in number or fused together. Vacuoles are found in the endoplasm and mitochondria. In the mucous membrane, neutrophilic and mast cell infiltraiton is present. The endothelial cells become markedly swollen and vacuolated. In some cases, necrosis or exposure of the basement membrane is seen. The junctions of the endothelial cells become widened with gap (Fig. 8.9) and type II epithelial cells show vacuole formation involving mitochondria and endoplasmic reticulum (Fig. 8.10). A proportion of the type I epithelial cells show marked edema and a large number of vacuoles, which often contain myelin figures (Fig. 8.11). Some of the type I cells are fragmented.

After 24 h, infection is the major factor determining the later course of inhalation injury. Peribronchial pneumonic infiltration is usually widespread.

Fig. 8.9 (*above*). Endothelial cells become markedly swollen and contain vacuoles in ▶ the lung tissue 6 h postburn in sheep with smoke inhalation injuries. Edema fluid was present at the interstitial space. The fibrin was degraded and the junctions of endothelial cells are widened with gaps. *Ep*, epithelial cell; *En*, endothelial cell; *Alv*, alveolus; *BM*, basement membrane

Fig. 8.10 (*below*). Type II epithelial cells showing vacuole formation involving mitochondria and endoplasmic reticulum 6 h postburn in the lung tissue of sheep with smoke inhalation injury. *Alv*, alveolus; *LB*, lamellar body; *N*, nucleus; *En*, endothelial cell; *Cap*, capillary

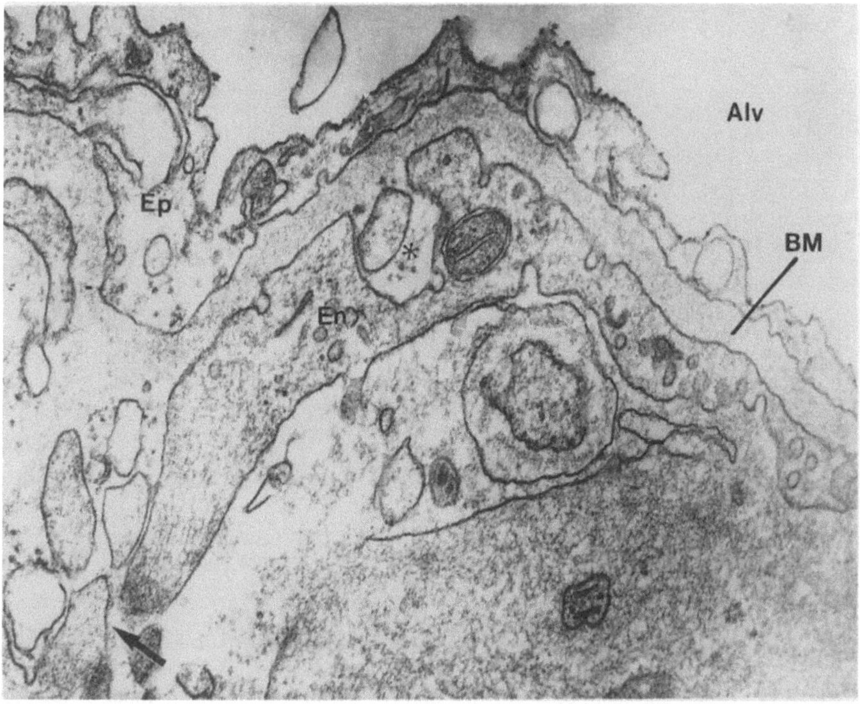
Alv
Ep
BM
*
En

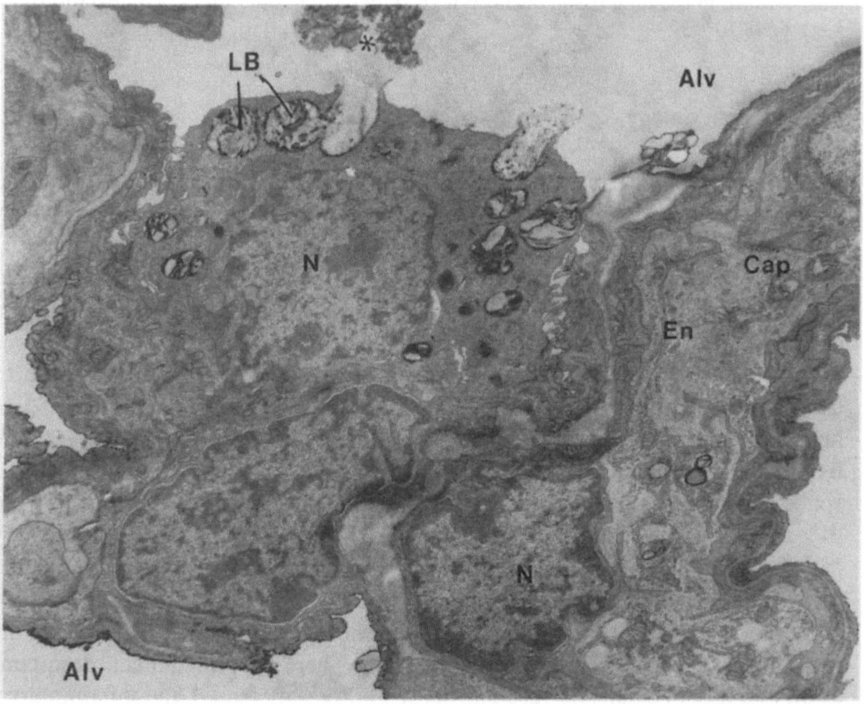
LB
*
Alv
N
Cap
En
N
Alv

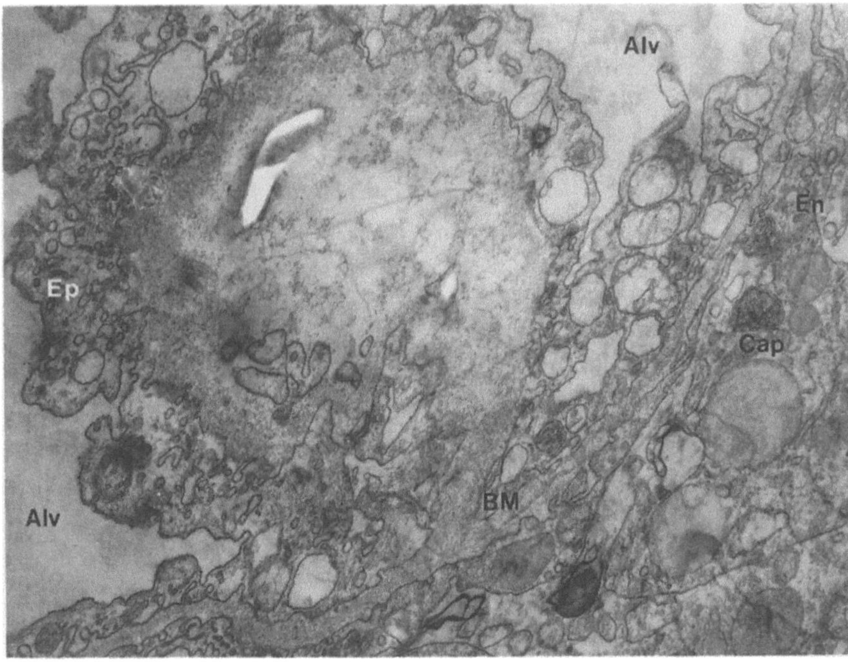

Fig. 8.11. Type I epithelial cells showing marked edema and a large number of vacuoles 6 h postburn in the lung tissue of sheep with smoke inhalation injury. Abbreviations, see Figs. 8.9, 8.10

8.3 Pathophysiology

As the causative factors of inhalation injuries are quite varied, the pathophysiological changes also very greatly. However, the basic changes are relatively uniform.

At the scene of the fire the predominant feature is asphyxiation due to either oxygen-poor air being inhaled or carbon monoxide poisoning. The affinity of carbon monoxide for hemoglobin is 257 times stronger that of oxygen [17]. It was found that 0.01% carbon monoxide inspired will convert 14% hemoglobin to carboxyhemoglobin. A level of 0.05% carbon monoxide will bind 44% of hemoglobin and 0.1% will bind 62% of hemoglobin [17]. Moreover, the oxyhemoglobin dissociation curve is shifted to the left. Combustion in a closed space consumes oxygen and decreases the ambient oxygen concentration from 21% to 10%–15%. In addition, air is displaced by fire-generated gases, principally carbon monoxide, which may reach 75 000 ppm [18]. All of these factors contribute to clinical hypoxia.

Soon after inhalation injury, the early pathological changes can be seen in the respiratory epithelium and microcirculation. There is epithelial cell desquamation and loss of cilia. The vascular permeability is increased and inflammatory reactions may be superimposed. These changes severely influence the function of air exchange. In severely injured cases, inadequate ventilation and respiratory function may result. Even respiratory failure may follow prolonged and progressive hypoxemia.

8.3.1 Airway Obstruction

The most deleterious effects of heat and noxious smoke are largely due to the formation of edema, which limits the rate of air flow and produces respiratory obstruction. Edema of the upper airway occurs frequently. In most cases injury is mainly limited to the supraglottic area. The vocal cords seldom swell because their structures are composed largely of avascular collagens. The structures above the vocal cord, however, are made up of loose tissue and can easily become edematous, resulting in obstruction. Though edema of the bronchi and trachea is more frequent, tracheobronchial obstruction is relatively uncommon, but it may occur due to mucosal slough and profuse secretions. Small airway obstruction can be caused by smoke inhalation, or inhalation of high-pressure steam, especially in cases of blast injury. Usually it is less severe. However, the chemicals may result in reactive bronchospasm, which may aggravate the severity of small obstruction. Airway obstruction may subside when the edema fluid is reabsorbed. However, remission may occur in severe cases because of recurrent detachment of mucosal slough into the airway.

8.3.2 Inadequate Ventilation/Perfusion Ratio (V/Q) and Shunt [19]

In the early period after inhalation injury, hypoventilation usually occurs, being caused by several factors. The airway can be obstructed by mucosal swelling, bronchospasm, and/or large amounts of tenacious secretion accumulated in the lumen; small airway obstruction may lead to alveolar expansion, resulting in atelectasis. The chest wall may be restricted by constructive chest eschar and pain. In addition, a prolonged supine position and doses of analgesics are also predisposing factors for hypoventilation.

The fluid content in the lungs has been studied [20] and in our studies has been measured in animals inflicted with inhalation injury by the dry weight method, Pierce's method, and the thermal green-dye double indicator dilution method. All the results show that pulmonary water volume increases rapidly as early as 2 h after inhalation injury, peaks at 24 h, and then declines gradually [9] (Fig. 8.12). However, the course might be prolonged and severer if sepsis is superimposed. It has been found that pulmonary edema is primarily caused by the increased vascular permeability after inhalation injury. The microcirculation in lung tissue has been continuously monitored using a lung lymph preparation in sheep and goats. The results demonstrate that the lung lymph flow and lymph:plasma protein ratio increase markedly [9] (Fig. 8.13), while the pulmon-

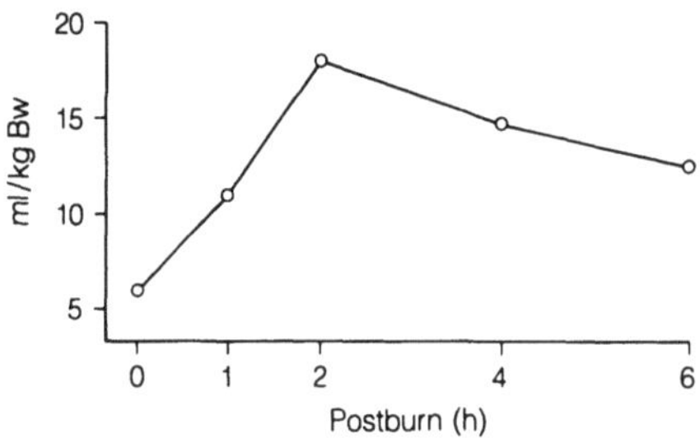

Fig. 8.12. Pulmonary extravascular water volume measured by the thermal green-dye double indicator dilution method

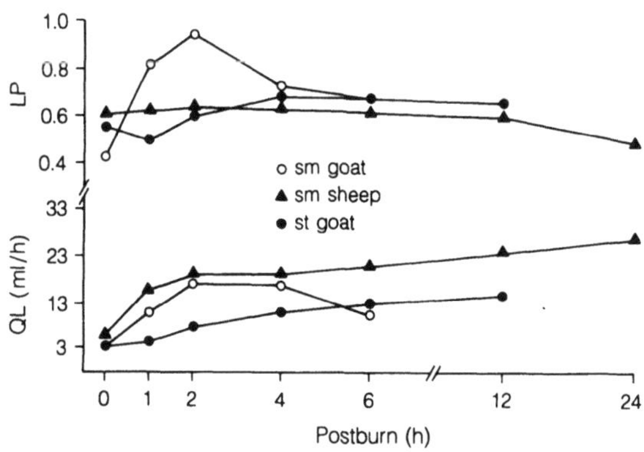

Fig. 8.13. Dynamic changes in lung lymph flow and lung lymph/plasma total protein ratio (*L/P*) after inhalation injuries. *st*, steam inhalation; *sm*, smoke inhalation

ary arterial pressure is increased only slightly shortly after injury, and then declines rapidly to its normal value.

Alveolar collapse or atelectasis presents another important pathological alteration. It might either be caused by the collapse of tissue distal to bronchial occlusion resulting from accumulation of mucosal slough or mucus in its lumen, or by changes in pulmonary surfactant. Our experimental study confirmed that surfactant activity is reduced in rabbits inflicted with steam inhalation injury [21].

The rapid shallow breathing usually observed in inhalation injury reduces the tidal volume; hence the average vital capacity is usually reduced.

All these factors will result in an increase in lung shunt. On the other hand, inadequate lung perfusion might also develop after inhalation injury. In the early stage, inadequate perfuson occurs mostly in the area of hypoventilation. This may result from vasoconstriction. The decreased blood flow may play some compensatory role in attenuating the degree of venous admixture. Later, microthrombosis in the lung supervenes, and mechanical blockage of the small pulmonary vessels increases the dead space, resulting in the retention of carbon dioxide.

8.3.3 True Diffusion Limitation

True diffusion limitation is the third factor contributing to hypoxia. In addition to the marked thickening of the alveolar capillary septum, there appears to be a reduction in the capillary volume per unit tissue. However, because of the high diffusion efficiency of both oxygen and carbon dioxide, carbon dioxide elimination and oxygen extraction do not present a problem in the early stage. Only in the later phase of pulmonary edema, when hyaline membranes develop and abnormal gas exchange evolves, do hypoxia and hypercapnia consequently appear. This results in an increase in dead space and reduction in effective alveolar ventilation, impairment of elimination of carbon dioxide, and elevation of $PaCO_2$.

Besides the direct effect of inhalation injury itself, other concomitant physiological alterations can complicate and participate in the deterioration of lung function, such as a decrease in compliance resulting from circumferential constriction of chest eschar, an increase in the need for carbon dioxide clearance, a decreased capability of oxygen transport resulting from carbon monoxide poisoning, an increased demand for oxygen utilization, a decreased number of red blood cells, a leftward shift in the hemoglobin dissociation curve due to alterations in the 2,3-diphosphoglyceric acid level, a decreased ATP level, acidosis, and other alterations after severe burn which is usually associated with inhalation injury.

8.4 Clinical Features

The clinical manifestation usually parallels the severity of the injury and the response of the patient to the injury, and demonstrates great difference between patients. In mild cases, symptoms may be absent, while acute respiratory failure may result in severe cases. Injuries are placed into three classes according to their severity and extent.

8.4.1 Mild Inhalation Injury

Usually the pathological lesions are confined primarily to oral, nasal, and pharyngeal areas. Most are associated with facial burns. The presence of carbon particles in the sputum, singed vibrissae, blistering of the mouth, oropharyngeal inflammation, a sooty tongue or pharynx, rapid breathing, and a hacking cough are common symptoms and signs. In addition, there is pain and a dry sensation in the laryngeal area. Hoarseness is less obvious and respiratory distress is absent. The chest is often normal under physical examination. Congestion and swelling of the mucous membrane of the nasal cavity and posterior wall of the phyarynx are not unusual, and in some cases even mucosal erosion and desquamation may be found.

8.4.2 Moderate Inhalation Injury

Lesions involve mainly the laryngeal, pharyngeal, and tracheal regions. In other words, the extent of injury is confined to the area above the carina. Besides the clinical manifestations found in mild inhalation injury, there is hoarseness and signs of upper airway obstruction. An irritative cough with carbonaceous sputum is often present and sometimes sloughed mucous membrane may be coughed up. Redness and edema of the upper airway are prominent and the swelling will progress to such an extent that narrowing and ultimate occlusion of the airway may occur. The breathing sound becomes weak and rough. A high-pitched crowing sound can be heard on inspiration when the upper airway obstruction is present. Rarely wheezing and dry rales can be detected, but moist rales are usually absent. Chest X-ray findings are usually normal. Fiberoptic bronchoscopy may reveal edema of the supraglottic area, congestion, edema, hemorrhagic spots, or even erosion and desquamation of the tracheal mucosa. The carina is usually normal or slightly widened due to edema.

8.4.3 Severe Inhalation Injury

The injury extend below the carina, involving the bronchi and bronchioles, and even as far as the alveoli. Besides the clinical features seen in mild and moderate inhalation injury, there is diffuse bronchospasm, occlusion of the small airway, and pulmonary edema. Severe respiratory distress and progressive hypoxemia can appear rapidly. Blood-tinged or bloody frothy sputum and sloughed mucous membrane are commonly seen. Restlessness, confusion, stupor, or even coma usually indicate that the degree of hypoxia is very severe. Wheezing, and dry and moist rales can be heard all over the chest. Fiberoptic bronchoscopic examination reveals congestion, edema, hemorrhage, and erosion of the mucous membrane of the small bronchioli. Different roentgenographic patterns of pulmonary edema can be shown as early as 2 h after injury. The xenon-133 scintiphotographic lung scan is usually positive. Although the clinical course of patients with inhalation injury is a continuum of events, an arbitrary definition of four phases is useful for a better understanding of the changes.

8.4.3.1 Initial Phase

The duration of the initial phase varies and depends on the severity of injury. Usually it lasts approximately 6 h, to just before the edema peak. In most severe cases, asphyxia or even death may occur at the scene of the fire, and pulmonary edema, diffuse bronchospasm, and small airway obstruction may appear shortly after injury, being followed by acute respiratory distress. But in patients with mild or moderate inhalation injury, the symptoms are mild during this period. Sputum with carbon particles and an irritative brassy cough may be present. It must be noted that the pathological changes are usually progressive. In some moderate cases, the superglottic edema may develop so severely that upper airway obstruction ensues.

8.4.3.2 Edematous Phase

Patients, except those with very mild injury, will proceed to the edematous phase. This phase usually lasts from 6 to 48 h, during which period the papillary permeability is markedly increased, and marked edema of the tracheobronchial mucous membrane and interstitial and alveolar edema become obvious. Marked supraglottic edema is usually the most significant early threat. Airway obstruction may also occur secondary to mucosal slough resulting from necrotizing pseudomembranous inflammatory changes. Small airway obstruction secondary to desquamative bronchiolitis can also occur in this phase. This obstruction may result in atelectasis. Compliance decreases steadily partly because of atelectasis. Decreased compliance concurrent with the still raised vascular resistance leads to an altered ventilation-perfusion ratio and a continuing increase in the alveolar-arterial PaO_2 difference. This may result in acute respiratory failure.

8.4.3.3 Septic Phase

As a result of pathological change in the airway mucous membrane, the local immunological function is depressed. Bacterial invasion can occur early in this phase. We demonstrated in steam respiratory burn studies that pulmonary infection could develop earlier than 6 h postburn. Bronchopneumonia was demonstrated in almost all patients with severe inhalation injury at 49 h. Usually infection starts near the injured bronchi, then spreads and rapidly become confluent. In some cases, blood-borne pneumonitis may also occur, mostly with organisms originating from the burn wound. Areas of alveolar edema and atelectasis are particularly fertile breeding grounds for pathogenic organisms. Uncontrolled pneumonitis can result in acute respiratory failure. In cases without pulmonary edema, the incidence of bronchopneumonia is less frequent and the development of respiratory failure is also less common.

8.4.3.4 Desquamative and Repair Phase

If the patient can survive the edematous phase and septic phase, he or she will proceed to the desquamative and repair phase, which may run a protracted course. Pseudomembranous tracheobronchitis is a predominant feature. The lesions vary from a mild, superficial desquamation of one or more homogenous, swollen and acidophilic epithelial cells to a complete disruption of the epithelial lining with focal necrosis and formation of a pseudomembrane composed of mucous cellular debris, fibrinous exudate, polymorphonuclear leukocytes, and clumps of bacteria. The submucosa shows severe congestion and edema, scattered with hemorrhage. The necrotic mucous membrane may be sloughed repeatedly. Mucosal slough could produce airway obstruction or evoke bronchospasm. Denuded friable granulation tissue may develop in severe cases and hemoptysis may supervene. Severe hemoptysis may prove fatal. The patient may die from profuse bleeding or suffocation due to blockage of the airway by blood clots. In addition, the denuded sloughed mucosal surface is particularly suitable for bacterial proliferation. The sloughed area is repaired with cuboid-type pneumocytes which will narrow the lumen of the airway produce excessive mucus. These factors also predispose to infection. Infection may invade the surrounding tissue, and lung abscess or multiple abscesses may supervene. Patients may become septic again, die from it, or may run a chronic course, showing continuous fever, deterioration, and cough with profuse amounts of thick sputum. Repair of the injured mucous membrane and restoration of the pulmonary function could be expected after 1 month or more in most patients. However, in some cases, as a result of the destructive injury to the airway and chronic infection, bronchiectasis, endobronchial polyposis, or tracheobroncial stricture may occur. Even in patients showing an apparently uncomplicated recovery, pulmonary function tests reveal lasting abnormality. A decrease in pulmonary compliance and an increase in pulmonary resistance are common.

8.5 Diagnosis

The establishment of the diagnosis of inhalation injury is not difficult. However, an accurate assessment of the severity of the injury may not be easy. Therefore continuous monitoring and repeated diagnostic interventions are needed. The diagnosis of inhalation injury should be considered if the following conditions are present on admission: (a) burn accident occurring in a closed space where a high concentration of carbon monoxide and potentially irritating toxic gases have been allowed to accumulate and to be continuously introduced into the respiratory tract, especially in patients associated with depressed mentality or blast injuries; (b) face, neck, and anterior thoracic burns, especially deep burns around the mouth and nose; (c) singed vibrissae, swollen lip, blistering of the mouth, oropharyngeal inflammation; (d) presence of carbon particles in the sputum, which is supposed to be pathognomonic for inhalation injury, but can also be seen in the absence of major airway injury due to backflow of secretions from the nasal passage to the pharynx; (e) hoarseness and stridor, indicating damage to the laryngeal structure, compromising the airway; and (f) dyspnea and wheezing, in case the injury extends to the small airway. However, it should be pointed out that inhalation injury can also occur in the open area and in patients without facial burn injury. It is estimated that 70% of inhalation-injured patients have facial burns, but 70% of patients with facial burns do not have significant respiratory burns [22].

Since impairment of pulmonary function does not occur immediately following the injury, immediate symptoms are uncommon even in cases with lethal injury. Therefore, it is unwise to rule out inhalation injury on account of normal pulmonary function at the time of admission. Repeated evaluation of the patient is required throughout the clinical course.

Initial physical findings are often related to upper airway injury. Restlessness, confusion, and rapid shallow labored breathing suggest airway obstruction. Swelling of the airway can alter the normal airflow pattern. Dyspnea is the most consistent symptom in inhalation injury, but should not be mistaken for anxiety or a sign of pain. Tachypnea is also frequent. Flaring of the nasal alae, the use of accessory muscles for respiration, and intercostal retraction are occasionally observed. Although severe hypoxemia is often present, cyanosis is not the rule, for it can be masked by the cherry red color of carboxyhemoglobin. The emergence of stridor or a high-pitched, crowing sound is a sign calling for urgent treatment. A brassy cough, bronchorrhea, and hemoptysis are often seen in patients with small airway obstruction.

Hypoxia is an important and consistent symptom after inhalation injury. Patients may die immediately at the site of conflagration from asphyxia because of the acute decrease in oxygen in the air or the rapid increase in carbon dioxide in the air and the liberation of other noxious gaseous substances, such as carbon monoxide. A small amount of inspired carbon monoxide may cause significant deleterious effects on the oxygen-carrying capacity of blood, as well as cellular enzyme systems, resulting in severe tissue hypoxia. Generally the carboxythemoglobin level in the case of inhalation injury is about 1%–5%, and the patient is asymptomatic. Levels exceeding 15%–20% cause mild symptoms, such as headache, nauses, vomiting, and/or dyspnea. At progressively higher levels (40%–60%), there will be myocardial toxicity, visual disturbance, ataxia, and seizures, followed by coma and death. Diagnosis may be reached tentatively by clinical manifestation and history. Definite diagnosis can only actually be made by measurement of the blood carboxyhemoglobin level. It is worth mentioning that the severity of inhalation injury is generally proportional to the level of carboxyhemoglobin in burn victims.

Hypoxemia can only be ascertained by blood gas analysis. Therefore repeated blood gas analysis is necessary. If the PaO_2 falls below 75 mmHg in patients without severe burn shock, inhalation injury should definitely be suspected. Soon after smoke inhalation, there might be a sharp fall in the PaO_2 because of asphyxia and/or inspiring low concentration oxygen, a rise in the $PaCO_2$, and the presence of acidosis. After breathing fresh air or a high concentration of oxygen, hypoxemia may become ameliorated and acidosis thus minimized. As a result of hypoxemia, hyperventilation may develop, and respiratory alkalosis may appear. After carbon monoxide is expelled, the cardiovascular system returns to normal, the alveoli become perfused and ventilated, excessive carbon dioxide is expelled, and the physiological dead space returns to near its normal size. However, in severe cases, these beneficial effects appear only transiently because of the superimposed interstitial pulmonary edema, which may lead to alteration of the ventilation-perfusion ratio and a continuous increase in the alveolar-arterial PO_2 difference. Hypoxemia will be aggravated. The value of $PaCO_2$ varies with the efficiency of ventilation. In most cases, hypocapnia usually prevails, and only in the terminal period does hypercapnia appear.

In the early phase of inhalation injury, X-ray examination is not very helpful in diagnosis. The chest roentgenograms may be essentially normal even when serious injuries are present. However, radiological studies must be planned sequentially in patients suspected of having inhalation injury. Abnormal findings can be found several hours later. Most of the early lesions are homogeneous and appear as ground glass-like patches. Sometimes fine reticular shadows can be seen in pathes. In advanced cases, patchy cloudiness of varying size and large areas of consolidation might appear. The above-mentioned signs are due to the accumulation of extravascular lung water. But, soon after, infection becomes superimposed. The X-ray appearances of pulmonary infection are similar to those of the pulmonary edema, but more dense in shadow. When dense miliary shadow appears on top of the preexisting cloudiness, pulmonary infection must be highly suspect. The emergence of diffuse pulmonary infiltration is a very serious X-ray sign, indicating that respiratory failure will follow. Besides the findings of edema and infection, not infrequently atelectasis can be seen. X-ray manifestations of atelectasis are scattered patchy shadow which cannot be well differentiated from those of edema or infection. Characteristic shadows of lobar atelectasis are uncommon. Narrowing of the tracheal lumen with thickening of the tracheal wall indicating the presence of tracheal damage can be seen several hours after injury, especially in the right oblique view of the chest film.

Fiberoptic bronchoscopic study is very helpful in the diagnosis of inhalation injury, and, if possible, can be performed repeatedly [23]. Usually local anesthesia is used. Before the examination, it is better to have the patient inhale pure oxygen for several minutes. In patients suspected of having upper airway obstruction, an endotracheal tube should be placed over the bronchoscope. When there is a need, the endotracheal tube can then be inserted quickly under direct vision. Positive findings of injury include mucosal and extramucosal lesions. There may be edema, erythema, blebs, and sloughing of mucosa. Carbonaceous debris and bronchorrhea constitute the extramucosal findings. The laryngeal region must be examined first to evaluate the airway patency. In mild upper airway injury, slight erythema and edema may be present but the airway is patent, while in severe upper airway injury the edema is so serious that the false vocal cord is bulging into the lumen and the true vocal cord is not visible. Usually airway obstruction is impending. Meanwhile marked erythema and mucosal slough may also be seen. To examine the major airway, the bronchoscope should be advanced through the cord. In these cases, the larynx is extremely sensitive, and reapplication of local anesthesia to the cord is necessary before the bronchoscope is further advanced. The severity of inhalation injury can usually be assessed by fiberoptic bronchoscopic study. Lesions limited to the pharyngeal area with normal cord are classified as mild inhalation injury. If the glottic injuries are obvious and tracheal damage can be seen and the case can be defined as moderate inhalation injury. In severe inhalation injuries, there are distal bronchial abnormalities, and the depth of the mucosal lesions can be directly seen and identified at the same time. Serial bronchoscopic studies help not only in the diagnosis but also in the prognosis. However, bronchoscopy has its limitation because the field viewed extends only to the third bronchi, and damage beyond this can only be reached by other means such as ^{133}Xe scintiphotographic lung scan and CT scan.

Xenon-133 scintiphotographic lung scan is another valuable means in the evaluation of patients with severe inhalation injuries [24]. Its diagnostic accuracy reaches 90% or above and is greater than 96% when combined with fiberoptic bronchoscopy. ^{133}Xe, when injected into a vein, will be carried via the circulation to the lung, and then volatilized and exhaled. Normally the injected ^{133}Xe can be eliminated completely by 90 s. In patients with severe inhalation injuries, the clearing time will be prolonged over 90 s, and an abnormal uneven scan might be observed. It can revert to normal by the fourth postburn day in most patients. Therefore it can only be used within 3 days after inhalation injury. False-positive results may be caused by preexisting illness, such as pneumonia, asthma, and chronic obstructive pulmonary disease. Moreover, there is the need to transport the patient from the burn intensive care unit to a nuclear medicine department, which will increase the burden on the already seriously ill burn patient.

8.6 Treatment

Early management of inhalation injury must begin before confirmation of the diagnosis. The basic goals of early treatment are maintenance of an adequate airway, prevention of atelectasis and subsequent pneumonia, and prompt management of pulmonary edema in an attempt to prevent respiratory failure.

8.6.1 Oxygen Therapy

Oxygen should be administered at the site of the accident as early as possible with the purpose of counteracting carbon monoxide poisoning and lessening hypoxia. Inspired 100% oxygen will lower the half-elimination time of carbon monoxide (COHb) from 250 to less than 50 min. Usually several hours later, the level of blood COHb has declined to near normal value. The inspired oxygen concentration must be reduced to 40% or less. Oxygen should always be preheated and humidified in order to prevent local drying of the mucosa, and to make bronchial secretions less sticky. However, it must be noted that humidification can provide as much as 500 ml/day water in positive balance. If oxygen therapy is continued for more than several days, the possibility of absorptive atelectasis and oxygen toxicity arises. As a general rule, it is essential to keep the inspired oxygen concentration as low as possible to maintain adequate oxygenation.

8.6.2 Management of Airway Obstruction

Whenever there are signs of impending airway obstruction, measures should be taken to maintain a patient airway. Indications for intubation generally include inhalation injury accompanied by coma or respiratory depression, posterior pharyngeal swelling, nasolabial full-thickness burns, prolonged hypoxia necessitating mechanical ventilation, and repeated suction or irrigation [25]. Nasotracheal intubation is preferred. However, it is very difficult to perform tracheal intubation or tracheostomy in those patients with facial or deep neck burns complicated by severe edema. In such cases, direct visualization is necessary with the aid of a fiberoptic bronchoscope ensheathed in the endotracheal tube.

Controversy exists over the use of long-term endotracheal intubation as opposed to early tracheostomy. Tracheostomy provides comfort to the patient, ease of pulmonary toilet, and ease of oral alimentation. Endotracheal intubation offers the advantages of nonoperative intervention, easier discontinuation, and a less direct route for bacterial contamination of the lung. Complications of tracheostomy such as bleeding, subcutaneous emphysema, pneumothorax, tube malposition, tracheal ulceration, and tracheitis are not uncommon [26]. On the other hand, endotracheal intubation may also lead to complications of subglottic stenosis, vocal cord damage, and necrosis of the nasal cartilage. The length of intubation apparently determines the incidence of such complications. Current trends appear to be in favor of long-term endotracheal intubation [27]. In our experience, it seems better to perform endotracheal intubation initially in the majority of cases. The situation is reviewed on the 2nd or 3rh day postburn, since the incidence of severe laryngeal complications increases after 48 h. If the intubation is prolonged more than 3 days, tracheostomy is better performed.

8.6.3 Ventilatory Support

Despite the aggressive treatment mentioned above, patients with severe inhalation injury may deteriorate, noted by the appearance of progressive hypoxemia, pulmonary edema, and even respiratory failure. Without doubt, in patients with fully developed respiratory failure, mechanical ventilation is imperative. However, there is difficulty in determining when to use ventilatory support in patients with a risk of developing respiratory failure, or having early signs of respiratory failure in the presence of lung edema, in which a vicious cycle will usually form, i.e., lung edema → decrease of vital capacity → appearance of hypoxia → more lung edema. It is therefore more profitable to start assisted mechanical ventilatory support early rather than late.

The criteria for ventilatory support are as follows:

1. Respiratory rate over 40/min
2. PaO_2 lower than 70 mmHg after a high FiO_2
3. $PaCO_2$ lower than 25 mmHg or over 45 mmHg
4. Tidal volume less than 15–20 ml/kg

5. Physiological shunt increased to over 30%, or A-aDO_2 to over 350 mmHg after inspiring 100% oxygen
6. Physiological dead space (V_d/V_t) increased to over 0.6

The use of positive end expiratory pressure (PEEP) plays a well-documented vital role in the management of patients with severe inhalation injury [28, 29]. PEEP is indicated if the PaO_2 remains below 60 mmHg despite the proper application of mechanical ventilation with a high FiO_2. It may start with a pressure of 5 cm H_2O, then is gradually increased as necessary. The beneficial effect of PEEP is mainly attributable to the increase in functional residual capacity (FRC) [30]. The improved ventilation to gas exchange units, which are the previous sites of shunting or marked VA/Q abnormalities, will increase PaO_2 and reduce A-aDO_2. In addition, PEEP can improve gas exchange by expanding the alveoli which were filled with edematous fluid, thus helping to increase vital capacity and improve lung compliance. PEEP may also conserve pulmonary surface tension. However, it is not yet clear whether PEEP would alter the course in preventing respiratory failure or decreasing the mortality of inhalation injury. Therefore, the therapeutic value of PEEP remains controversial. It is better to use an intrapulmonary shunt fraction of 15% or 20% or a PaO_2/FiO_2 of over 300 as the clinical therapeutic end point. The use of PEEP is not without hazard. Cardiac output frequently tends to decline as PEEP is increased from 5 to 10 cm H_2O. When it is above 10 cm H_2O, the fall in cardiac output will be more liable to occur and more pronounced. But in patients with severe inhalation injury, their lungs often become quite stiff, and little the end expiratory airway pressure can be transmitted to the intrathoracic vessels. Therefore there will be less effect on the venous return, and cardiac output decreases only slightly. In addition to the decrease in cardiac output, it has also been observed that PEEP can induce pulmonary hypertension and reduce subendocardial and bronchial mucosal blood flow. Other complications encountered are pneumomediastinum, subcutaneous emphysema, and pneumothorax.

There are no rigid rules to determine the exact time to wean a patient from mechanical ventilatory support. However, premature weaning may be dangerous. An adequate oxygen supply is needed before weaning. Usually the PaO_2 should be over 70 mmHg at an FiO_2 of 0.4–0.5 and an A-aDO_2 of less than 30–50 with a $PaCO_2$ between 30 and 40 mmHg. A vital capacity of 15 ml/kg is necessary. The maximal inspiratory pressure generated against an occluded airway should be greater than -20 cm H_2O.

8.6.4 Clearance of Secretions and Lavage

The main aims of this therapy are to make the secretion thin, to encourage cough, and to institute postural drainage. Hydration of the patient and humidification of inspired air are necessary. If the patient is breathing through an artificial airway, continuous humidification is essential. Cough must be stimulated. Chest percussion and vibration not only help to move secretion into the large bronchi but also often stimulate coughing. These must be performed at frequent intervals throughout 24 h. Patients with severe inhalation injury often have complications of pseudomembranous inflammation of the airway. There is a marked increase in quantity and viscosity of the secrtion which cannot easily be cleared by coughing. It must be supplemented by mechanical suction. However, in some severe cases, in the presence of a huge amount of persistent secretion, pseudomembranous exudates and necrotic debris in either small and large airways, suction might not be effective. Helpful in these cases is fiberoptic bronchoscopy, which should be performed repeatedly, and which is better performed through an endotracheal tube or tracheostomy stoma. In some patients neither suctioning nor fiberoptic bronchoscopy is able to clean the airway. Then bronchial lavage is necessary. At first, the suction tube is passed into the right or left bronchus through the tracheostomy tube and 5–10 ml warm sterile saline is injected through the suction tube. As soon as coughing is initiated, suction is performed. Several minutes later, this procedure can be repeated. Then the suction tube is reinserted but into the other bronchus and lavage is reperformed. If necessary, the volume of lavaging saline can be increased by as much as 30–50 ml provided the patient can tolerate it, and lavage can be repeated every 4–6 h. Effective irrigation can prevent atelectasis, maintain the airway patency, facilitate gas exchange, hasten the removal of sloughs and necrotic mucous membrane, and decrease the severity of septic inflammation.

8.6.5 Extracorporeal Membrane Oxygenation

Extracorporeal membrane oxygenation (ECMO) is feasible and effective in providing temporary support for patients in whom the pathological changes of the lung require a prolonged period to heal [31]. However, the equipment is not perfect, and it is only used in a few burn patients, and no improvement in survival with ECMO is observed. Furthermore, lung pathology is not changed by ECMO. Further study in this direction is necessary.

8.6.6 Fluid Management

Because of the usual presence of pulmonary edema, early fluid resuscitation of it is traditionally apt to limit the amount of early fluid resuscitation. It is generally believed that elevation of the capillary hydrostatic pressure engendered by vigorous administration of fluid for resuscitation will enhance the escape of capillary fluid and make the lung worse. Since severe inhalation injury is often associated with large area body surface burns, restoration of adequate perfusion is critical for all the important organs including the lung itself, because as is well known, inadequate perfusion of lung tissues will also cause pulmonary edema because of hypoxemia. In patients with severe burns, pulmonary edema could develop very soon after injury, sometimes long before resuscitation. Our experimental studies have shown that the volume of fluid calculated with our formula or the Parkland formula given to dogs with 30% TBSA burns and severe steam respiratory burns does not aggravate the existing pulmonary edema [32]. Therefore it is thought inappropriate to recommend the limitation of fluid therapy in inhalation injury, suffice to say that volume replacement should be carried out judiciously, considering only the state of perfusion, and it is not necessary to restrict the amount.

8.6.7 Steroids

The use of adrenal corticosteroids is controversial. Theoretically it benefits the reduction of mucosal edema and bronchospasm and helps maintain surfactant function. The results of experimental animal studies show tremendous variation. Some demonstrated an increase in mortality in animals treated with daily doses of adrenal steroids [33], while others showed improved mortality in animals when a high dose of methyl prednisolone or dexamethasone was administered [34]. Clinically, no definite beneficial results have been obtained in inhalation injury patients. Generally administration of corticosteroids is not recommended in the treatment of inhaltion injury except in those patients with severe pulmonary edema.

8.6.8 Treatment of Infection

When infection is suspected, intensive efforts should be made to identify the specific pathogens. This can usually be accomplished by culture of wound exudate, aspirated pulmonary secretion, sputum, and lavage fluid. The organisms most commonly found are of the *Pseudomonas*, *Proteus*, and *Klebsiella* groups. However, other organisms such as *Staphylococcus* or several species of fungus colonizing the face and neck burn wound surfaces may also invade the respiratory tract. Once a specific organism is identified, appropriate antibiotic therapy should be initiated. Prophylactic use of antibiotics usually shows no benefits. However, as secondary infection often supervenes early, it is advisable to institute antibiotics at an early burn phase.

8.6.9 General Care of the Airway

Pulmonary hygiene is of great significance in the treatment of inhalation injury. It is necessary usually to change the position of patients, to encourage deep breathing and coughing, and to suck and clear the secretions in the airway. Because the larynx is often swollen, swallowing in these patients is difficult. Cleaning the mouth and nasal cavity is important. In unconscious patients or patients with complications of gastric stasis, it is better to introduce gastric intubation. The functions of the upper airway are normally to filter, warm, and moisten the inspired air. These functions are markedly reduced in cases of inhalation injury. Humidification of inspired air is necessary to maintain the pulmonary function and tissue oxygenation. Hemodynamic stability should be assured. Bronchodilators may be given either by intermittent injections every 4–6 h or by a continuous infusion. Aminophylline, salbutamol, and dexamethasone are the drugs of choice.

References

1. Moylan JA, Chan CK (1978) Inhalation injury – an increasing problem. Ann Surg 188: 34–37
2. Di Vincenti FC, Pruitt BA Jr, Reckler JM (1971) Inhalation injury. J Trauma 11: 109–117
3. Foley FD, Moncrief JA, Mason AD (1968) Pathology of the lung in fatally burned patients. Ann Surg 167: 251–264
4. Putman CE, Loke J, Matthay RA, et al. (1977) Radiographic manifestations of acute smoke inhalation injury. Am J Roentgenol 129: 865–870
5. Schlag G, Redl H, Traber L et al. (1984) Impaired respiratory mechanisms in smoke inhalation (abstract). Circ Shock 13: 78
6. Shook CD, Macmillan BC, Altimeir WA (1968) Pulmonary complications of the burn patients. Arch Surg 97: 215–224
7. Silverstein P, Dressler DF (1970) Effect of current therapy on burn mortality. Ann Surg 171: 124–129
8. Herndon DN, Langner F, Thompson P et al. (1987) Pulmonary injury in burned patients. Surg Clin North Am 7: 31–46
9. Li N, Yang ZC, Jiang KP et al. (1987) Roles of some inflammatory mediators in the pathogenesis of early pulmonary edema in steam respiratory burn. Chin Med J 100: 132–141
10. Huang WH (1985) Decline of serum complement hemolytic activities following thermal injury. Proceedings of the 1st Sino-American conference on burn injuries. Chongqing, p 8
11. Zhou SC (1985) The dynamic changes of the contents of left ventricular plasma C_{3a} in dogs after steam inhalation injury. In: Li N (ed) Research in burns, Chongqing Press, Chongqing, p 194
12. Huang YH, Yu SL, LU JH et al. (1986) The effects of antihistamines on the histamine content of blood in dogs with thermal injury of respiratory tract. Chin J Plast Surg Burns 2: 54–56
13. Huang JH, Li N, Yang ZC et al. (1988) Changes of thromboxane and prostacyclin after smoke injury in goats. J Med Coll Chin PLA 3: 41–45
14. Zhao ZD, Li N, Yang ZC (1988) The relationship between early lung injury and active oxygen radicals after smoke inhalation injury in goats. J Med Coll Chin PLA 3: 206–213
15. An J, Li N, Yang ZC (1987) Dynamic changes of platelet aggregation and serum fibrin degradation product after smoke inhalation injury in rabbits. J Med Coll Chin PLA 2: 236–240
16. Wang CZ (1988) An experimental study of the pathogenesis of acute respiratory failure after smoke inhalation. Acta Acad Med Milit Tertiay 10 [Suppl] 1–34
17. Fein A, Leff A, Hopewell PC (1980) Pathophysiology and management of the complications resulting from fire and the inhaled products of combustion. Crit Care Med 8: 94–98

18. Chu C (1982) Special burn injury and burns of special area in China. J Trauma 22: 574–580
19. Robinson NB, Hudson LD, Roberson HT et al. (1981) Ventilation and perfusion alterations after smoke inhalation injury. Surgery 90: 352–383
20. Tranbaugh RF, Lewis FR, Christensen JM et al. (1980) Lung water changes afte1 thermal injury. Ann Surg 192: 479–490
21. Liu ZY, Li AO, Yang ZC (1986) Changes in the pulmonary surfactant activity in rabbits with severe steam inhalation injury. Burns 12: 330–336
22. Moylan JA (1981) Inhalation injury – a primary determinant of survival. JBCR 3: 78–84
23. Moylan JA (1980) Smoke inhalation and burn injury. Surg Clin North Am 60: 1533–1540
24. Moylan JA, Wilmore DW, Mouton DE et al. (1972) Early diagnosis of inhalation injury using Xenon^{133} lung scan. Ann Surg 176: 477–484
25. Bartlett RH, Niceole M, Travis MJ et al. (1976) Acute management of the upper airway in facial burns. Arch Surg 111: 744–749
26. Moylan JA, West JT, Nash G et al. (1972) Tracheostomy in thermally injured patients: a review of five years experience. Am Surg 38: 119–123
27. Tranbaugh RF, Lewis FR, Christenson JM et al. (1980) Lung water changes after thermal injury. Ann Surg 92: 479–490
28. Davis LK, Poulton TJ, Modell JH (1983) Continuous positive airway pressure is beneficial in treatment of smoke inhalation. Crit Care Med 11: 726–729
29. Herndon DN, Adams T, Traber LD et al. (1984) Inhalation injury and positive pressure ventilation in a sheep model. Circ Shock 12: 107–113
30. Herndon DN, Thompson PB, Traber DL (1985) Pulmonary injury in burned patients. Crit Care Clin 1: 79–96
31. Brown M, Traber DL et al. (1987) The use of venovenous extracorporeal membrane oxygenation in sheep reciving severe smoke inhalation injury. Burns 13: 34–38
32. Li N, Yang Z, Jiang et al. (1983) Effect of intravenous infusion on development of pulmonary edema after inhalation injury. Burns 9: 394
33. Stone HH, Rhame DN, Corbitt JO et al. (1967) Respiratory burns: a correlation of clinical and laboratory results. Ann Surg 165: 157
34. Dressler DP, Skornik MS, Kupersmith S (1975) Corticosteroid treatment of experimental smoke inhalation. Ann Surg 183: 46

9 Management of Local Burn Infection

Ge Sheng-de

9.1 Occurrence and Importance of Burn Infection

Skin is the largest organ in the body and serves as an extensive protective covering of the body surface. It is multilayered, with the cornified cells as the outermost layers on top of the viable epithelial cells to form the superficial protective layer, while the epithelial cells, which are closely bounded, form the deep protective layer. The protective function of the skin as maintained by its multilayered structure is as a mechanical barrier to keep out the invading microorganisms. The natural flora of the skin serves as a preventive measure against the colonization of pathogenic microorganisms. The integrity of the mechanical barrier of the skin is disrupted by burn injury, when the wound surface is inevitably contaminated by microorganisms, with ensuing infection of the local burn wound.

As a result of advances in knowledge and measures of burn resuscitation during the last 4 decades, burn infection has now become the most common complication and dominates the clinical features in the remaining postburn course after shock. Local infection not only interrupts epithelialization for permanent coverage, but also deepens the wound. In addition, it may cause failure of skin grafting. These unfavorable effects will result in delayed wound healing with a prolongation of hospital stay.

Breach of the skin's mechanical barrier by burn injury makes penetration by microorganisms possible. Invasive infection supervenes when the virulent pathogens proliferate, spread, and invade the surrounding or underlying normal tissue, resulting in burn wound sepsis with obvious clinical features of toxemia. Furthermore, vascular invasion of microorganisms will result in bacteremia, and septicemia ensues when the mechanism of host resistance is compromised.

Until recently, systemic infection has been the predominant cause of burn death. Generally speaking, systemic infection accounts for 40%–50% of burn deaths. Analysis of 20 years of clinical data from 5448 burn patients seen by Tien Fu-Quan showed that the main cause of 139 out of 308 deaths (or 45.1%) was systemic infection [1].

The main source of invasive microorganisms is the burn wound, although there are other sources. It is well known that bacterial invasion by the intravenous route is usually life threatening, and systemic infection due to pulmonary complication following inhalation injury is also a serious condition.

In general, burn infection is still a major problem not only in clinical practice, but also in laboratory research. Burn injury makes the patient vulnerable to infection by lowering the systemic resistance due to a compromised immunological mechanism and homeostasis disorder. Contamination of the local burn wound may lead to bacterial colonization which can result in superficial infection, cellulitis, wound sepsis, and septicemia. Since sepsis is responsible for 40%–50% of burn deaths, it is, therefore, of great importance to establish some basic principles for local burn care. Moreover, preventive and therapeutic measures for systemic infection are of greater importance. These principles should be used as guide lines in the management of burn infection.

9.2 Route of Burn Infection

9.2.1 Local Burn Infection

Bacteria usually reside on the skin surface and up to the depth of the skin, i.e., in the hair follicles and sweat glands. Thus local burn would may be readily contaminated by the originally existing bacteria. Bacterial contamination may be from the bacteria which harbor different parts of the body, e.g., oral and pharyngeal cavity, tracheobronchial tree, and gastrointestinal tract. All these are defined as self-contamination.

Bacteria present in the local environment may contaminate the burn wound through direct contact. The commonly seen vectors of bacterial transfer are clothing, bed linen, pillow covers, gowns of medical personnel, and medical instruments, while the hands of medical personnel are the commonest source of contamination. Many other carriers of bacteria such as aerosol gels, droplets, and floating particles in the air are less important than the factors mentioned above. Local burn infection may be caused by fungi in a relatively highly humid local environment, and rarely by virus.

9.2.2 Respiratory Tract Infection After Inhalation Injury

Thermal injury may cause respiratory burn, when hot air or steam is inhaled, and more severe damage may be produced by inhalation of noxious gases, which in essence is a chemical burn of the respiratory tract. It is readily contaminated not only by the microorganisms which inhabit it, but also by those carried by aerosol gels, droplets, and floating particles in the air during inhalation. It is obvious that infection of the respiratory tract is inevitable in inhalation injury.

9.2.3 Systemic Infection

The major route of systemic infection is invasion by pathogenic bacteria in or near the burn wound through the vascular wall, giving access to the blood circulation. Lymphatic drainage is another infection route. Occasionally, the common inhabiting flora in the gastrointestinal tract may gain access to the blood circulation by penetrating through the mucosa and the vascular wall of the gut. Bacterial invasion in the respiratory tract and several other areas is an alternative source of systemic infection.

As for systemic fungus infection, especially intravascular disseminated candidiasis, the pathogenic *Candida albicans* invades the gastrointestinal tract due to its vigorous proliferation resulting from disorders of the intestinal flora. *Candida albicans* can cause superficial infection of local burn wound but rarely invades the bloodstream in the burn wound. However, other species of fungus can invade through the vascular wall, being disseminated by the intravascular route.

Deitch et al. (1987) in their work on bacterial translocation [2] reported that bacteria could pass through the epithelial mucosa to the mesenteric lymph nodes, liver, spleen, and bloodstream causing systemic infection. Their recent work showed that protein malnutrition and endotoxemia would enhance bacterial translocation. The authors supported the concept that bacteria could translocate from the gut to other organs, becoming a potential source of lethal infection after thermal injury, and protein malnutrition could not promote bacterial translocation from the gut.

9.3 Origin of Burn Infection

9.3.1 Endogenous Origin

The oral cavity, nasal cavity, and naso- and oropharynx are heavily inhabited by bacterial flora. Numerous bacteria inhabit the entry of the gastrointestinal tract, especially when there is infection in the oral cavity such as peridentitis. The epithelial lining of the mucosa forms a physical barrier which prevents penetration and invasion of pathogenic microorganisms. Saliva contains lysozyme, an enzyme that splits the muranic acid B (1,4)-*n*-acetyal glucosamine linkage in bacterial cell walls, and IgA, an immunoglobulin also contained in nasal secretion which can prevent some bacteria from adhering to the epithelial cell surface and neutralizing viruses. Normal flora may compete with pathogens and thus prevent their attachment to epithelial cells.

Phagocytic cells found in nasal secretions and saliva can prevent the entry of pathogenic microorganisms into the body. A reduction in salivary flow, whatever the cause, may result in a marked increase in the number of oral bacteria.

A huge amount of resident bacteria are found at the exit of the gastrointestinal tract. This large population of bacteria constitutes 25% of the fecal mass, with a bacterial count of 10^{11} microorganisms/g feces.

Most microorganisms inhaled are nonpathogenic airborne bacteria and fungi, amounting to 10000–20000/day. Nasal hairs, mucous secretion, and ciliated epithelium of the respiratory tract trap the majority of the inhaled microorganisms offering a local defense against infection. Secretory immunoglobulins are also found in the tracheobronchial secretion which provide a similar function to those in the nasal secretion. The macrophages can ingest and remove fungi.

Several factors such as smoke inhalation, dehydration, and fluid accumulation within the alveoli predispose the respiratory tract and alveoli to infection.

9.3.2 Exogenous Origin

A number of bacteria are located on the body surface. The skin is exposed to the surrounding environment, particularly those areas near the nose, mouth, and anus. A dry skin surface is unfavorable for bacterial growth, while moist areas such as the axilla and genital regions have markedly higher numbers of bacteria. The acid pH of normal skin and the long-chain fatty acids secreted by the sebaceous glands have a bactericidal effect. Nevertheless, contamination of burn wound by environmental microorganisms is a serious condition. Furthermore, bacterial contamination through medical instrumentation is more dangerous, since bacteria of a resistant strain can be transferred from one patient to another.

Prevention of bacterial infection of external origin can be achieved by good personal hygiene, an aseptic technique in burn treatment, and nursing care.

9.4 Classification of Burn Infection

Burn infection may be classified by the microorganisms which produce infection or by pathophysiological and clinical features.

9.4.1 Pathogenic Microorganisms in Burns

9.4.1.1 Bacteria

Local or systemic burn infection, which occurs early or late, may be caused by various species of pathogenic bacteria. Gram-positive bacteria are *Staphylococcus*, *Streptococcus*, enterococcus, pneumococcus, pepsin coccus, pepsin streptococcus, *Clostridium tetani*, *Clostridium perfringes*, etc. and gram-negative bacteria are *Pseudomonas aeruginosa*, *Acinetobacter multiformis*, *Aerobacter cloacae*, *aerogenes*, *Alcaligenes*, *Escherichia coli*, *Citrobacter*, *Bacillus subtilis*, *Serrratia*, *Klebsiella pneumoniae*, *Bacteroides fragilis*, *B. melaninogenicus*, and *B. fusiformis*.

Streptococcus hemolyticus is an important pathogen in burns, which can cause severe infection in early postburn days, showing a clinical picture of surgical scarlet fever. Its infection in deep burns will cause failure of skin grafting. Infection of burns by *Staphylococcus aureus* occasionally produces toxic necrosis, i.e., deepening of the local burn wound associated with systemic toxic syndrome. This rarely seen complication may have a fatal outcome. In extensive burns, particularly deep burns, infection is mostly caused by gram-negative bacteria. The most commonly seen pathogenic species is *Pseudomonas aeruginosa*, which is usually predominant. Nevertheless, its incidence is decreasing, but is not very obvious, as are *coli*, *Citrobacter*, etc. *Serratia*, *Aerobacter cloacae*, and several other bacteria species are becoming more and more common in causing burn infection in some burn centers. This changing picture of invading bacteria is probably due to the increasing use of potent antibiotics, particularly the third-generation products of both the penicillin and cephalosporin groups.

9.4.1.2 Fungi

Fungal infection is a commonly seen complication, particularly when exposure treatment of the local burn wound is used, especially in an environment with a relatively high humidity.

Most of the pathogens of fungal infection belong to the genus *Aspergillus*, i.e., *Aspergillus flavus*, *niger*, *ruber*, etc. The infected area shows a colored focus. The depth of tissue injury of the infected area is increased and full-thickness damage, which appears to be gray or brownish-gray in color, may ensue.

A rarely seen pathogenic fungus is *Mucor*. Mucomycosis of the burn wound shows a continuous deepening of the local wound with possible involvement of the bone. Mucomycosis of maxillofacial burns, particularly burn of the nose, may cause intracranial infection due to its penetration and invasion through the basal plate of the cranium, and it can have a fatal outcome.

Candida albicans is the most commonly seen pathogenic fungus, causing intravascular disseminating candidiasis, which is produced by the invasion of *Candida* from the gut. *C. albicans* may produce infection of the local burn wound. Although it has been demonstrated to be able to invade tissues underneath the wound, it has not been cause systemic infection by this route.

9.4.1.3 Viruses

A prospective study of viral infection in burns in children using both serological and viral culture techniques showed that cytomegalovirus, herpes simplex, and adenovirus infection developed in 33%, 25%, and 17% of the children, respectively. Cytomegalovirus infection is likely to develop in severely burned children. Its pathogenesis is not known. Depressed cellular immunity may play a role in its infection in burn patients.

Autopsy records of 156 burned patients that died showed that infection in 19 patients was due to either herpes simplex virus or cytomegalovirus [3]. The number of infections caused by cytomegalovirus, herpes simplex virus, and both were 7, 11, and 1, respectively. Incidence of viral infection in severely burned patients was 12%, as shown by autopsy. Analysis of the clinical data showed that cytomeglovirus was more frequent in those patients who had received multiple transfusions. Internal organ involvement was more common in cytomegalovirus infection than herpes simplex virus, the latter being more frequently found in the skin.

Some of the unexplained fevers commonly seen with pediatric burns may be due to cytomegalovirus infection, which is characterized by prolonged fever and lymphocytosis without abnormal lymphocytes. Immediate virological examination may be of use in differential diagnosis, once cytomegalovirus infection has been considered. There is no obvious harm induced by cytomegalovirus. Local burn wounds usually heal well in the course of the infection. Consideration and recognition of cytomegalovirus is important in the treatment of burn infection, otherwise one may hesitate to use antibiotics with a higher toxicity, resulting in inadequacy of treatment and a possible fatal outcome.

9.4.2 Clinical Features

9.4.2.1 Local Infection

Burn injury of the body surface causes disruption of the skin with death of the epithelium and damage to the dermis. Devitalized tissue and fluid exudation offer a culture medium for bacterial proliferation which predisposes the local burn wound to colonization and infection.

9.4.2.2 Invasive Infection

9.4.2.2.1 Burn Wound Sepsis

Pathogenic bacteria of local burn infection may invade normal tissue surrounding and beneath the wound. This is probably due to the break down of the local and systemic defense mechanism.

9.4.2.2.2 Burn Septicemia

Bacteria of local burn wound, tracheobronchial tree, particularly after inhalation injury, and several other routes, may invade the blood circulatory system due to local and systemic resistance being compromised.

9.5 Local Burn Infection

Burn wound with bacterial contamination is prone to local infection. Although prophylactic measures such as wound protection, early debridement, definitive local care, operative therapy, topical antimicrobial agent, and systemic antibiotics are usually applied, burn infection is still inevitable.

9.5.1 Diagnosis

Clinical diagnosis of local burn infection can be made mainly by signs and symptoms, and also laboratory examinations may be of great importance.

When a burn wound is infected, the patient may complain of local pain with restriction of movement. An offensive odor is noted which is sometimes typical for certain bacterial infections. There may be exudation on the wound surface, soiling dressings. The surrounding skin may show erythematous changes. There may be secondary necrosis with deepening of the local wound with delay of wound healing. The devitalized dermis can undergo autolysis, and granulation tissue is formed when the local burn is full thickness. Wound healing is usually delayed due to the interruption of epithelialization and failure of skin grafting.

During the course of local burn infection, the patient may have a fever, a rapid pulse, tachycardia, fatigue, coating of the tongue, and a poor appetite. Laboratory study shows an increase in polymorphonuclear granulocytes in the differential count. Swab culture of the local exudation or pus may identify the pathogenic bacteria and verify an increase in bacterial number. A sensitivity test will show effective antibiotics for the pathogenic bacteria.

9.5.2 Treatment

Treatment of local burn infection is achieved by local management and systemic therapy. As for mild infection of minor burns, only local management is needed.

9.5.2.1 Local Management

Local management of an infected burn wound is carried out by performing dressing changes. A dressing change is a heavy burden and a painstaking task for the attending surgeons and nurses. It should be done with meticulous care, for it brings about not only local pain but also mental excitement, and rough handling causes mechanical injury to the wound. Analgesia is sometimes needed to relieve the pain, which also helps to gain cooperation from the patient. Meperidine and phenergan are usually used for this purpose. However, its use is limited to guard against drug addiction. Occasionally, acupuncture is used for relieving pain caused by a dressing change with some success. Anesthesia using ketamine is not indicated for this purpose in China.

A dressing change is usually carried out in the burn ward. Surgeons and nurses taking part should follow the requirements of aseptic technique. A dressing change for extensive burns, particularly in the early postburn days, may be performed in the operating theater. A better or ideal place for performing a dressing change is the operating room equipped with laminar flow. However, such equipment has not yet been widely adopted.

The first step of the dressing change procedure is to remove the bandage and the gauze when the occlusive method is employed. The inner layer gauze is soaked with normal saline before its removal. This is more easily achieved by immersing the infected local area in a water bath with a whirlpool.

The wound surface is gently cleaned with cotton sponges. For superficial burns, antimicrobial agent either in solution form, such as chlorhexidine, which is still used in our center and some burn units [4], or cream is used. In some burn units herbal medicine paste is applied. In deep burns, autolysis of the devitalized dermis is enhanced by lysozyme produced in the course of infection. Hence, dressing changes are usually associated with sequential debridement. Some burn surgeons prefer hydrotherapy, and the separated necrotic tissue is removed during the bath.

In China, topical agents containing herbal medicine are widely used. Some are effective in promoting autolysis of burn eschar or devitalized tissue and in enhancing granulation formation or wound healing. However, wound infection is inevitable during the course of autolysis of burn eschar. Lysozyme released from either pathogenic bacteria or leukocytes will further accelerate the course of autolysis. Burn paste (comprising frankincense, calcite powder, *Phellodendronum*, *Rehmannia glutinosa*, sesame oil, and yellow wax) and "Wound Healing No. 10" paste (comprising calamine, gypsum fibrosum, calcite powder, pearl powder, borneolum, aethyparabenum, Vaseline, adeps lanae, and liquid paraffin) [5].

The above-mentioned therapeutic measures and agents are important in promoting wound healing in deep dermal burns and in forming granulation wound which is finally closed by gradual epithelialization from surrounding skin, or skin grafting.

Preparation of topical enzymatic medicine such as elastase and collagenase have been used. However, their clinical application is limited and far from becoming popular, since they are not as effective as claimed in the medical literature.

9.5.2.2 Systemic Treatment

In addition to local management of the burn wound, systemic treatment is also important, particularly in moderate and major burns with severe infection. Systemic treatment of severe burn infection comprises a series of effective therapeutic measures which form a complex treatment.

9.5.2.2.1 Antibiotics

Clinical use of antibiotics is an important component in the principles of surgical treatment of burns. There is still controversy surrounding its reasonable use in clinical burn management. Timely diagnosis, which is based on careful study and accurate determination of clinical criteria, is a reliable basis for the clinical administration of antibiotics. Although the prophylactic use of systemic antibiotics has not been widely accepted, it is still routinely used in some burn units, particularly in burn centers where extensive burns are dealt with.

Twenty years ago, we ventured for a limited period to treat minor burns without the administration of prophylactic penicillin in th early postburn days and before and after skin grafting. We found that hemolytic *Streptococcus* infection occurred more frequently, with delay of wound healing, failure of skin grafting, and prolonged hospital stay (S.D. Ge 1974, Prophylactic use of antibiotics in burn treatment, unpublished work).

In the current clinical practice of our Burn Center, systemic use of antibiotics is for prophylactic and therapeutic purposes, and they are administered in the early postburn days, before and after skin grafting and several other related operations, as well as when infections complications occur.

9.5.2.2.2 Systemic Support

In order to obtain homeostasis in a burn patient, maintenance of the water, electrolyte, and acid-base balance is of great importance. In addition, nutritional support is also important, which is mainly achieved by increasing caloric supply. Intravenous transfusion of blood, plasma, and some nutrient fluid is required in some patients. A high-protein, high-calorie, and elementary diet will have a beneficial effect in improving the patient's general condition and increasing systemic resistance against pathogenic bacteria.

9.6 Burn Wound Sepsis

Burn wound sepsis is the most serious, life-threatening local burn infection. Its incidence was very high 2 decades ago. Since escharectomy and tangential excision of deep burns have gradually popular, the topical application of effective chemical antimicrobial agents and systemic antibiotics has become widely accepted, and systemic support has been adopted, burn wound sepsis is rarely encountered in big city hospitals, particularly burn units or burn centers. But in rural areas and community hospitals where burns are not satisfactorily treated, burn wound sepsis still appears as a major problem in burns and has a relatively high mortality rate.

Burn wound sepsis is sometimes classified as a kind of systemic infection. Since it is closely related with and follows local infection, therefore, it is better to discuss the problem in the present chapter for the convenience of evaluating the principle of local burn management.

9.6.1 Diagnosis

Most burn patients with complications of wound sepsis have a history of inadequate treatment either due to lack of knowledge and incorrect management or delay in management for various reasons. An inadequately resuscitated patient will have a compromised homeostatic state and the inappropriately managed burn wound will be readily infected. The unfavorable systemic and local conditions characterized by inadequate body resistance against pathogenic bacteria and the presence of wound infection predispose the patient to wound sepsis or even septicemia.

Burn wound sepsis is characterized by proliferation and invasion of the pathogenic bacteria out of the area of the devitalized burn tissue into the normal tissue beneath the wound and in its periphery. In other words, burn wound sepsis is referred to as invasion of the pathogenic bacteria into the normal surrounding tissue [6]. Hence, it is termed as an invasive infection. The patient may have further complications of septicemia if the pathogenic bacteria have passed through the blood vessel wall into the bloodstream.

The clinical picture of burn wound sepsis consists of profuse amounts of local wound exudation which might be associated with an offensive smell. The wound may show secondary necrosis, which gives an appearance of hemorrhagic necrosis in burn eschar. The area of necrotic lesion soon enlarges or covers the whole burn wound. Occasionally, the necrotic lesion can go beyond the border of the burned wound to the surrounding normal skin.

The patient usually has obvious signs of toxemia, including high and septic fever, rapid pulse, tachycardia, rapid respiration, disorientation or confusion, coated tongue, and loss of appetite. In severe cases with further development and worsening of the local infectious focus, there may be signs and symptoms of endotoxemia. The patient may have a low body temperature, pallor, rapid and weak pulse, dyspnea, flatulence, loss of consciousness, and eventually coma and septic shock.

Laboratory studies show an increased WBC count and a decreased platelet count. Although the patient's clinical picture resembles that of septicemia, the blood culture gives a negative result. The limulus tests for endotoxin determination is helpful. Biopsy of the local lesion is important for further study.

Sequential observation of bacterial invasion in rat full-thickness burns inoculated with *Pseudomonas aeruginosa* immediately after the injury indicated that subeschar colonization was established within 6 h, local invasive infection was present within 24 h, and systemic infection, e.g., extensive invasive infection and septicemia, was present within 48–72 h [7].

Quantitative bacterial culture of subeschar tissue has been used for diagnosis of burn wound sepsis. Generally, a bacterial count exceeding 10^5/g subeschar tissue is of diagnostic significance. Tian FQ et al. (1985) suggested that a bacterial count 10^6 is of critical diagnostic value. However diagnosis should not rely solely on the laboratory data but should consider concurrently the clinical signs and symptoms of systemic infection [8].

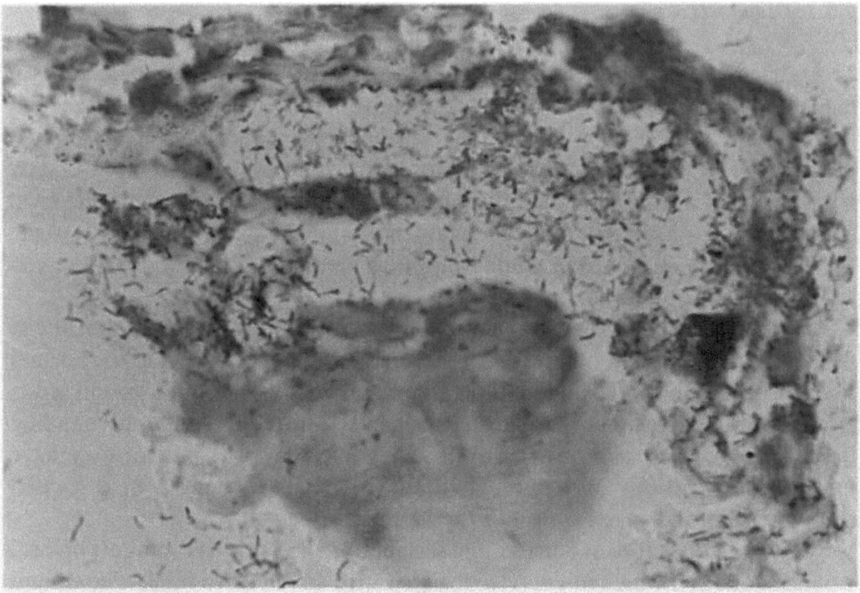

Fig. 9.1. Subeschar invasion of gram-negative bacteria (*Pseudomonas aeruginosa* by bacterial identification) in a patient with a 34% TBSA burn, 26% being third degree, complicated by wound sepsis. Original magnification × 800

Bacterial culture is useful for the identification of specific microorganisms and has been used for a long time for differential diagnosis of burn wound infection, particularly for confirmation of burn wound sepsis. A bacterial count using a stained smear of burn tissue homogenate was found to correlate well with the tissue quantitative culture technique [9]. Therefore, aggressive treatment could be instituted using the homogenated smear technique without waiting for the quantitative culture report. However, quantative culture can only give the amount of bacteria proliferated within the burn tissue, and cannot be used to differentiate bacterial colonization from bacterial invasion. Therefore, it is not a valuable guide for clinical management.

Histological examination of a burn wound biopsy sample permits the differential diagnosis of bacterial invasion from colonization, and has proved to be the best means of diagnosing burn wound sepsis [10] (Fig. 9.1).

Histological examination is better performed by a combination of frozen section and rapid section technique [11, 12]. The former, which takes about 30 min after the biopsy is taken, is the fastest method for laboratory diagnosis and the latter, which takes about 4 h, is used for diagnostic confirmation.

Burn wound biopsy should be freshly obtained and processed within 30 min after the biopsy is taken. Each specimen should be divided into two portions, one for frozen section technique and the other for rapid section.

Histological diagnosis is classified into two grades on the basis of nonviable tissue and viable tissue. Each grade is further divided into three subgrades. Grade I denotes bacterial colonization and Grade II bacterial invasion. Hence the junction between Grade I, subgrade C, and grade II, subgrade D, is of diagnostic importance in differentiating bacterial colonization and invasion. Grade II, subgrade F, is bacterial invasion through the blood vessel wall into the bloodstream.

There is good agreement between the frozen section technique and the rapid section technique. The former has a slight decrease in accuracy in making histological diagnosis compared with the latter. However, the rapidity of the frozen section technique makes it useful not only for making a timely diagnosis but also for guiding prompt therapy.

It should be emphasized that Sabouraud's agar is used as the culture medium when it is desirable to detect fungal infection. Recently diagnostic technique has been improved using the fluorescence microscope, and also cultivation of tissue biopsy to obtain rapid diagnosis of fungal infection in burns.

9.6.2 Management

Although many laboratory studies are very important in diagnosing burn wound sepsis, management should not be delayed waiting for the laboratory reports. In other words, therapeutic measures should be instituted as soon as the clinical diagnosis is made. Sometimes, vigorous treatment is initiated even when such a clinical diagnosis is suspected. Since the frozen section technique has proved to be a reliable and rapid measure in diagnosing invasive infection, it is recommended as a good laboratory technique for the purpose.

9.6.2.1 Local Management

9.6.2.1.1 Dressing Change

Since burn wound sepsis is a kind of invasive infection and the local wound is deepened, vigorous local antimicrobial treatment is mandatory. An effective agent like mafenide (Sulfamylon) is the first choice, because it can readily penetrate the burn eschar or necrotic tissue and play an important role in controlling proliferation, colonization, and invasion of the pathogenic bacteria, which are usually *Pseudomonas aeruginosa.* Frequent dressing change using its 10% cream or solution is carried out every 8 h. When mafenide is used, one must be careful when the wound area exceeds 5% TBSA, because metabolic acidosis sometimes ensues due to its absorption, and carbonic anhydrase is inhibited. Special attention should be paid when it is used in children. Silver sulfadiazine is not indicated in the treatment of deep burn infection. A preliminary clinical trial of topical application of silver norfloxacin was demonstrated to be effective and gave promising results [13, 14].

9.6.2.1.2 Exposure Method

When local infection is under control, the devitalized tissue will undergo autolysis which is usually associated with bacterial infection resulting in the second episode of wound sepsis. The exposure method is favored in the prevention of recurrent local infection, which offers the chance of general stabilization and subsequent surgical intervention when indicated.

The semi-exposure method may be used by leaving the layer of dressing gauze undisturbed next to the wound. Close inspection of the wound is mandatory at least at the intervals of the dressing changes.

9.6.2.1.3 Surgical Intervention

Invasive infection of burn wound or an infected focus is a source of further spread of infection. The principle treatment for an infected focus is surgical intervention. Escharectomy is usually performed so that the necrotic lesion can be excised as a whole to eliminate the infected focus and create a clean surgical wound. Skin substitute is used for immediate and temporary closure of the open wound, which prevents local infection and stabilizes the general condition. Transplantation of skin autograft can be performed when the general condition permits. However, surgical operation may fail for several systemic and local reasons, and another episode of wound sepsis ensues.

If the invasive infection of the septic focus cannot be controlled or excised, or it surgical treatment fails death is inevitable.

Although the operation is usually performed when the infection has been relatively or completely controlled and the patient is in a relatively good condition, it may be carried out on other occasions. Following the principle of treating the infected focus, emergency surgical intervention is sometimes indicated. However, preoperative treatment is necessary for systemic control of infection, and measures to maintain the water, electrolyte, and acid-base balance, and necessary nutritional support are given.

9.6.2.2 Systemic Treatment

9.6.2.2.1 Antibiotics

Since the pathogenic bacteria of burn wound sepsis are usually resistant to the more commonly used antibiotics, new antibiotics with a potent antimicrobial effect are administered in combination in order to obtain a synergistic effect in the treatment.

For controlling infection produced by *Pseudomonas aeruginosa*, a third-generation product of cephalosporin, either cephotazidime or cephotriaxone, is usually administered. Although cephoperazone is also indicated, in our experience it is not as effective as the two former products. For broad-spectrum coverage, a combination of cephatazidime and cephradine is administered with fairly good effect in our clinical practice.

Potent antibiotics should be given by the intravenous route in an adequate dose to obtain timely control of the invasive infection. Treatment is initiated when it is needed; one should never delay the treatment by waiting for the relevant laboratory reports.

Systemic treatment consists of preoperative administration of antibiotics. However, the administration of antibiotics during the operation is more important. Perioperative means before, during, and after the operation. Of course, postoperative administration is also important, because manipulation of infected tissue during the operation can cause the local infection to spread. Administration of antibiotics is usually initiated soon after the induction of anesthesia, and it is continued throughout the whole or main course of the operation. This type of administration is thought to be effective in obtaining a coverage of pathogenic bacteria during surgical manipulation.

9.6.2.2.2 Maintenance of Homeostasis

Maintaining homeostasis is of great importance in keeping up body resistance against critical burn infection. Close inspection of the patient's general condition with the follow-up of several laboratory determinations will help physicians and surgeons be aware of the slight changes that occur during the course of burn treatment. For example, water, electrolyte, and acid-base balance should be carefully maintained. Patients with a major burn complicated by wound sepsis often sustain a certain amount of insensible fluid loss by evaporation from either the body surface and/or the respiratory tract and fluid loss from either local wound exudation and/or vomiting, diarrhea, as drainage of the gastrointestinal tract, and from diuresis due to either excretion of excessive solute and/or administration of diuretic agents. Hyponatremia and hypopotassemia are often encountered in the course of burn treatment due to excessive loss and/or inadequate supply, as well as metabolic disorders. Systemic infection caused by gram-negative bacteria is often associated with hypernatremia or non-ketogenic hyperglycemia and hyperosmolar coma, which are not readily amenable to treatment, and, therefore, close observation and prompt and appropriate management of systemic infection in association with the maintenance of the water and electrolyte balance is mandatory. Tachypnea, which causes excessive loss of carbon dioxide, often follows systemic infection, and may result in respiratory alkalosis.

Some of the therapeutic measures, either systemic administration of topical application, may bring with them several problems in association with their therapeutic effects. Administration of some antibiotics, particularly those against gram-negative bacteria, may result in renal damage. Metabolic acidosis occurs due to impairment of renal function and several other factors. Inappropriate administration of alkali will lead to metabolic alkalosis. A mixed-type respiratory and metabolic alkalosis will occur if the above-mentioned respiratory alkalosis exists beforehand. It is a serious condition and may have a fatal outcome [15].

9.6.2.2.3 Nutritional Support

Nutritional support is very important and plays a significant role in burn management. The nutrients are the elementary materials replenished for reconstruction of tissue and enhancement of body resistance.

Since patients are in a critical state and some have flatulence and a poor appetite, nutritional supply cannot rely on rich food and an elementary diet. Parenteral nutrition must of course be used. Several kinds of blood preparation and nutrient solution are used besides fresh blood and plasma transfusion, e.g., lyophilized human plasma, human albumin, amino acids, and Intralipids (intravenous fat emulsion containing 10% soybean oil stabilized with egg-yolk phospholipids). When total parenteral nutrition is used and the patient is supported with hyperalimentation through a central venous route, care must be taken to prevent infection such as suppurative thrombophlebitis, septicemia, and intravascular disseminated candidiasis.

9.6.2.2.4 Immunotherapy

For the enhancement of nonspecific body resistance of the patient, in addition to fresh blood and plasma transfusion, γ-globulin is administered. Since burn wound sepsis is mostly caused by *Pseudomonas aeruginosa*, specific measures to improve body resistance are used. These are convalescent plasma and polyvalent serum against *P. aeruginosa*.

9.6.2.2.5 Traditional Chinese Medicine

Traditional Chinese medicine (TCM) is sometimes used to strengthen the effects of comprehensive treatment of burn wound sepsis. It is well known that TCM is a mixture of several kinds of herbs, minerals, insects, etc., and has multiple effects in clinical treatment. The mixture is prescribed according to the diagnosis, and treatment is based on an overall analysis of the illness and the patient's condition. Antipyretics, medicines of a "cold" nature to treat acute febrile diseases, antidotes, and medicine to relieve "internal heat" or fever are usually prescribed. It is worth mentioning that some of the antipyretics and antidotes possess an antimicrobial effect. Medicines to promote the patient's appetite and suit the patient's taste are prescribed in combination, while in critical cases medicines to maintain homeostasis and enhance body resistance are added. As for patients with disorientation and coma, medicines to enable them to regain consciousness are indicated.

9.7 Topical Agents

Topical agents are widely used in clinical burn management. Most possess an antimicrobial effect, while others are characterized by their astringent and dissolution effects.

An ideal topical agent meets the following criteria:

1. Is effective in protecting the wound
2. Has an antimicrobial effect
3. Has a broad antibacterial spectrum
4. Is able to penetrate the burn eschar with adequate antibacterial concentration in the subeschar tissue
5. Is nontoxic to normal tissue and visceral organs when absorbed
6. Is nonallergic and free of side effects
7. Should not inhibit sloughing of eschar and growth of the granulation wound
8. Is easily applied
9. Is readily removed
10. Is readily available and inexpensive

The simplest local management of burn wound, particularly superficial second-degree wound, is not to use any topical agent after early debridement. The wound may be wrapped with sterilized absorbent gauze and cotton pads, the so-called occlusive method, or simply left open, what we call the exposure method. However, in order to obtain a better therapeutic result, topical agents of various kinds are applied in most cases.

9.7.1 Silver Sulfadiazine

Silver sulfadiazine is an antimicrobial agent which is most effective against *Pseudomonas aeruginosa* [11, 12]. It is widely used in most burn units in China. Since it does not readily penetrate burn eschar, it is better used in fresh burns.

Silver sulfadiazine has a low solubility and is commonly applied in a cream in a thickness of about 0.5 mm. The treated area can be either wrapped or exposed. Dressing change should be carried out once to twice daily. The wound is cleaned and the residual cream is removed before its next application.

Although Silvadene (silver sulfadiazine) has been supplied worldwide for decades, Dermazin (silver sulfadiazine), a Yugoslavian product, has been available since the 1970s [16]. It is prepared with microparticles of silver sulfadiazine in a hydrophilic base. Further clinical trails are needed to clarify its therapeutic effect in China.

Silver sulfadiazine has proved effective in treating fresh, particularly superficial, burns. However, it is also used to treat deep burns.

In China, most extensive deep burns are treated by the exposure method, which is followd by staged surgical excision, either down to the fascia or tangentially. Therefore, local management beneficial in protecting the dry eschar will be preferable. Suspension of silver sulfadiazine meets the requirement when topically applied.

The depth of burn and its subsequent change should be assessed. The area to be subjected to surgical treatment and the mode of operation should be decided in advance, because the silver content of the suspension will give the wound surface a dark gray color which will hinder subsequent judgment of changes in burn depth.

9.7.2 Zinc Sulfadiazine

Zinc sulfadiazine cream has recently been commercially available in China. Although it has been proved to be effective in treating burn infection, it is not as potent as silver sulfadiazine [17]. Zinc sulfadiazine is preferred by some surgeons because of its beneficial effect in promoting wound healing, particularly in extensive burns where zinc may be depleted due to excessive loss and inadequate replacement during the course of treatment. Hence, it is sometimes indicated in treating residual wound with delayed healing.

9.7.3 Mafenide

Mafenide (Sulfamylon) is a potent antimicrobial agent with a wide antibacterial spectrum [18]. It can penetrate through burn eschar, which makes it more potent in the prevention and treatment of severe burn infection, particularly burn wound sepsis. But its clinical use is limited, because of its inhibiting effect of renal excretion of hydrogen ion and reabsorption of bicarbonate as carbonic anhydrase. Its extensive and frequent use can result in metabolic acidosis. However, it is still the agent of first choice when effective treatment of suspected and/or confirmed burn wound sepsis is to be achieved.

9.7.4 Povidone-Iodine

Povidone-iodine is a complex compound of iodine polyvinylpyrrolidone (PVP) [19]. It is a kind of local disinfectant for skin sterilization. Its bactericidal effect is proved when used on skin or mucosa. It has a wide antimicrobial spectrum which covers not only gram-positive and negative bacteria, but also fungi and viruses. It is nonirritant, not affected by blood, plasma, secretion, and pus, and is nontoxic. It is water soluble.

When povidone-iodine is topically applied to the burn wound, the amount of iodine absorbed is directly related to the size of burn treated [19]. Serum iodine levels continue to rise until application is discontinued and remain elevated for as long as 7 days thereafter. Iodine excretion is related to renal function. The drug is contraindicated in patients with impaired renal function. The high serum levels imply potential toxicity.

9.7.5 *Silver Salts of Quinolone*

The second- and third-generation of quinolone, such as pipemidic acid and norfloxacin, are highly effective antimicrobial agents. Their silver salts have proved to be effective in controlling *Pseudomonas aeruginosa* infection in burns. Silver norfloxacin has been demonstrated to be superior to silver pipemidate. However, we have just started its clinical application with limited experience. Therefore these products are still far from being widely accepted in China, although they show promise.

References

1. Tian FQ, Cuei JY, Yu FZ (1987) The major reasons of fatality in burns – analysis of 308 cases. Chin Emerg Med 7(3): 6–10
2. Dietch EA, Berg R, Specian R (1987) Endotoxin but not malnutrition promotes bacterial translocation of the gut flora in burned mice. Arch Surg 122: 185–190
3. Kim SH, Mason AD, Okerberg CV et al. (1989) Viral infection in burn patients: a review of seven-year autopsies. Proceedings of the 2nd Sino-American conference on burn injury and trauma, p 82
4. Yang FX (1989) Clinical observation of cold wet soaking using chlorhexidine on burn wound. J Pract Surg (Chin) 9: 52–54
5. Xu FX (1985) Management of deep burn wound. In: Fang ZY et al. (eds) Handbook of burn treatment, 3rd edn. Shanghai Publishers of Science and Technology, Shanghai, pp 118–119
6. Woolfrey BF et al. (1981) An evaluation of burn wound quantitative microbiology. I. Quantitative eschar culture. Am J Clin Pathol 75(4): 532
7. Zhang YP, Li A, Wang DW et al. (1988) Dynamic observation of invasive pyocyaneous infection in scalded rat. Chin J Exp Surg 5: 109–110
8. Tian FQ, Cuei JY, Yu FZ et al. (1985) Clinical and laboratory study of bacterial invasion in deep burn tissue. Chin J Plast Surg Burns 1: 289–291
9. Qin XJ, Wang DW, Zhang YP et al. (1989) Evaluation of forecasting bacterial count of burn tissue homogenate using smear staining technique. Chin J Plast Surg Burns 5: 45–46
10. Pruitt BA Jr, Foley FD (1973) The use of biopsies in burn patient care. Surgery 73: 887–897
11. Kim SH (1985) A rapid section technique for burn wound biopsy. JBCR 6: 432–435
12. Kim SH, Hubbard GB (1985) Frozen section technique to evaluate early burn wound biopsy: a comparison with the rapid section technique. J Trauma 25: 1134–1137
13. Holder IA (1986) Norfloxacin and silver-norfloxacin as topical anti-microbial agents: results of in vitro susceptibility testing against bacteria and candida SP isolated from burn patients. JBCR 7: 479
14. Ge SD, Huo ZL, Tu SZ et al. (1987) The effect of quinolones as topical antibiotics on the prevention and treatment of *pyocyaneous* infection following burn. Chin J Plast Surg Burns 3: 10–13
15. Ge SD, Huo ZL, Gu B et al. (1989) Evaluation of water, electrolyte, and acid-base imbalance in major burns. Proceedings of the 2nd Sino-American conference on burn injury and trauma, Beijing, p 5
16. Brcic A (1978) The value of topical chemotherapy with Dermazin in the treatment of extensive burns by primary necrectomy. Lek Pharmaceutical and Chemical Works, Ljubljana

17. Ge SD, Fang ZY, Tu SZ et al. (1982) N′-metal sulfa drugs and zincpolyanemine and its derivatives in prevention of burn wound sepsis. Chin J Surg 20: 264
18. Lindberg RB (1965) The successful control of burn wound sepsis. J Trauma 5: 601
19. Hunt JL, Sato R, Heck EL et al. (1980) A critical evaluation of povidine-iodine absorption in thermal injured patients. J Trauma 20: 127–129

10 Systemic Infection and Its Management

Liu Shi-kang and Fang Zhi-yang

The mortality of burn patients with infections improved recently as new topical chemotherapeutic agents and systemic antibiotics were instituted. Sepsis, however, remains the most frequent cause of death in thermal injury due to serious infection of local burns and infection of the organ system, as well as infected cannulated vein [1–3]. An understanding of the etiology of the septic processes is essential for their possible prevention, early diagnosis, and effective treatment once they are established.

10.1 Incidence of Burn Infected and Mortality of Septicemias

Infections of the burn wound usually develop 48 h or more after thermal injury. The mechanical barrier of the burned skin and mucosa is lost and the wound serves as a rich culture medium, becoming colonized with microbes. When the systemic host defense mechanisms of the burn patient are profoundly suppressed, the microbes, such as gram-negative bacilli, enterococci, and *Candida albicans*, may translocate through the gastrointestinal tract epithelial mucosa to the mesenteric lymph nodes (MLNs) and other systemic organs, and lead to systemic infection, especially if the normal ecology of the gut microflora has been changed.

Several decades ago, streptococcus and staphylococcus were the predominant pathogenic organisms causing burn infection. Since the late 1950s, gram-negative bacteria, primarily *Pseudomonas* species, have emerged as the dominant organisms causing serious wound infections in burn patients due to the extensive use of systemic antibiotics. With the topical use of mafenide and silver sulfadiazine in the past 2 decades, the incidence of major infection such as burn wound sepsis and septicemia has decreased in some groups of burn patients.

Infection, however, is still a significant problem in burns. Local infection can often be prevented by adequate local burn care while invasive infection continues to be a difficult problem. The prognosis is poor if the burn is associated with inhalation injury complicated by pulmonary infection.

Statistical data from 9329 burned patients from the Burn Centers of the Second, Third, and Fourth Military Medical University showed that 51.87% of overall deaths following burns are related to serious infection, while in the Burn Center of Shanghai, Ruijin Hospital, the mortality from septicemia and burn wound sepsis was as high as 68.96%.

In China the incidence of burn wound sepsis and septicemia has decreased probably due to adequate resuscitation of burn shock, early use of topical antimicrobial agents, prophylactic and therapeutic use of systemic antibiotics, and surgical excision of deep burn wound.

10.2 Occurrence of Septicemia

10.2.1 Early Septicemia

Early septicemia tends to occur in patients sustaining extensive deep burns. Particularly patients with an eventful or turbulent shock phase will more frequently develop systemic infection [4]. Delayed early management with inadequate fluid resuscitation followed by water, electrolyte, and acid-base imbalance, compromised immune system, decreased local and systemic resistance, and bacterial colonization may result in septicemia with a vicious clinical course and possibly lead to a fatal outcome. This type of systemic infection is referred to as fulminating septicemia, which has a relatively high incidence.

The burn septicemia episodes often develop in the 1st week postburn days. The occurrence of early septicemia in our burn center is 58.9% in the development of overall septicemia, which reflects the combined effect of both the burn-related impairment of host resistance and microbial invasive capacity of burn wound.

1. Microbial colonization of burn wound may lead to systemic invasion. Both local factors (e.g., wound maceration, acidosis, and lack of competitive bacterial pressure as a result of either antibiotic therapy or topical antimicrobial therapy) and microbial factors (e.g., endotoxin, a number of exotoxins and enzymes with tissue destructive potential, produced in variable amounts by different microbes, and bacterial motility [5]) influence the rate of bacterial proliferation [1]. The denatured protein of the burn eschar provides a culture media for microbes, and the avascularity of the burned tissue places the microbes within conditions beyond the reach of both host defense mechanisms and systemically administered antibiotics of low diffusibility [6].
2. An extensive burn injury affects the function of all other components of the immune system. Circulating levels of immunoglobulins such as IgG are depressed [7, 8], and the functional activity of the complement system, such as C3, C4, and C5 is impaired [9]. Circulating levels and/or the function of all the cellular elements of the immune system are also altered. The early postburn leukocytosis is followed by secondary leukopenia [10]. Lymphocyte subpopulations are altered with the emergence of suppressor cells occurring 5–7 days postburn [11, 12]. All aspects of granulocyte function are impaired with the suppression of chemotaxis as well as phagocytosis and bactericidal activity [13–16], especially the patients with burn covering more than 20% of the body surface area. Incidence of systemic infection shows another peak usually at the 2nd week postburn, since the devitalized tissue tends to autolyse and local infection is inevitable.

10.2.2 Late Septicemia

The incidence of septicemia is relatively low after 3rd week postburn, because deep second-degree wounds tend to heal and third-degree wounds form granulation tissue which serves as a barrier against microbial invasion. Although granulation wound of burns could be repaired by skin grafting, the patients may develop serious malnutrition and systemic infection with a possible fatal outcome. In addition, suppurative thrombophlebitis, pulmonary infection, suppurative chondritis, and gastrointestinal tract infection, etc., might lead to sepsis or septicemia. Multiresistant bacterial strains or opportunistic bacteria are common pathogens during this period.

10.3 Pathogens of Invading Infection

Pathogens causing systemic invading infection include bacteria, fungi, and viruses.

10.3.1 Pathogenic Bacteria

The variations of predominant gram-positive cocci and gram-negative bacilli on local wounds of burn patients treated at our burn center during a period of 11 years are shown in Table 10.1, in which the changes in annual frequency of recovery of main bacteria species illustrate well the magnitude of year to year variability. Although members of the genus *Staphylococcus* appear to persist at a more or less constant level in the burn wound flora, members of the gram-negative flora show pronounced temporal variations in prevalence, while *Streptococcus hemolyticus* has almost been eliminated. In our series of 20 patients with burn involving greater than 60% TBSA, the six predominant organisms isolated from the burn wounds, i.e., *Pseudomonas aeruginosa, Staphylococcus aureus, Escherichia coli, Acinetobacter anitratum,* fungi, and *Enterobacter* species, showed incidences of 21.58%, 18.34%, 14.42%, 11.54%, 4.36%, and 2.29%, respectively.

10.3.1.1 Streptococcus

Prior to the introduction of penicillin, *Streptococcus*, especially *S. hemolyticus*, was the most frequently isolated organism from burn wounds. It can proliferate rapidly and is often present in the hair follicles and sweat glands. When streptococcal colonization of the burn wound occurred, the patient had fever, cellulitis of the unburned skin surrounding the wound, and late development of lymphangitis.

Table 10.1. Main microbes discovered from burn wound cultures

Organism	Annual percentage of total isolates										
	1974	1975	1976	1977	1978	1979	1980	1981	1982	1983	1984
Staphylococcus aureus	14.46	25.83	21.26	21.81	29.35	7.69	13.20	25.36	17.44	29.32	10.53
Staphylococcus epidermidis	3.80	0	1.57	0.53	2.49	2.56	1.20	2.39	2.13	0	0
Streptococcus hemolyticus	0	3.33	0.79	1.86	0	0.85	0	0.48	0	0.40	0
Pseudomonas aeruginosa	15.20	26.67	22.05	18.62	24.88	17.95	28.40	29.19	32.36	28.11	21.81
Escherichia coli	8.86	4.17	9.45	13.30	10.45	14.53	22.40	14.35	6.59	11.24	19.55
Enterobacter species	13.92	13.33	12.60	11.17	6.47	2.56	4.80	0.48	4.78	17.67	25.56
Proteus species	1.27	10.00	0.79	0.53	1.00	0	0.80	1.44	0.19	0.80	1.50
Acinetobacter anitratum	12.66	9.17	11.02	6.94	3.98	10.26	1.20	2.39	1.55	8.84	7.50

10.3.1.2 Staphylococcus

Staphylococcus aureus is one of the most important organisms causing infection in burn patients. It has moderate virulence and is easily transmissible. Staphylococcal carriers among personnel are an important source of pathogenic bacteria, and the most important mode of transmission from patient to patient is usually via personnel in an environment that is not strictly controlled.

Epidemiological surveillance of *Staphylococcus* in our burn center has shown that the epidemic virulent strains of *S. aureus* seen in 1965 were of phagotypes 80 and 52/52A/80/81 while those seen in 1982 were of types 52/52A/80 and 85. Recent studies of *S. aureus* isolates from patients with toxic shock syndrome (TSS) have shown the dominance of phage type 29/52, with a 95.7% capacity for producing pyrogenic exotoxin C and enterotoxin F.

Outbreak of burn wound infection due to methicillin-resistant *S. aureus* (MRSA) is particularly serious. It accounted for 73.9% of the *Staphylococcus* in Shanghai Ruijin Hospital from 1986 to 1987.

10.3.1.3 Pseudomonas

Pseudomonas aeruginosa is an opportunistic pathogen which causes infection in burn, particularly extensive deep burns. It proliferates readily in necrotic tissue. The serotype of *P. aeruginosa* seen in our burn ward, serotype I, may be an epidemic strain with a stronger antibiotic resistance.

10.3.1.4 Opportunistic Pathogenic Bacteria Other than Pseudomonas

Besides *P. aeruginosa*, a large number of opportunistic pathogenic bacteria other than *Pseudomonas* such as *Escherichia coli, Klebsiella, Proteus, Acinetobacter, Enterobacter cloacae*, and *Providencia stuartii* have been found to be clinically important. These organisms appear generally on a burn wound as a consequence of contamination. However, the most important factor that renders them pathogenic is the selective elimination of their competing gram-positive cocci from the burn wound by antimicrobial therapy. The antibiotic-resistant strains may transfer their resistance factors to nonresistant strains, which leads to nonsocomial infection caused by antibiotic-resistant bacteria.

The opportunistic pathogenic bacteria of enteric origin have low pathogenicity. They are pathogenic because the burn patient is immunologically compromised.

10.3.1.5 Anaerobic Spore-Forming Bacilli

Patients with burn injury most be considered at risk from clostridial species infection, and appropriate prophylactic therapeutic measures should be instituted. Early contamination with clostridial species including *Clostridium perfringens* and *C. tetani* is relatively common. The potential for clostridial infection is greatest in patients sustaining severe electrical contact burn or crush injuries [17].

10.3.1.6 Non-Spore-Bearing Anaerobes

During the past decade anaerobic bacteria, especially nonsporing ones, have been found to be important causative organisms of infection in burns. The major source of non-spore-bearing anaerobes in humans is the large bowel and wounds at the periphery of the anus, which prone to contamination. Wang et al. [18] reported that the incidence of non-spore-bearing anaerobic infection was 14.7%, and 12 genera had been isolated, in which the predominant anaerobes were *Bacteroides melaninogenicus*, *Peptococcus*, *B. fragilis*, *Peptostreptococcus*, and others [18]. The non-spore-bearing anaerobes may play an important role in causing generalized burn infection [19].

10.3.2 Fungi

Significant invasive fungal infection by *Candida*, *Aspergillus*, *Mucor*, and *Geotrichum* species has been reported.

10.3.2.1 Candida Species

Invasive infection caused by *Candida* species, especially C. *albicans*, is frequently seen, most commonly in the gastrointestinal tract; surface colonization with low potential invasion has been observed in extensive and debilitating burn injuries. Such patients have usually received broad-spectrum antibiotics for long periods. In 1961, we reported four patients with burns associated with fatal disseminating candidiasis. Nash et al. [20] reported a tenfold increase in fungal colonization on burn wounds following the topical use of mafenide acetate cream. MacMillian et al. [21] reported positive *Candida cultures* in 5.1% of a group of 427 burn patients and in 21.5% of 65 autopsies.

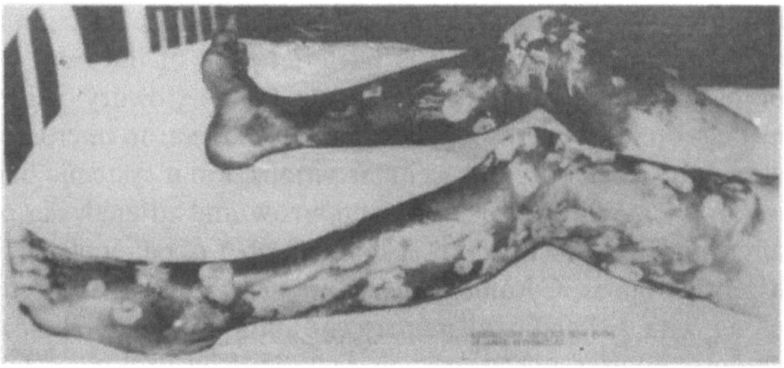

Fig. 10.1. Aspergillus infection of local burn wound

10.3.2.2 Aspergillus Species

Aspergillus flavus, *A. fumigatus*, *A. niger*, and *A. albicans* have been found in 88% of *Aspergillus* infections. *Aspergillus* species are localized in burn wound (Fig. 10.1), seldom spreading across the fascial planes, and can be adequately dealt with by local excision in most patients. *Aspergillus* has been reported to invade the lung, gut, brain, heart, kidney, and liver in cases of disseminated aspergillosis in which penetration of the vessel wall resulted in dissemination via the bloodstream.

10.3.2.3 Phycomycetes

The most frequent pathogens among the Phycomycetes are *Mucor and Rhizopus*, which are aggressive invaders and show a propensity to spread rapidly along and across fascial planes and invade arteries, resulting in rapidly progressive ischemic necrosis. It is emphasized that phycomycetic infection is characterized by centrifugally advanced ischemic necrosis and rapid spread along the fascial planes. The areas preferentially invaded by Phycomycetes are the nose, brain, deep soft tissue, bone, and gastrointestinal tract. The incidence of phycomycetic infection appears to be greatest in patients with uncontrolled diabetes mellitus and acidosis. Liu [22] studied three patients with extensive burn who all died from profound *Mucor* infection. Recent studies showed that burned patients might have associated *Alternaria* wound sepsis.

10.3.3 Viruses

Viruses infections in local burn wound have been reported. Such infections are most commonly caused by herpes simplex; infections by cytomegalovirus have rarely been reported. Microscopic examination of either lesion scrapings or lesion biopsies is the most reliable means of diagnosing cutaneous viral infections in burns. The vesicles typical of cutaneous herpetic infection are easily ruptured and rapidly colonized by the bacterial flora of the burn wound, which may obscure or obliterate the characteristic type A Cowdry bodies; these are usually evident on light microscopic examination. Electron microscopy should then be employed to identify intracellular virions. Fatal systemic herpes infection with involvement of liver, spleen, bone marrow, and adrenals has been identified even after burn wound closure in a small number of patients, particularly those with extensive burns. Cytomegalovirus infections may also occur in burn patients along with a significant increase in antibodies. The clinical manifestation of cytomegalovirus infection is characterized by prolonged fever, lymphocytosis without atypical lymphocytes, and occasionally anicteric hepatitis.

10.4 Invading Routes of Pathogens

10.4.1 Burn Wound

One of the principal functions of intact skin is to act as a microbiological barrier to bacteria, fungi, or viruses. Thermal injury breaks this barrier. Most burn wounds are initially free of bacterial colonization, since the heat, which has destroyed the cutaneous elements, also kills surface microorganisms, with the exception of the gram-positive cocci located in the depths of the sweat glands and hair follicles. If topical antimicrobial agents are not used prophylactically to reduce the rate of bacterial proliferation, the wound may become colonized with up to 10^5 CFU gram-positive cocci/g tissue within 48 h. The rapid development of gram-positive cocci overgrowth is now rarely observed because of the application of potent topical chemotherapeutic agents.

Gram-negative bacilli often appear in the wound between 3 and 21 days, but topical chemotherapeutic agents inhibit gram-negative growth, and bacterial concentrations of less than 100 organisms/g tissue can be maintained. If the bacterial concentration increases by more than 10^5 CFU organisms/g tissue, invasion of the viable subcutaneous tissue usually develops, with subsequent dissemination in the bloodstream. This syndrome is called deterioration of the burn wound and the late appearance of systemic sepsis. When cellulitis appears in unburned skin surrounding the wound or localized hemorrhagic necrosis within the burn wound occurs, the possible development of burn wound sepsis should be considered.

The clinical characteristics of burn wound infections are consistent with differences in microbial motility. Infections caused by gram-positive organisms infrequently penetrate the fascial layers and are commonly confined to the skin and subcutaneous tissue. Gram-negative bacilli appear proliferate more rapidly in necrotic tissue and invade underlying and adjacent viable tissue, even blood vessels, to produce progressive ischemia and permit hematogenous dissemination of the infecting pathogens to remote tissue and organs [23]. (See Chap. 10 for diagnosis and care of burn wound sepsis.)

10.4.2 Lungs

With improved methods of managing the burn wound, pulmonary infection with subsequent respiratory failure has now emerged as the most frequent cause of septic death in burn patients. Before the utilization of topical chemotherapeutic agents to control the proliferation of bacteria, about the two-thirds of pulmonary infections in burn patients represented hematogenous dissemination from wound to lungs. Hematogenous pneumonia is now relatively rare and most pulmonary infections are bronchopneumonias secondary to the inhalation injury by airborne organisms. In addition, serious pulmonary compromise is often observed in patients with major burn secondary to the inhalation injury of smoke, resulting in severe chemical tracheobronchitis, which manifests itself by the destruction of the lower respiratory epithelium, with loss of ciliary action, severe bronchospasm, and the development of mucous and cellular plugs within the tertiary bronchi. All of these factors favor the proliferations of bacteria introduced into the lung by airborne organisms.

10.4.3 Indwelling Venous Catheter

Suppurative thrombophlebitis is almost always associated with the peripheral insertion of synthetic catheters for venous infusion of fluids, this complication representing the third most common infection in burn patients [24, 25]. The incidence of these infections in patients with burn exceeding 20% TBSA is approximately 5%. This disease is rarely accompanied by any local or systemic signs prior to the development of bacteremia. Local tenderness over the involved vein, distal edema, or a positive Homan's sign is unusual. Late in the course of the thromobophlebitis, local abscesses may be noted surrounding the affected vein and involving the soft tissue. Suppuration within a thrombosed peripheral vein may occur as long as 3 weeks after the removal of an indwelling venous catheter [24].

The diagnosis of thrombophlebitis should be considered whenever systemic signs of sepsis are apparent or blood cultures are positive in the absence of obvious local infection. Our clinical experience has shown that septicemia occured in two cases due to suppurative thrombophlebitis of the upper great saphenous vein, and the thrombi was immediately removed by means of negative pressure suction.

10.4.4 Urinary Tract

Patients with major burns require an indwelling Foley catheter to allow careful monitoring of urinary output and renal function during early fluid resuscitation. Periurethral and prostatic abscesses or trigonitis and cystitis occasionally occur, and dissemination subsequently takes place.

10.4.5 Enteric Translocation

The gut has been proposed as a potential source of secondary infections. Patients undergoing enteric decontamination with oral antibiotics have decreased colonization of the oropharynx and a decreased incidence of pneumonia. Herndon et al. [26] reported that in the ovine burn model mesenteric arterial blood flow markedly decreased following thermal injury, with a slow return to baseline levels. In rats receiving a scald injury, blood and splenic cultures were positive in 65%, while pretreatment with bombesin (trophic hormones) resulted in a positive culture in only 9%, because trophic hormones may alter the response of mesenteric blood flow to injury as a mechanism that abrogates translocation. Deith et al. [27] believed that movement of indigenous bacteria from the gut to the mesenteric lymph nodes and other organs occurs after a major burn (40% TBSA), but not a moderate thermal injury (20% TBSA), and disruption of the normal gastrointestinal flora by antibiotics or by bacterial overgrowth resulted in the systemic spread of enteric tract organisms. More recently, by Ma et al. [28] reported that 74% of Balb-c mice receiving 25% burns exhibited viable bacteria in their MLNs 24 h after the thermal injury (Fig. 10.2 a, b); in antibiotic-decontaminated mice, *Escherichia coli* at higher incidence and greater numbers translocated to the MLN, spleen, liver, and blood of the burned mice, and 80% of mice receiving 2 mg endotoxin showed variable levels of bacteria in their MLNS.

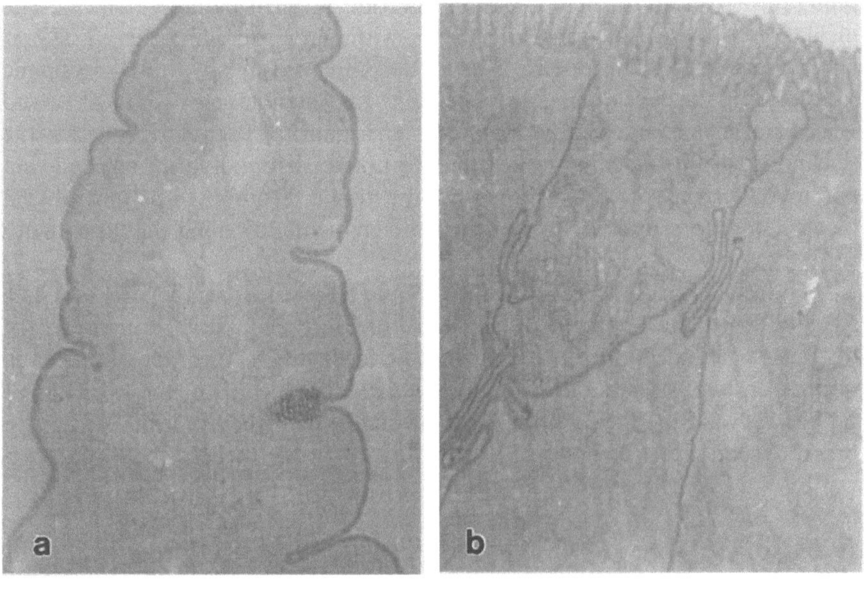

Fig. 10.2 a, b. Translocation of bacteria through the gastrointestinal tract in Balbc mice burns. **a** Viable indigenous bacteria pass through the tight junction between the epithelial cells of the gastrointestinal mucosa. **b** Bacteria penetrate down to the submucosal layer into the mesenteric lymph nodes

The combination of malnutrition plus endotoxin was associated with a higher incidence of bacterial translocation to the systemic organs and higher numbers of bacteria per organ than were seen in normally nourished mice receiving endotoxin only. Lan et al. [29] have noted that the enteric bacilli penetrated the mucosal gut barrier from three types of lesion including: (a) focal necroses of intestinal mucosa, (b) epithelial defects, and (c) gaps between epithelial cells.

10.4.6 Other Routes

Miscellaneous infections in other organs including suppurative chondritis, bacterial endocarditis, intraperitoneal infection, cancrum oris, intracranial infection (e.g., brain abscess, meningitis), osteomyelitis or arthritis, and infusion of the contaminated blood or solution may result in bactericemia or septicemia.

10.5 Systemic Infection

10.5.1 Burn Wound Sepsis

Burn wound sepsis is a typical form of invasive infection in local burns with obvious systemic manifestations [30]. It is classified as systemic infection although it is characterized by local changes and wound care and its systemic manifestation and treatment resembles that of septicemia. Therefore, the topic of burn wound sepsis is described in Chap. 9, which deals with local burn infection.

10.5.2 Septicemia

Before describing septicemia in detail, it is better to repeat a few words on bacteremia in burns as noted previously. Bacteremia occurs in burns due to wound manipulation in 20.6% of cases, its incidence rising in direct relationship to both size and extent of the wound manipulated [31]. It usually clears promptly without specific therapy.

10.5.2.1 Clinical Diagnosis

The signs and symptoms of septicemia may be subtle. Early clinical diagnosis should be made and initial treatment must be started empirically [32]. The clinical features of the sepsis or septicemia are as follows: (a) septicemia caused by *Staphylococcus aureus* often shows hyperpyrexia with continued fever or intermittent fever, while that caused by *Pseudomonas aeruginosa* usually shows a high fever followed by hypothermia or occasionally remittent fever; (b) disorientation or gradual loss of consciousness, the latter being commonly seen in

Table 10.2. Clinical features of septicemia caused by *Pseudomonas aeruginosa*, *Staphylococcus aureus*, and fungal infection in burns

Parameters	*Staphylococcus aureus*	*Pseudomonas aeruginosa*	Fungal infection
Onset	Insidious, 2–6 days	Rapid, 12–36 h	Delayed
Temperature	Hyperpyrexia	Hypothermia	Hyperpyrexia
Disorientation	Severe	Mild	Mild
Ileus	Severe	Severe	Occasional
Diarrhea	Unusual	Common	Common
Hypotension	Late	Early	Late
Wound	Early dissolution of granulation tissue	A shaggy green exudate with typical odor and later progress to form patchy black areas of necrosis	Dry and flat with yellow or orange color
Leukocyte count	Neutrophilia	Neutropenia	Neutrophilia
Platelet count	Normal	Low	Low
Prothrombin time	Normal	Increased	Normal
Fibrinogen	Normal	Low	Normal

septicemia caused by *P. aeruginosa* while the former is observed in septicemia caused by *S. aureus*; (c) abdominal distention with paralytic ileus, which is a frequent sign of late septicemia; (d) bleeding tendency manifested by petechiae, ecchynoses, oozing from the burn wound, and ecthyma gangrenosum is commonly seen in *P. aeruginosa*; (e) white blood cell count greater than $20\,000/mm^3$ or lower than $5000/mm^3$ with a shift to the left; (f) thrombocytopeia is common in gram-negative septicemia; and (g) multiple positive blood cultures (Table 10.2).

In addition, although the ability of neutrophil to phagocytose bacteria is normal leukocyte chemotaxis and intracellular killing of bacteria are markedly depressed during septicemia. Nitro blue tetrazolium (NBT) reduction [32], neutrophil chemiluminescence (PMN-CL), and opsonic index (OI) values were significantly depressed; especially PMN-CL was lower in cases of sepsis caused by *P. aeruginosa* than by staphylococci. Therefore, PMN-CL may provide a rapid, sensitive, and noninvasive method of detecting impending sepsis in burn patients [15]. The plasma fibronectin level shows progressive decrease; however, several other complications may also exhibit a low plasma fibronectin level [33].

A blood culture is essential in making a clinical diagnosis of septicemia. However, a single positive blood culture is inadequate and particularly difficult for the purpose. A single positive blood culture in the absence of any change in clinical signs of sepsis should be followed by subsequent blood cultures repeated two to three times for confirmation or elimination of the diagnosis. Gram-negative organisms are more likely to be isolated than gram-positive ones.

10.5.2.2 Treatment of Septicema

An accurate bacteriological study is essential for proper treatment. Once the diagnosis of septicemia has been established clinically, an initial effective therapeutic program must be started empirically.

10.5.2.2.1 Local Treatment

Focal and even multifocal burn wound infection that involves less than 2% TBSA may be treated by a subeschar infusion of antibiotics. The effectivenss of the antibiotic used for the subeschar infusion is related to its ability to diffuse into tissues. A semisynthetic penicillin such as carbecillin is sometimes used for the purpose [5]. The antibiotic infusion is given twice a day until the septic process is under control. In addition, mafenide acetate cream, in which the antimicrobial component is diffusable, and can penetrate burn eschar, should be topically applied.

Excision of the infected burn tissue is indicated if the infection involves more than 2% TBSA, especially if the lesions are quite extensive, if new foci of infection follow, if there is dissemination of the infection to unburned tissue, remote organs, or if there is persistent systemic sepsis [1]. The diagnostic criteria of foci of infection are as follows: (a) marked infection or sloughing of the eschar; (b) maceration of the eschar with subeschar hemorrhage; (c) patchy necrosis of the wound; (d) necrosis of the underlying musculature; and (e) infected open wound escharotomy or fasciotomy performed for decompression.

Following surgical excision of an infected burn wound, wound care is dictated by the status of the tissue in the excised wound. If the adequacy of the excision is uncertain, the excised wound should be covered with dressing soaked with an antimicrobial solution, reexamined in 24 h, and debrided further as necessary. If the ability of the wound bed is questionable for accepting skin transplantation, a biological dressing such as fresh pig skin or lyophilized glutaraldehyde-treated pig skin should be applied and skin autografting delayed until the wound appears to be ready for skin grafting. If the excision is thought to be adequate and the wound bed viability is certain, the wound should be definitively closed by skin autografting. In fungal wound infection where the subcutaneous tissue is involved, extensive local excision should be performed with the wound left open for daily examination. Fungal infection of the neck, head, and trunk, extending below the fascia, is treated by massive excision, and that of the extremities may require amputation.

10.5.2.2.2 Systemic Treatment

Major burn patients usually have hypermetabolism during their main course of treatment and are inevitably in a catabolic phase with a negative nitrogen balance. It is obvious that major burn patients should receive vigorous nutritional support for calorie and protein deficits. A high-calorie and high-protein diet is ordered if the patient is well able to cope with the oral route, which is the most physiological method of dietary supplementation. Tube feeding with a liquid diet is indicated in most patients.

An elementary diet is usually given by this route in China. Of course, nutritional support by the intravenous route is also important when the gastrointestinal is unable to tolerate anything. However, nutritional support may rely mainly on the intravenous route due to anorexia or paralytic ileus (see Chap. 15).

There will be a marked increase in the gluconeogenic response and catabolic response in severe burn septicemia, especially with apparent utilization of branched-chain amino acids (BCAAs) as an energy source. Thus, BCAAs appear to be theoretical benefit for nutritional support in the treatment of septicemia. Adequate amounts of glucose, amino acids, and Intralipid solutions are supplied simultaneously. Electrolytes, trace elements, and multivitamins are supplied daily together with the nutrient, but extra potassium may be needed because of excessive urinary losses and utilization of potassium.

Maintenance of the fluid and electrolyte balance is important in the treatment of critical burns particularly in those with septicemia. Gross errors in fluid management must be avoided. Frequent measurements of plasma electrolyte concentrations and blood urea nitrogen (BUN) level are an essential guide to therapy. Urine and gastrointestinal fluid should be collected, monitored, and analyzed for sodium, potassium, chloride, and urea nitrogen content. The loss of these ions must be replenished. Water requirements may be extraordinarily high for burn septicemia, and the tendency of hypernatremia to occur should be carefully monitored.

Blood transfusion requirements depend upon the hemolytic properties of the offending microorganism. One of two transfusions daily are often necessary to maintain a normal hemoglobin level. If the plasma protein content is lower, fresh or frozen plasma must be administered. Oxygen is indicated in patients who have marked tachypnea and tachycardia. If the burn is associated with severe inhalation injury with hypoxemia, artificial ventilation should be employed as necessary. In septicemia patients who have developed hypotension, therapeutic measures for treating septic shock are used as indicated.

10.5.2.2.3 Antibiotic Therapy

Prophylactic and therapeutic antibiotic regimens play an important role in the prevention and control of systemic invasive infection in seriously burned patients [34]. For several decades, penicillin has been used prophylactically to prevent the occurrence of acute invasive streptococcal infection of the burn wound. Hence, α-hemolytic streptococcal cellulitis is found infrequently at present. However, penicillin causes the emergence of resistant microbes and a deleterious change in

Table 10.3. Anti-*pseudomonas* penicillin

	Carbenicillin	Ticarcillin	Piperacillin	Azlocillin
Active	β-Lactamase-negative gram-negative rods and gram-positive cocci and rods; *Pseudomonas* sp. (β-lactamase-negative)	β-Lactamase-negative gram-negative rods and gram-positive cocci and rods; *Pseudomonas* sp. (β-lactamase-negative)	β-Lactamase-negative gram-negative rods and gram-positive cocci and rods; *Pseudomonas* sp. (β-lactamase-negative) *Klebsiella* sp.	β-Lactamase-negative gram-negative rods and gram-positive cocci and rods; *Pseudomonas* sp. (β-lactamase-negative)
Peak serum concentration after iv doses	200–300 μg/ml (5 g)	150–300 μg/ml (3 g)	220 μg/ml (3 g)	300 μg/ml (3 g)
Serum elimination half-life	1.0 h	1.2 h	1.0 h	0.8 h
Dosing schedule	4–8 g q 4 h	3–6 g q 4 h	3 g q 4 h	3 g q 4 h
Sodium (mmol)/g drug	4.7	5.2	1.98	2.17
Distinguishing features	Platelet abnormality	Platelet abnormality	Extends spectrum of anti-pseudomonal penicillins (*Klebsiella* especially)	Primarily used with aminoglycosides against pseudomonal infection
	Large sodium load; primarily used with aminoglycosides against pseudomonal infections	Primarily used with aminoglycosides against pseudomonal infection		

Table 10.4. Third-generation cephalosporins

	Moxalactam	Cefotaxime	Cefoperazone	Ceftazidime	Ceftriaxone
Active	Most Entero-bacteriaceae, *Pseudomonas*, *Serratia*, *Bacteroides fragilis*	*Escherichia coli*, most Entero-bacteriacea, *Neisseria* sp.	*Neisseria* sp., many Entero-bacteriaceae, *Pseudomonas*, *Salmonella*	*Neisseria* sp., *E. coli*, many Entero-bacteriaceae, *Pseudomonas*, *Serratia*, *B. fragilis*	*Neisseria* sp., *E. coli*, many Entero-bacteriaceae, *E. cloacae*, *B. fragilis*
Peak serum level after i.v. dose	200 μg/ml	80–90 μg/ml	250 μg/ml	200 μg/ml	260 μg/ml
Serum elimination half-life	2 h	1 h	1.8 h	2 h	7–9 h
Dosing schedule	1–2 g q 8–12 h	2–4 g q 4–6 h	1–2 g q 8–12 h	1–2 g q 8–12 h	1–2 g every 12–24 h
Cerebrospinal fluid Penetration	0.5–4 μg/ml 10%–20% serum	0.8–18 μg/ml 10%–20% serum	0.5–12 μg/ml (not reliable)	1–20 μg/ml	Up to 15 μg/ml 2%–10% serum
Route of elimination	90% renal	Renal and hepatic	Renal, hepatic, and biliary	Renal	Renal, hepatic

the ecology of the burn wound flora. Thus, careful monitoring of the burn wound and nasopharynx should be carried out for the detection of bacterial flora and the early existence of colonization or infection.

In patients with invasive burn wound infection in whom there is systemic sepsis and/or evidence of microvascular lesion, systemic antibiotics should be administered. The initial choice of antibiotic should be guided by the results of the Burn Unit's microbial surveillance program, with subsequent change based on the sensitivity of the specific organisms discovered from the patient. Since the patient's outcome after a septicemia episode is critically dependent on selection of the appropriate antibiotic, a drug or combination of drugs which is active against all potential pathogens and is able to exert this antibacterial effect at the site of infection is desirable.

The principles of antimicrobial therapy in septicemia include: (a) the initial therapy must be comprehensive, covering the likely pathogens that could be responsible for clinical findings; (b) the initial therapy should be started rapidly, and in hypotensive patient this should take place within minutes; (c) the drugs should be administered intravenously, unless the drug is particularly well absorbed by another route; (d) bactericidal agents should be used, and combining a bacteriostatic with a bactericidal agent should be avoided; (e) a dose to maximize initial antibacterial effect should be selected; (f) patients should be carefully monitored (particularly with aminoglycosides) and dosing should be altered depending on blood level measurements and organ function; (g) evidence of systemic fungal infection or progressive local extension of such infection warrants systemic antifungal treatment using both amphotericin B and 5-fluorocytosine or ketoconazole; and (h) long-term antibiotic therapy of severe septicemia may be limited by drug toxicity, e.g., the β-lactam antibiotics may cause a number of immunomediated reactions including type I (immediate hypersensitivity reactions), type II (hemolysis, leukopenia, thrombocytopenia), type III (Arthrus reaction), and type IV (cell-mediated dermatitis and interstitial nephritis). Cross-resistance between cephalosporins and penicillins develops occasionally. Aminoglycosides also cause ototoxicity and nephrotoxicity.

The pharmacology and microbiological activity of anti-*pseudomonas* penicillin and third-generation cephalosporins is summarized in Tables 10.3 and 10.4. Ciproxin (ciprofloxacin) is a new broad-spectrum antibiotic for oral or iv administration and in the treatment of some gram-negative infections, especially of antipseudomonal septicemia.

10.5.2.2.4 Immunotherapy

Active Immunization. Polyvalent *Pseudomonas* vaccine is a highly purified and a high molecular weight polysaccharide. Pierson and Feller [35] reported that the incidence of *Pseudomonas* septicemia decreased to 43% and the mortality rate decreased to 27% in patients immunized by monovalent *Pseudomonas* vaccine. A heptavalent purified soluble *Pseudomonas* vaccine containing representative antigens from seven major highly virulent serotypes of *P. aeruginosa* isolated from major or fatal burns with septicemias has been administered to burn patients. In China, the heptavalent *Pseudomonas* vaccine has been used safely in large doses in burns and has elicited marked rises in hemagglutinating antibody titer up to 1:16–1:256. A beneficial clinical effect was demonstrated by a comparative study between a therapeutic group with vaccinated patients and a control group before the vaccine became available.

A polyvalent vaccine prepared from the cell walls of 16 different serotypes of *P. aeruginosa* afforded complete protection within 3 days of vaccination.

Every milliliter of *Staphylococcus aureus* somatic protein-toxoid mixed vaccine contains 10 U toxoid and 500 μg somatic protein. A course of mixed vaccine treatment consists of an initial dose of 0.2 ml, followed by 0.3, 0.4, 0.5, and 0.5 ml daily. The first dose is given intramuscularly within the first three postburn days, followed by doses at weekly intervals. Twenty-five vaccinated *S. aureus* infected patients with an average burn area of 43.1% were compared with 11 patients with an average burn area of 37.9% as controls; after two course of vaccination therapy the detectable level of bacteria from the burn wound of the vaccinated patients decreased, hemagglutinating antibody titer rose to peak values at 14 and 28 days postburn and then gradually decreased, serum antitoxic titer increased from 1:8 to 1:98 at 14 and 28 days postburn respectively, and the neutrophil phagocytic index percentage increased.

Passive Immunization. The ED_{50} (50% effective dose) of *Pseudomonas*-immunized plasma is 1:20, and that of *Pseudomonas*-immunized globulin is 1:190. Results of animal experiments indicate that the efficacy of these agents (Chengdu Biological Production Research Institute) is 14 to 15 times greater than that of gentamicin therapy. Of 36 severely burned patients, 27 were given an average of 740 ml immunized plasma for prophylactic purposes; 22 (81.5%) did not develop severe *pseudomonas* wound infection or septicemia. The remaining nine patients were given immunized plasma (600–1200 ml) only after severe *Pseudomonas* wound infection or septicemia had developed, and seven cases were brought under control. Therefore, *Pseudomonas*-immunized plasma or γ-globulin may be used as a beneficial adjunctive agent in the prevention and treatment of *Pseudomonas* infection in burns patients [36].

Stinnett et al. [37] stimulated an (nonspecific) immune response with *Corynebacterium parvum* and have shown improved survival in dogs with deep burns covering one-third of the body surface.

Hyperimmune plasma obtained from patients who had recovered from sepsis caused by *P. aeruginosa* had a protective effect on other patients with sepsis caused by the same strain of *P. aeruginosa* with an increase in survival rate. Administration of this hyperimmune plasma to patients (250 ml daily to adults, 125 ml daily to children) with major burns (care being taken to ensure ABO donor-recipient compatibility) reduced its mortality from 25% to 6%, and the incidence of sepsis from 29% to 6%. The hyperimmune plasma has no bactericidal activity against the immunizing strains, but may reduce the rate of growth of the organisms when they are cultured in vitro in media containing the hyperimmune plasma. Fractionation of the hyperimmune plasma showed that the protective factor was a macroimmunoglobulin (IgM).

Human endotoxin protein (EP) hyperimmune plasma (Shanghai Transfusion Center, Shanghai, China) contained 1155–1690 mg/dl IgG, 132–200 mg/dl IgA, and 57–82 mg/dl IgM, and its anti-EP antibody titer was 1:256 and more. Prophylactic use of hyperimmune plasma may lead to an increase in chemotactic, phagocytic, and killing activity of the neutrophils and a marked reduction in the mortality from *P. aeruginosa* infection.

The frozen human plasma opsonic protein agent produced by the Shanghai Biological Production Research Institute is an opsonin (e.g., cryoprecipitate). The agent is administered intravenously at a dosage of 500–1000 ml daily. The cryoprecipitate has several characteristics which improve the pulmonary shunt and dead space, increase blood flow and oxygen consumption, and markedly improve creatine clearance index and renal filtration rate.

10.5.2.2.5 Environmental Control

Protection of the burn wound from cross-contamination is promoted by maintaining the patient in an isolated environment such as a bacterially controlled nursing unit (BCNU). The personnel in charge of patient care are allowed access to the BCNU. All visitors allowed into the unit should strictly adhere to the rules used by the personnel, including wearing caps, masks, shoe covers, and special garments. Particular attention should be given to the control of fomites and the care of supporting equipment such as ventilators and nebulizers.

The indications for strict, complete isolation of burn patients include colonization with α-hemolytic streptococcus, group A, staphylococcus resistant to methicillin anaerobic bacterial spore formers, viral diseases, presence of immunosuppression, and third-degree burns covering more than 30% TBSA. We noted that cross-contamination did not occur in the laminar airflow room but gave no protection against self-contaminated microbes. The mortality rate for patients in the laminar airflow room was 25% compared with a mortality rate of 55% for patients in the extensive care unit.

References

1. Pruitt BA Jr, McManus AT (1984) Opportunistic infections in severely burned patients. Am J Med 76(3A): 146–154
2. Gu B, Wang LN (1987) A retrospective survey of burn treatment in recent five years (1981–1985). Chin J Plast Surg Burns 3(2): 84–87
3. Fang ZY (1989) Burn infection. In: Fang ZY, Wu ZL, Gao XS et al. (eds) The theory and practice in burns, 1st edn. Liaoning Science-Technology Press, Shengyang, pp 295–345
4. Xu WS, Shi JX (1985) Invasive infection in burns. In: Yang ZJ, Xu WS, Shi JX (eds) The treatment of burns, 2nd edn. Shanghai Science-Technology Press, Shanghai, pp 87–120
5. McManus AT, Moody EE, Mason AD (1980) Bacterial motility: a component in experimental *Pseudomonas aeruginosa* burn wound sepsis. Burns 6: 235–239
6. Pruitt BA Jr (1979) The burn patient I: initial care. Curr Probl Surg 16: 8–11
7. Munster AM, Hoagland HC, Pruitt BA Jr (1970) The effect of thermal injury on serum immunoglobulins. Ann Surg 172: 965–969
8. Liu SK (1978) The change of serum immunoglobulins in severely burned patients (special issue of burn). Acad J 2nd Milit Med Coll 3: 34–36
9. Bjornson AB, Altemeier WA, Bjornson S (1977) Changes in humoral components of host defense following burn trauma. Ann Surg 186: 88–96
10. Eurenius K, Brouse RO (1973) Granulocyte kinetics after thermal injury. Am J Clin Pathol 60: 337–342
11. Li BG, Feng SJ, Jin ZM et al. (1983) Dynamic changes of T-lymphocyte and $T\mu$, $T\gamma$-cells in burned patients. Chin J Surg 21: 493–497
12. Miller CL, Baker CC (1979) Changes in lymphocyte activity after thermal injury: the role of suppressor cells. J Clin Invest 63: 202–210
13. Xu DZ, Xu YP, Shi JX et al. (1983) Relationship between the chemotaxis of neutrophil and the infection in burned patients. Chin J Surg 21: 134–137
14. Guo ZR, Sheng ZY, Zhuo ZM et al. (1982) Change of leukocytic phagocytosis in burned patients. Chin J Surg 20(7): 417–420
15. Dong YL, Sheng ZY, Zhang ZY (1985) Measurement and significance of neutrophil chemiluminescence in period of infection following thermal injury. Chin J Plast Surg Burns 1(2): 17–20

16. Curreri PW, Heck EL, Browne L et al. (1973) Stimulated nitroblue tetrazolium test to assess neutrophil antibacterial function: prediction of wound sepsis in burned patients. Surgery 74: 6–13
17. Liu SK, Fang ZY (1982) Infection due to anaerobic sporeforming bacilli in severely burned patients. Acad J 2nd Milit Med Univ Chin PLA 3 [Suppl]:76–78
18. Wang DW, Li N, Xaio GX et al. (1985) Anaerobic infections of burns. Burns 11: 192–196
19. Xiao GX, Zhang YP, Wang DW et al. (1987) Non-Sporing anaerobic septicemia in burns. Chin J Plast Surg Burns 3: 219
20. Nash G, Foley FD, Goodwin MN et al. (1971) Fungal burn wound infection. JAMA 215: 1664–1666
21. MacMillan BG, Law EJ, Holder IA (1972) Experience with *Candida* infections in the burned patient. Arch Surg 104: 509–514
22. Liu SH, Sheng ZY (1980) Infection due to phacomycetes in major burns (three case reports). J Med CPLA 5: 354–356
23. Pruitt BA Jr (1984) The diagnosis and treatment of infection in the burn patient. Burns 11: 79–91
24. Jia XM, Guo ZR, Kong et al. (1987) Catheter-induced septicemia in severely burned patients. Chin J Plast Surg Burns 3: 6–8
25. Sterin JM, Pruitt BA Jr (1970) Suppurative thrombophlebitis. A lethal iatrogenic disease. N Engl J Med 282: 1452–1455
26. Herndon DN, Morris SE, Desai MH et al. (1989) Enteric translocation of microorganisms in cutaneous thermal injury. Proceedings of 2nd Sino-American Conference on Burn Injury & Trauma, Beijing, p 87
27. Deitch EA, Berg R (1986) Translocation of the gut flora: a mechanism of nosocomial infection in the burn patient. Proceedings of 1st Sino-American Conference on Burn Injury & Trauma, Chongqing, p 43
28. Ma L, Ma JW, Deitch ED et al. (1989) Genetic susceptibility to mucosal damage leads to bacterial translocation in a murine burn model. J Trauma 29: 1245–1251
29. Lan FS, Shi AG, Yu Y et al. (1989) A pathological study of the endogenous infection caused by the translocation of intestinal bacteria after burn. Proceedings of 2nd Sino-American Conference on Burn Injury & Trauma, Beijing, p 76
30. Yang XD, Zhou YP (1988) Patterns of outbreaks of burn sepsis. Chin J Plast Surg Burns 4: 271–273
31. Sasaki TM, Welch GW, Herndon DN et al. (1979) Burn wound manipulation-induced bacteremia. J Trauma 19: 46–50
32. Xu FX, Wei T, Fang ZY et al. (1964) Clinical early differential diagnosis for *Pseudomonas aeruginosa* and *Staphylococcus* septicemia in burn patients. J Med CPLA 1: 254–257
33. Fang ZY, Xiang XE, Sun JL (1984) The NBT reduction response of polymorphonuclear leukocytes in burn patients. Proceedings of 10th Chinese PLA Conference on Burn Injury & Plastic Surgery. pp 84
34. Xu WS (1986) The use of antibiotics in burn patients. Chin J Plast Surg Burns 2: 84–89
35. Pierson C, Feller I (1970) A reduction of *Pseudomonas* septicemia in burned patients by the immune process. Surg Clin North Am 50: 1377–1384
36. Xiao GX, Li N et al. (1985) Clinical therapeutic effect of *P. aeruginosa* immunized plasma. In: Li N, Yang ZC (eds) Research in burns. Chongquing Press, Chongqing, pp 69–74
37. Stinnett JD, Alexander JW, Morris MJ et al. (1981) Improved survival in severely burned animals using intravenous *Corynebacterium parvum* vaccine post injury. Surgery 89: 237–242

11 Multiple Organ Failure

Sheng Zhi-yong, Dong Yuan-ling, and Liang Yan-jie

Progressive failure of several organ systems as the final pathway in critical surgical illness was first described by Skillman et al. in 1969 [1] and Tilney et al. in 1973 [2]. It remained for Baue in 1975 to define the syndrome [3]. Fry [4] correlated the syndrome to uncontrolled infection. Since then, it has been recognized that multiple organ failure accounts for most intensive care unit stays of over 5 days and is the cause of death in over 90% of surgical intensive care unit (SICU) patients [5]. In China, Liu and Sheng [6, 7] first reported its occurrence in extensive burn patients.

An array of complications may occur in a case of major burns. Way back in the 1940s, hypovolemic shock took a large toll. With progress in the understanding of burn shock and improvements in replacement therapy, patients now rarely die of shock per se. However, occasionally a case of acute renal failure is still seen, especially when the replacement therapy is not carried out efficiently for extensive full-thickness burns. With the prolongation of the patient's life through the initial shock period, infection has become and has remained a predominant cause of death. In the 1970s, we began to recognize that sequential functional failure of a series of organs or systems also occurred in cases of major burns. In 1988, we again examined a series of 2390 burn patients admitted from January 1970 through January 1988, using specific criteria to define organ failure; multiple organ failure (MOF) was found in 68 patients, an incidence of about 2.8% [8]. It was also found that this syndrome accounted for 75.9% of all deaths during that period. The above data clearly show that MOF has now become the major killer in patients suffering from extensive deep burns.

11.1 Clinical Features

The clinical course of MOF may be quite typical. Usually it is seen in patients with extensive and deep burns. The patient is sent to hospital a few hours after the injury, and may have traveled for several hours in an ambulance or other vehicle. Very little has been done after the injury and during the journey. Immediate resuscitation with fluids according to a definite fluid replacement regimen is instituted at the time of admission. The patient appears to rally from burn shock uneventfully. The hemodynamic parameters are apparently near normal values, and the urinary output satisfactory. A new days up to 2 weeks later, the wound becomes infected. Or multiple excisions are performed on the patient, in an attempt to eliminate the full-thickness burn surface, and unfortunately followed by grafting failure, either autogenous or allogenous. An obvious secondary infection of the burn wounds then occurs. Along with infection of burn wounds, the heart rate increases and respiration quickens. Soon both the PaO_2 and $PaCO_2$ values decrease, followed by the appearance of hazy infiltration of the lungs. The patient gradually becomes dependent on a ventilator for adequate oxygenation. Efforts to eradicate the infectious foci are made, antibiotics are administered, and repeated attempts to cover the wounds are made. However, the patient becomes cloudy in sensorium, and the abdomen is distended with much retention in the stomach. Sometimes evident jaundice ensues, and there is coagulopathy. Though the urinary output is normal in quantity, blood creatinine level rises. Bleeding from the upper gastro-intestinal tract occurs. Blood sugar increases continually despite the use of increasing amounts of insulin. There may be hypernatremia and hyperchloremia. Finally, septicemia, which is usually multimicrobial, is identified. Very soon thereafter, there are manifestations of cardiovascular and renal failure, and the patient dies with anuria.

Illustrative Case. A male patient 37 years of age sustained a propane gas burn of 60% TBSA, with 50% full-thickness injury. He was brought to the hospital after a 3-h ambulance ride from a distant city. He complained of some oppression in the chest and difficulty in breathing, and had no urine output. The burn covered mainly the head, neck, trunk, and upper and lower extremities. There was also an apparent respiratory burn. Fluid resuscitation was immediately instituted, and a tracheostomy was performed. The response to fluid resuscitation was apparently good, and he excreted 1530 ml urine; 9670 ml fluids, including crystalloids, colloids, and whole blood, were infused in the first 24 h after the burn injury. The urinary output was 1170 ml, and the quantity of fluid given was 7430 ml in the second 24 h. His breathing became more and more labored, and the PaO_2 fell to 58 torr on the 3rd day. He was put on a ventilator. The respiratory support was necessary throughout the course of the illness.

Excisions of third-degree burn eschar were performed in stages on the 4th and 13th days and were first carried out on the chest and upper extremities, followed by the back and lower extremities. Every time the resultant wounds were covered completely with large sheets of allograft, small bits of autograft inserted into the small apertures preformed in the former.

Parenteral alimentation was given from the 3rd day on, with glucose, amino acids, and fat emulsion. Multiple antibiotics were used, including penicillins, aminoglycosides, macrolides, and cephalosporins.

On the 16th day, thrombophlebitis of the right saphenous vein became obvious, and the right lower extremity became swollen with a large amount of transudation from the grafted wound. A high ligation of the saphenous vein was performed, erroneously leaving the infected vein in situ. Blood cultures on the 15th, 18th, 19th, 20th, and 25th days all grew *Staphylococcus aureus*, which was identical to that isolated from the infected vein.

Beginning from the sixth postburn day, the patient passed large amounts of tarry stools. The abdomen became distended on the 7th day. Arrhythmia

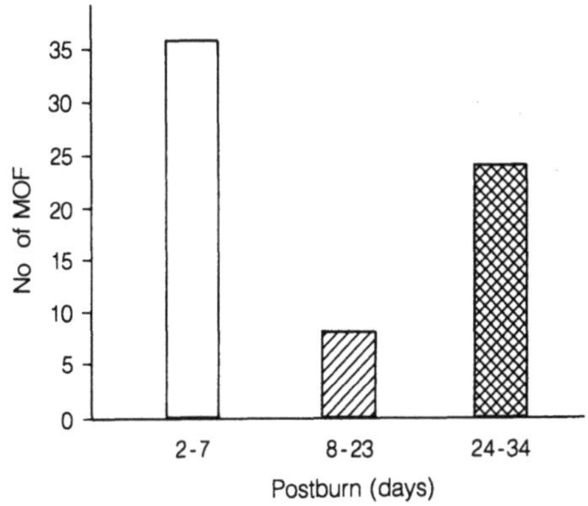

Fig. 11.1. Time of onset of MOF

appeared on the 17th day, with a heart rate of 180/min. On the 25th day, the blood creatinine level rose to 2.6 mg/dl and blood urea nitrogen (BUN) to 57 mg/dl. On the 25th day, the patient became disoriented, which was followed by coma. He died 26 days after the injury with failure of the lung, digestive tract, heart, kidney, and brain.

In analyzing our cases, we have found that the occurrence of MOF shows two peaks. Taking the day when the second organ begins to fail as the onset of MOF, 53% of patients developed MOF during two to seven postburn days, and 35% within the fourth postburn week. The remaining patients developed MOF between the 2nd and 3rd week (Fig. 11.1).

In our experience of 68 patients with MOF, 10 suffered burns of 30%–59% TBSA, 16 burns of 60%–79% TBSA, and 42 (61.8%) burns larger than 80% TBSA (Table 11.1). Thirty-one patients (45.6%) were brought to the hospital later than 8 h after the injury, and 27 (39.7) had had signs of hypovolemic shock at the time of presentation or some time during the course of their hospital stay. Forty-six patients had at least one epidose of septicemia, which was proved by blood culture (Table 11.2). The causative organisms of septicemia during the 1st week postburn were predominantly gram-negative bacilli, including *Pseudomonas aeruginosa* and colon bacilli (18/24), while *Staphylococcus aureus* was the more common culprit (13/22) in the 4th week (Table 11.3). Four patients developed MOF subsequent to pyogenic thrombo-phlebitis due to infection of the venous lines. In seven patients MOF appeared soon after a massive infection of the burn wound resulting from failure of allografts after the excision operation. Peritoneal infection as a consequence of peritoneal dialysis led to MOF in two patients. Long-distance transportation without adequate supportive measures precipitated MOF in 12 patients. This brief analysis demonstrates the importance of hypovolemic shock and systemic infection in the development of MOF in burn patients. It also illustrates that MOF may occur after iatrogenic errors, which should be preventable.

Table 11.1. Relationship between percentage TBSA burned and occurrence of MOF

% TBSA burned	No. of MOFs	%
30–59	10	14.7
60–79	16	23.5
80–100	42	61.8
Total	68	100.0

Table 11.2. Precipitating factors of MOF

Precipitating factors	No. of MOFs	%
Shock	33	48.5
Septicemia	21	30.8
Inhalation injury	10	14.7
Others	4	5.9
Total	68	100.0

Table 11.3. Agents of bacteremia in MOF

	Blood cultures	
	1st week postburn	4th weeks postburn
Pseudomonas aeruginosa	13	3
Escherichia coli	5	4
Staphylococcus aureus	3	13
Salmonella	1	0
Aerobacter	1	0

11.2 Diagnostic Criteria

In a broad sense, when an organ cannot support its function it is supposed to fail. But in clinical practice work, it is not so easy to judge whether there is a dysfunction or actually a failure. Especially so when we come to the liver. Since the liver has multiple functions, and it is known to have a strong regeneration potential, and since, up to the present, there has been no sensitive and specific test to evaluate its functions, it is difficult for us to pinpoint early hepatic function failure.

Nevertheless, the consensus of opinion is that criteria for diagnosis of MOF are important both to enable clinicians to recognize the syndrome as early as possible and to facilitate the comparison by clinicians of their experiences with an uniform understanding of the syndrome. Many authors have put forward their diagnostic criteria, and, among them, those described by Baue have been widely accepted. The following is a description of our criteria for diagnosis of MOF, which are essentially a modification of Baue's criteria.

11.2.1 Pulmonary Failure

Systemic hypoxemia requiring mechanical respiratory support for at least 5 days; $PaO_2/FiO_2 < 200–300$.

11.2.2 Renal Failure

Serum creatinine level higher than 2 mg/dl. In order to differentiate MOF from extrarenal azotemia, FeNa should be determined. Daily urinary output is a poor indicator because many patients may apparently output an adequate amount of urine while the kidneys are actually failing.

11.2.3 Hepatic Failure

Serum bilirubin level higher than 2 ml/dl, elevation of glutamic pyruric transaminase (GPT) or lactate dehydrogenase (LDH) values to twice normal. Recently, it has been postulated that the ratio between blood ketone bodies (acetoacetic acid: β-hydroxybutyric acid), which reflects the mitochondrial redox potential of the liver cells, is a good index of liver damage [9].

11.2.4 Gastrointestinal Tract Failure

Intractable distension of the gastrointestinal tract with abnormal motility and absorption; bleeding from the upper digestive system necessitating a blood transfusion of 1000 ml/24 h.

11.2.5 Cardiovascular Failure

Hypotension requiring support with ionotropic agents for over 48 h.

11.2.6 Central Nervous System Failure

Cloudy sensorium, disorientation, Glasgow coma scale below 7.

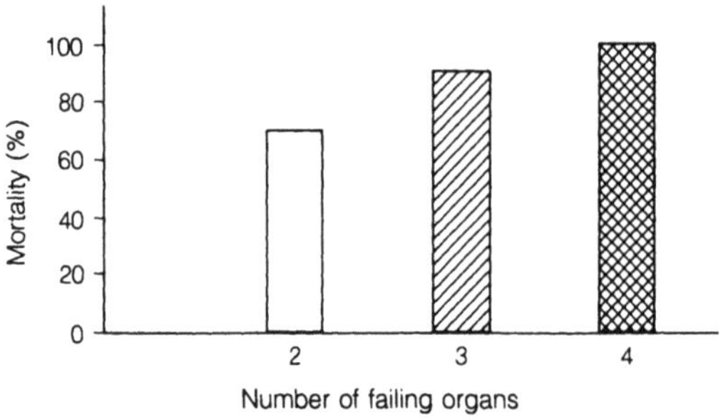

Fig. 11.2. Relationship between mortality and number of failing organs

11.2.7 Coagulation

Platelet count lower than $50 \times 10^9/l$ (50000/mm^3), or when a diagnosis of disseminated intravascular coagulopathy (DIC) is established.

11.2.8 Metabolism as a System

Uncontrollable hyperglycemia, with a blood sugar level above 400 mg/dl; plasma osmolality above 400 mOsm/kg H_2O; ratio of BCAA to AAA below 1.5, Phe/Tyr greater than 2.0; uncontrollable hypernatremia and hyperchloremia.

11.3 Prognosis

The development of MOF in a burn patient denotes a prognosis. The overall mortality from MOF in our series has been 88.2%, and it has accounted for 75.9% of all the deaths within the study period. It is not surprising to find that the mortality rate was directly related to the number of organs failed. In our series, 28 patients manifested failure of 2 organs, and 21 of them died, with a mortality rate of 75%. Of the 28 patients suffering from failure of 3 organs, 27 died, comprising a mortality rate of 96.4%. All 12 patients who had failure of 4 or more organs finally succumbed to the syndrome (Fig. 11.2). While the lung was usually the first organ to show functional failure clinically, renal failure frequently cast the last stone in the whole process, as our data showed the mortality rate was 100% when the kidnies failed.

11.4 Pathology

The fundamental histopathological changes in MOF seem to consist mainly of circulatory disturbances, i.e., congestion, hemorrhage, edema, microthrombi, etc., cellular degeneration and necrosis, and inflammatory reactions. However, these changes may vary in intensity depending on the causative factors of MOF, duration of underlying disease, time of appearance of failure of that specific organ, etc. It has also been found that there is often a disparity between the severity of functional failure and the degree of histopathological changes in the organ in question. With the advent of electron microscopy and histochemical staining techniques, new findings with regard to the finer structural changes have been made. According to our postmortem studies and animal experiments, the pathological changes in different organs are as follows.

11.4.1 Lung

Under light microscopy, the early changes are chiefly aggregation of neutrophils in the small blood vessels, interstitial edema with edema cuff formation around the small blood vessels, focal hemorrhage, and microthrombi formation. These are followed by the appearance of neutrophilic infiltration in the lung interstitium, resulting in widening of the alveolo-capillary septa, alveolar edema and hyaline membrane formation, focal atelectasis, bronchopneumonia, and minute abscess formation in advanced cases. Osmic acid sodium iodide (OsO_4-NaI) staining reveals in increase in type II pneumocytes, which becomes more marked with time. Electron microscopy reveals swelling of the capillary endothelium, interstitial edema, and edema of type I pneumocytes in the early stage. Alveolar edema and hyaline membrane formation, and hyperplasia of type II pneumocytes with emptying lamellar bodies appear later. With the freeze-etching technique, changes in intercellular tight junctions of the alveolar epithelium and capillary endothelium including a marked decrease in number, breakage, irregularity, free endings, and damage in the strands of the intercellular junctions can be seen. Distention of the meshes can also be discerned in the intercellular junctions of the epithelial cells. All the above pathological changes found in the lung contribute to the impairment of diffusion of gases, resulting in lowering of the PaO_2.

11.4.2 Myocardium

In the myocardium, there is interstitial congestion, focal hemorrhage, interstitial edema, mild fatty myofibril degeneration, and occasionally focal necrosis. With the electron microscope, changes like edema between the myofibril bundles and in the sarcoplasmic reticulum, separation of myofibrils, congestion, edema, and hemorrhage in the myocardial interstitium are found. Early in the disease process lanthanum deposits occur on the mitochondrial membrane with lanthanum nitrate staining, indicating that the damage in the plasma membrane of myofibrils may be the initial change which gives rise to myocardial lesions.

11.4.3 Kidney

The main finding in the kidney is congestion or ischemia of the glomerular capillaries. There is proliferation of the mesangial cells. Periodic acid-Schiff (PAS) stain reveals an increasing amount of eosinophilic material in the mesangial region. Degeneration of the tubular epithelium (including cloudy swelling, hyaline degeneration, and vacuolar degeneration) and mild necrosis can also be found. Hyaline casts are seen in the lumina. There is also interstitial congestion, and sometimes focal hemorrhage under the capsule and in the medulla. With chemohistological techniques, it can be shown that the acidic phosphatase (ACP) content is increased in the tubular epithelium, while there is an early and late decrease in ATP. The only early findings with electron microscopy are focal edema of the glomerular capillary endothelium, swelling and breakage or disappearance of the mitochondrial crest, an increase in the lysosomes of the epithelium of the proximal tubules, and focal edema of the cytoplasm of the distal tubular epithelium. Following these changes, there appear diffuse edema of the glomerular capillary endothelium, focal rarefaction of the basement membrane, swelling of the podocytes, vacuolation of the mitochondria, fusion of the foot processes, an increase in the mesangial cells and ground substance in the mesangial region, and marked edema of the tubular epithelium. Lanthanum nitrate staining shows there are lanthanum deposits on the mitchondrial membrane and its vicinity.

11.4.4 Liver

The early histopathological changes are essentially dilatation and congestion of the central veins and sinusoids, marked hyperplasia and swelling of Kupffer's cells, degeneration of the hepatocytes (cloudy swelling, rarefaction of the cytoplasm, eosinophilic change, fatty degeneration), and focal necrosis. Then necrosis of the central or intermediate zone of the hepatic lobules ensues, with necrotic cells found in the sinusoids, retrogression of hyperplasia of Kupffer's cells, and infiltration of inflammatory cells in the portal space and sinusoids. Histochemical study reveals an early increase in acidic phosphatase in the liver cells, while ATP is decreased in amount in both early and late stages. PAS staining of the hepatic cells is weak, whereas Kupffer's cells show a strong reaction. Electron microscopic examination in the early stage reveals margination of the chromosomes of the hepatocyte nucleus and pyknosis of the nucleolus, swelling and clustering of the mitochondria, a few fat droplets, an increase in lyzosomes, and degranulation of the endoplasmic reticulum. There are also edema of the cytoplasmic matrix of the sinusoid endothelial cells, hyperplasia and swelling of Kupffer's cells, and an increase in glycogen granules, lyzosomes, and phagosomes. Then damage of the nucleus and organelles of the hepatic cells ensues, and there is necrosis, hemorrhage, and infiltration of lymphocytes, swelling and desquamation of the bile ductule, microvilli, presence of necrotic cells and inflammatory cells in the sinusoids, swelling of Kupffer's cells, clustering of mitochondria, and a decrease in lysosomes and phagosomes. With lanthanum nitrate staining, an early finding is the presence of lanthanum deposits in the cytoplasm of the hepatocytes and on the membrane of the mitochondria. Bile ductules are also filled with lanthanum.

11.4.5 Brain

Findings are congestion and vasodilatation in the subarachnoid space and brain tissue, focal hemorrhage, brain edema, and degeneration and necrosis of the nerve cells. The nerve cells show swelling of the cell body and pyknosis of the nucleus. Some cells, in contrast, show shrinkage of the cell body, appearing slender in shape, with eosinophilic cytoplasm and pyknosis of the nucleus. These findings are verified by electron microscopy. In the early stage, edema is found in the capillary endothelium, with swelling and flocculation of the mitochondria, and swelling of the terminal foot of the extrabasement membrane astrocytes. Later on, there is degeneration and necrosis of the nerve cells. Both lucid and dim nerve cells can be seen. The former show swelling of the cell body, edema of the cytoplasmic matrix, degenerative changes in the mitochondria, and loss of mitochondria, with the cytóplasm becoming electron transparent. The cytoplasm shows slender cell bodies, pyknosis of the nucleus, and densification of the mitochondria, and the cytoplasm is electronically dense. Necrotic nerve cells are phagocytized by glial cells, resulting in the phenomenon of neuronophagia.

The above changes seen in the brain probably lead to retarded rosponsiveness and drowsiness.

11.4.6 Digestive Tract

No significant pathological changes are found in the stomach, unless stress ulceration occurs. It is in the small intestine that the main lesions are located. The mucosa is congested and edematous, and there is patchy or segmental hemorrhage and erosion in the mucosa. This gross pathology is verified by microscopic examination. Electron microscopy reveals a decrease in the microvilli of the intestinal mucosa, swelling of the cytoplasmic matrix of the mucosal epithelium, scarcity of organelles, submucosal congestion, swelling and hemorrhage, and leukocytic infiltration. These pathological changes probably contribute to the impairment of barrier function of the intestinal mucosa, allowing the escape of toxic materials into the systemic circulation to enhance the injury in the different viscerae.

11.4.7 Immune Organs

Lymph Nodes. Early changes in the lymph node consist of dilatation of the cortical lymph sinuses, which are filled with macrophages, and a decrease in the number of cortical lymphocytes. The lymph sinuses are later filled by a large number of plasma cells and neutrophils. There is also neutrophilic infiltration in the lymph cords and hyperplasia of the lymph follicles. Electron microscopy reveals degeneration of the cortical lymphocytes and proliferation of macrophages, showing phagocytosis of the fragments of dead cells. Plasma cells and neutrophils are also found in the sinuses.

Spleen. Findings are dilatation and congestion of the splenic sinuses, which are filled with macrophages, and atrophy of the splenic bodies. With the lapse of time, there is also neutrophilic infiltration and hyperplasia of the germinal centers of the white pulp. With neutral α-naphthylacetate esterase (ANAE) staining, one can see that the macrophages contain a large quantity of enzyme, indicating increased activity of the macrophages. Electron microscopy shows endothelial cell swelling, an abundant amount of macrophages and neutrophils in the sinuses, degeneration and necrosis of lymphocytes in the white pulp, proliferation of macrophages, and phagocytosis of dead lymphocytes.

Thymus. Similar to the lymph nodes and spleen, findings are also degeneration and necrosis of lymphocytes, leading to a decrease in the number of lymphocytes. On the contrary, there is an increase in the number of macrophages. Due to the decrease in lymphocytes in the medulla, there is a reversal in the amount of lymphocytes in the cortex and medulla. Electron microscopy reveals degeneration and necrosis of lymphocytes, proliferation of macrophages and active phagocytosis, and swelling of the capillary endothelium.

11.5 Mechanism of Organ Failure: Theoretical Considerations

The most prevalent hypothesis of the pathogenesis of MOF is that of bacterial invasion. Statistically, uncontrolled infection is definitely the variable that correlates with the emergence of MOF. Of our 68 patients, 78% were accompanied by well-documented septicemia, and many others exhibited obvious burn wound sepsis. In some patients, serious wound infection with *Pseudomonas aeruginosa* or *Staphylococcus aureus* occurred after wound excision, either because of poor-quality allograft or because of the presence of devitalized tissues which were not completely excised. Many authors have also incriminated bacterial invasion or the presence of an uncontrolled infectious focus as the most important causative factor. Fry et al. [4] reported that 87 out of 553 surgical patients developed MOF. Of these 87, only 4 were not septic. Hassett et al. [10] considered that one-third of these patients begin with a clear-cut infection, and two-thirds eventually develop bacteremia.

The septic response to bacterial invasion is a systemic one and is not specific to the type of invading microorganism, be it *P. aeruginosa*, *S. aureus*, or *Mucor*. The hypermetabolic response due to the primary injury becomes reactivated instead of abated. If the source of infection is not controlled, the hypermetabolism continues until such time as the source is controlled or the organ failure ensues [5].

With the onset of hypermetabolism, there is an increase in resting energy expenditure, reflected in the marked increase in oxygen consumption demand and a fall in systemic vascular resistance. To meet these physiological alterations, there is a corresponding increase in heart beat, and, in turn, cardiac output (CO). Thus, a typical hyperdynamic state with low peripheral resistance emerges. In the early phase of hypermetabolism, the arterial venous oxygen content difference (DVO_2) is quite normal, while in the late phase of organ failure there is marked narrowing of DVO_2, probably due to an extraction failure at the periphery.

A high CO does not infer that myocardial function is necessarily well preserved, as indicated by a lowering of SWI_{LV} by actual measurement. When the patient is unable to meet the cardiac demands because of impaired cardiac reserve, he or she may finally develop frank hypotension.

In the hypermetabolic state, there is oxidation of mixed substrate of carbohydrate, fat, and amino acids. In fact, there is a reduction in fractional energy expenditure that is being derived from the oxidation of glucose. On the other hand, it is attended by a significantly increased gluconeogenesis, which cannot be shut down by an exogenous supply of glucose. At the same time, owing to the presence of stress, the pancreatic glucagon level is higher than normal. There also appears a state of insulin resistance, probably due to the combined effects of a high level of catecholamine and decreased activity and number of insulin receptors on various cells, including erythrocytes and monocytes [11]. As a result, hyperglycemia is a usual occurrence, and the blood sugar level may reach as high as 800–1000 mg/dl.

Ketosis is markedly suppressed in a hypermetabolic state. With the development of organ failure, there is an increase in lipogenesis. The triglyceride clearance becomes reduced, and spontaneous lipemia or hypertriglyceridemia becomes a prominent feature.

With the onset of hypermetabolism, total body protein synthesis is decreased, though hepatic protein synthesis is increased. There is at the same time severe catabolism of the protein stores, particularly in skeletal muscles, with resultant rapid loss of skeletal muscle mass. There is also a marked increase in the total body oxidation of amino acids for energy production. The term "autocannibalism" has been coined to describe this phenomenon [12]. This marked proteolysis is probably mediated by interleukin [13].

The catabolic state enhances ureagenesis, with a corresponding increase in the prerenal azotemia. The latter is present throughout the hypermetabolism organ failure complex irrespective of whether exogenous amino acid support is given or not.

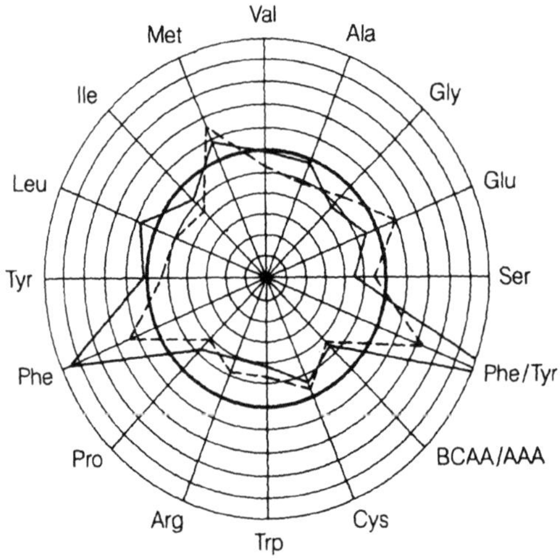

Fig. 11.3. Amino acid pattern 3 days after burn injury. —, MOF group (mean burn size, 83.9% TBSA; third degree, 54.3%); – – –, non-MOF group (mean burn size, 69.8%; degree, 29.8%)

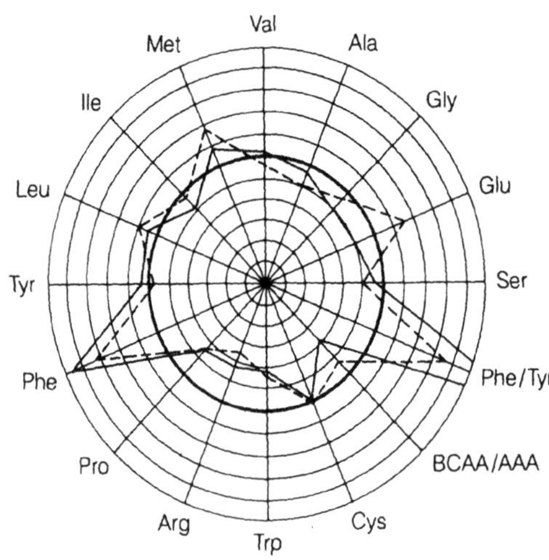

Fig. 11.4. Amino acid pattern 7 days after burn injury. —, MOF group (mean burn size, 83.9%; third degree, 54.3%); – – –, non-MOF group (mean burn size, 69.8%; third degree, 29.8%)

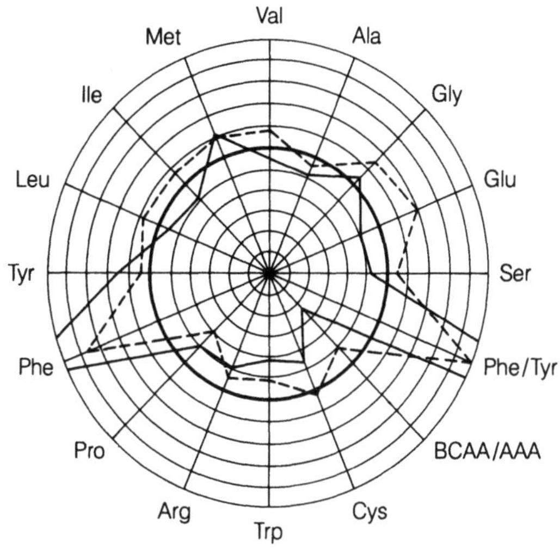

Fig. 11.5. Amino acid pattern 14 days after burn injury. —, MOF group (mean burn size, 83.9%; third degree, 54.3%); – – –, non-MOF group (mean burn size, 69.8%; third degree, 29.8%)

Table 11.4. Relationship between the AcAc/β-OHB ratio and occurrence of MOF

AcAc/β-OHB	No. of patients	No. of MOFs	No. of non-MOFs
–0.4	9	8	1
0.4+	8	4	4
0.8+	27	1	26

The hypermetabolism, which is perpetuated by a systemic septic response, inhibits pyruvic dehydrogenase in the liver. As a result, aromatic amino acids accumulate rapidly, and the ratio of branched-chain amino acids (BCAA) to aromatic amino acids (AAA) is markedly reduced (Figs. 11.3–11.5). When we examined our own cases, we found that, when the ratio of BCAA to AAA was greater than 2, only 3 to 11 patients developed MOF, while 8 out of 10 developed MOF when it was less than 1.5 [14]. Furthermore, it seemed that the ratio of phenylalanine and tyrosine also bore a certain predictive significance. When it was lower than 1.5, only 2 of 12 patients developed MOF, and when it was higher than 2, 6 of 7 developed MOF.

We have also found a decrease in the acetoacetate/β-hydroxybutyrate molar ratio. The ratio is more noticeably lowered in patients who finally developed MOF (Fig. 11.6, Table 11.4). Since this ratio is governed by the intra-mitochondrial $NADH^{+}/NAD^{+}$ molar ratio, this observation implies that there is an abnormality in the redox state within the cytoplasm, especially the liver cells.

In summary, in an extensive deep burn injury, sustained and unrelenting insults, consequent upon repeated surgical interventions, persistent wound

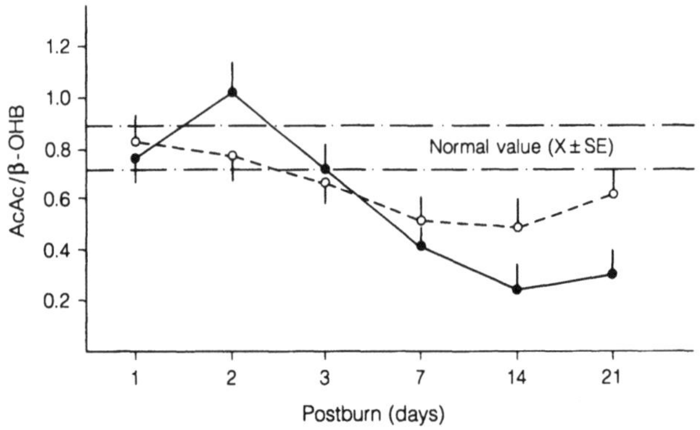

Fig. 11.6. Changes in AcAc/β-OHB in arterial blood of patients with MOF (●——●) and patients without MOF (○- - -○)

infection and episodes of bacteremia, and perhaps bouts of translocation of intestinal bacteria, cause an exaggerated and protracted course of stress response. As a result, the body protein reserves are diverted into gluconeogenesis and synthesis of acute-phase reactants rather than reparative synthetic processes or albumin, triggering the cascade of MOF.

Recently, conflicting reports have emerged concerning the role of invading infection as the cause of MOF, and a hypothesis maintaining that the underlying pathogenesis is a systemic inflammatory process, including invasive infection, has been proposed by some authors.

Goris, Schirmer, and Steinberg were separately successful in developing a bacteria-independent experimental model which simulated the patho-physiology and histopathology of the MOF syndrome [15, 16, 17], with a sterile intraperitoneal or intravenous injection of zymosan. The experimental results illustrate well that the systemic inflammatory process, which is meant to limit the spread of infection, may become deleterious to the organism if unchecked or may become uncontrollable. We have not only confirmed their experiments, but we have also found that cantharidin, which is a potent local irritant, can induce the development of MOF in rats when injected in small repeated doses into the peritoneal cavity (C.Y. Sheng et al., unpublished data). The predominant cells in the peritoneal cavity are the monocytes. It is, therefore, postulated that the possible mechanism of induction of noninfection MOF might be activation of complements by a systemic inflammatory process produced by these local irritants. This initiates a cascade of complement degradation, with the liberation of the cleavage product C5a. A high level of C5a in the circulation may result in microaggregation of cellular elements of the blood, especially leukocytes. Thus, these microaggregates secondary to systemic complement activation, triggered by zymosan or cantharidin in animal experimentation, or by necrotic tissue, bacteria, endotoxin, etc. in burn patients, may affect the nutrient blood flow of critical organs and may mediate tissue-level injury that heralds the clinical

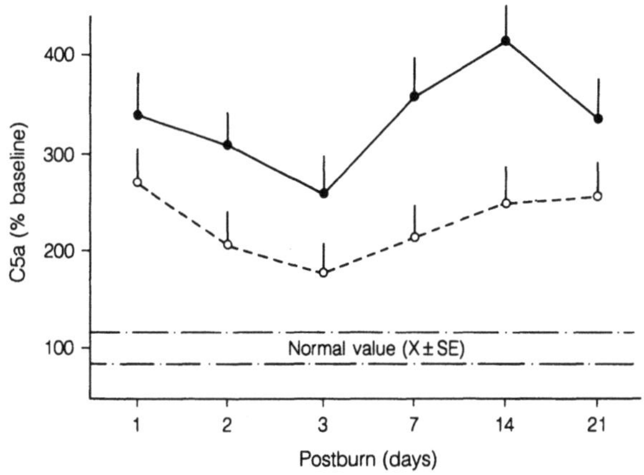

Fig. 11.7. Changes in C5a content in plasma of burned patients. ●———●, patients with MOF; ○---○, patients without MOF

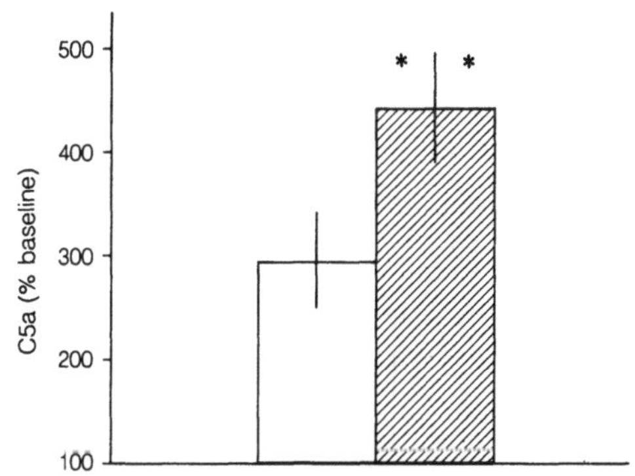

Fig. 11.8. Comparison of C5a content in plasma before septicemia (□) and after septicemia (▨)

evolution of MOF. In our own experiments, we have demonstrated that there are abundant microaggregates in the vessels especially in the lungs, and prior administration of C5a antibody could ameliorate the lung lesions [18]. Further, we documented a rise in C5a level in the blood on postburn day 1 in our burn patients, and its level was significantly higher in patients who developed MOF later (Fig. 11.7). C5a level was lowered on postburn day 3, but there appeared a second peak 2 weeks after the injury. It was especially high after an episode of septicemia (Fig. 11.8) [19].

Some authors emphasized the importance of humoral mediators in the pathogenesis of MOF. Among these, interleukin I, eicosanoids, free oxygen radicals, opinoids/neuropeptides, and false neurotransmitters are the most frequently mentioned [13].

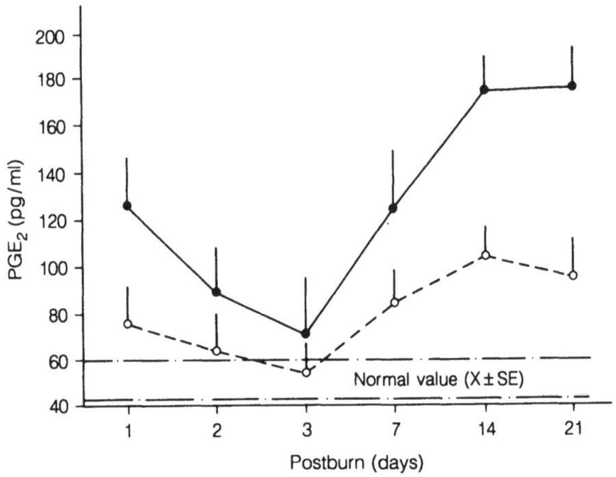

Fig. 11.9. Changes in PGE_2 content in plasma of burned patients. ●——●, patients with MOF; ○---○, patients without MOF

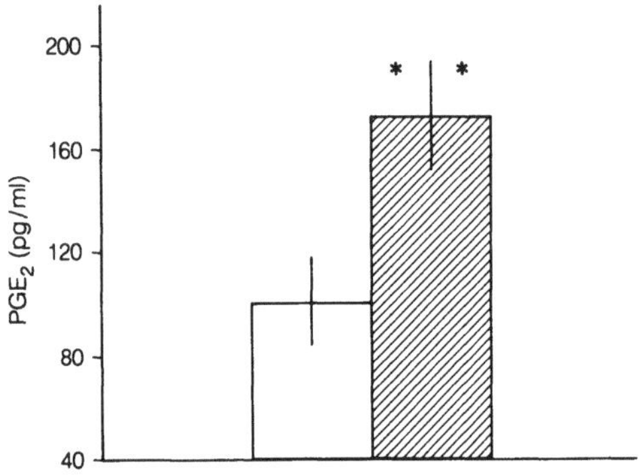

Fig. 11.10. Comparison of PGE_2 content in plasma before septicemia (□) and after septicemia (▧)

Interleukin I is a versatile compound (or a group of compounds) which is produced by macrophage. It acts on the hypothalamus to promote fever. It stimulates neutrophilia from the bone marrow. Neutrophils are activated by this compound to release lactoferrin. It reduces zinc levels; it promotes acute-phase proteins; it is presumed to increase muscle proteolysis; it increases peripheral amino acid oxidation; and it may promote production of immunoglobulins [13, 20]. The bulk of evidence in the literature suggests that interleukin I may very well be responsible for mediating many of the catabolic processes that result in protein-calorie malnutrition and may make the host vulnerable to MOF.

Another group of mediators which are of interest are the eicosanoids, specifically the prostaglandins. Of the latter, two compounds are basically the focus of an enormous amount of attention, i.e., prostacyclin and thromboxane.

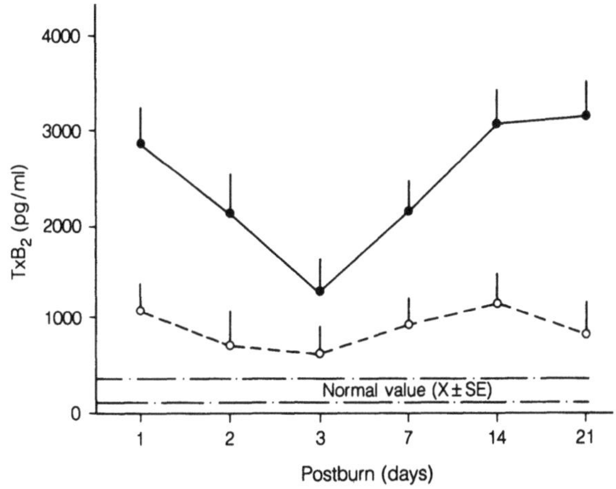

Fig. 11.11. Changes in TxB_2 content in plasma of burned patients. ●———●, patients with MOF; ○---○, patients without MOF

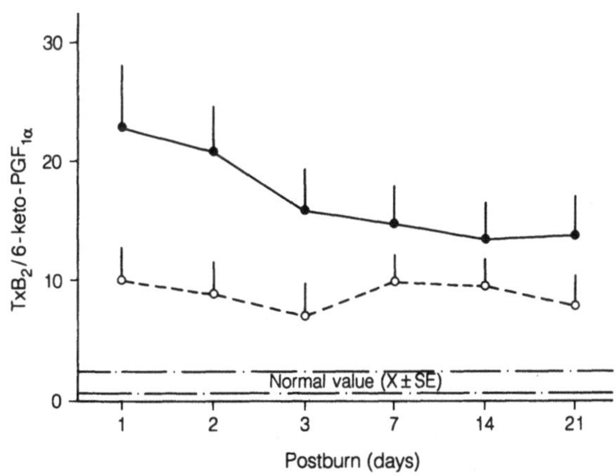

Fig. 11.12. Changes in the ratio of TxB_2 and 6-keto-$PGF_{1\alpha}$ in plasma of burned patients. ●———●, patients with MOF; ○---○, patients without MOF

Our clinical observations [21] showed there was an elevation of both TxB_2 and $PGF_{1\alpha}$ on the first postburn day, being more marked in the group of patients who developed MOF later. In addition, the elevation of TxB_2 was proportionally higher than that of $PGF_{1\alpha}$, and the ratio of $TxB_2/PGF_{1\alpha}$ was significantly higher in the MOF group (Figs. 11.9–11.13). Since thromboxane is a potent vasoconstrictor that aggregates platelets, it is postulated that it contributes to the formation of thrombi in the microvasculature of different organs, and thus precipitating functional failure.

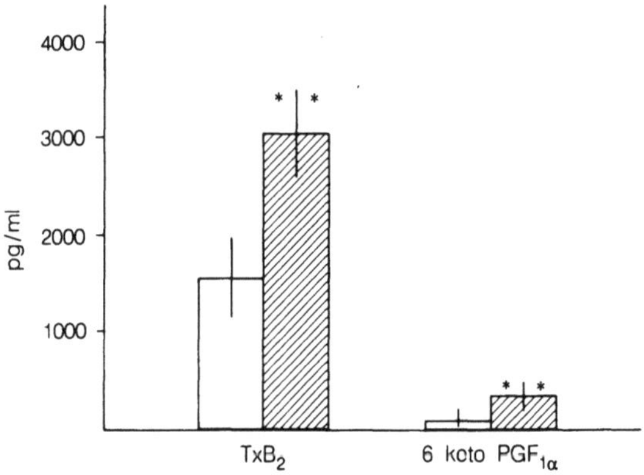

Fig. 11.13. Comparison of TxB_2 content and 6-keto-$PGF_{1\alpha}$ content in plasma before septicemia (□) and after septicemia (▧)

Free oxygen radicals are liberated in the process of reperfusion of various organs, as well as by respiratory bursts of neutrophils and macrophages. They bring about lipid peroxidation, leading to damage of the biological membranes, and have been shown both in vivo and in vitro directly to injure endothelial cells, pneumocytes, fibroblasts, and probably also other cells other cells and organelles [22]. The cell damage is probably the result of a massive intracellular influx of calcium ions subsequent to the damage of the cellular membrane. Further, through damage of the mitochondria, the production of ATP is markedly impaired, simultaneously with an increase in the consumption of ATP in an attempt to repair the damaged cells. Therefore, the cells are rendered energy starved and unable to protect themselves from further injury. Morphologically, the cells become rounded, releasing tight junctions with other cells. When free oxygen radicals encroach upon endothelial cells, a marked increase in permeability occurs, hence the interstitial edema and increase in weight consistently found in various failing organs.

Our clinical observations strongly suggest that organ failure following serious burn injury is attributable to lipid peroxidation, which can be detected both in the early stage and 2–3 weeks after the injury [19]. The data showed that there was a lowering of blood superoxide dismutase (SOD) levels and a rise in malondialdehyde (MDA) levels reaching a peak 7 days after injury. Interestingly, the lowering of SOD and rise in MDA were were significantly more marked in patients with emergence of MOF than those without. The alterations in values were particularly marked in those who finally died (Figs. 11.14–11.19). Zhao et al. [23], who also studied the role of free oxygen radicals in the pathogenesis of MOF subsequent to burn injury, found that the degree of functional derangement of organs was closely related to the lipid peroxidation process after extensive burns. In patients who had complications of MOF, the quantity of exhaled ethane and ethylene, which were the end products of lipid peroxidation,

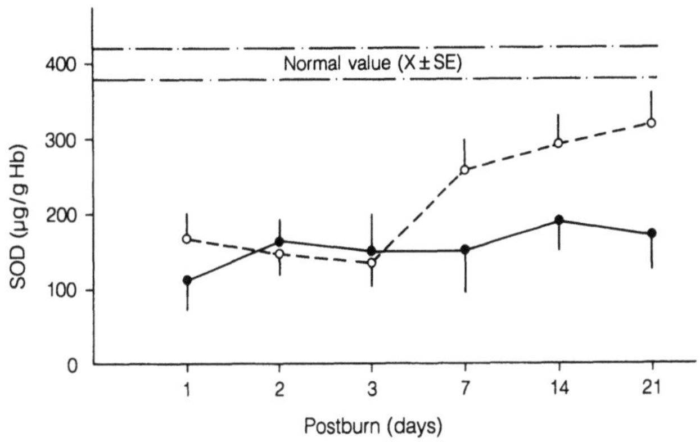

Fig. 11.14. Changes in superoxide dismutase (*SOD*) content in blood of burned patients with and without MOF. ●——●, patient with MOF; ○---○, patient without MOF

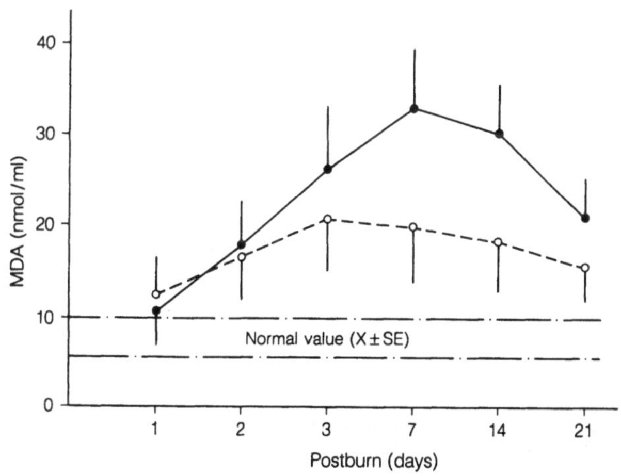

Fig. 11.15. Changes in MOA content in plasma of burned patients with (●——●) and without (○---○) MOF

Fig. 11.16. Changes in superoxide dismutase (*SOD*) content in blood of burned patients with septicemia. □, before septicemia; ▨, after septicemia. Comparison with pre-septicemia; **, $p < 0.01$

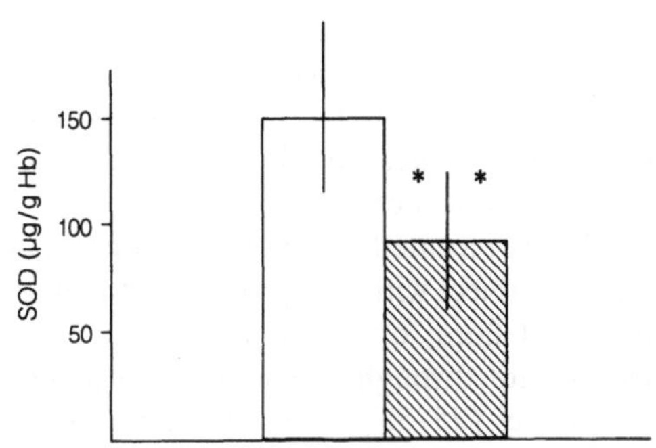

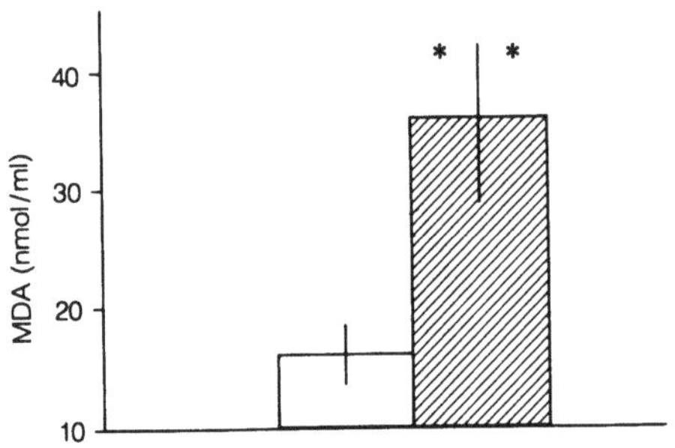

Fig. 11.17. Changes in malondialdehyde (*MDA*) content in plasma of burned patients with septicemia. ▢, before septicemia; ▨, after septicemia. Comparison with presepticemia: **, $p < 0.01$

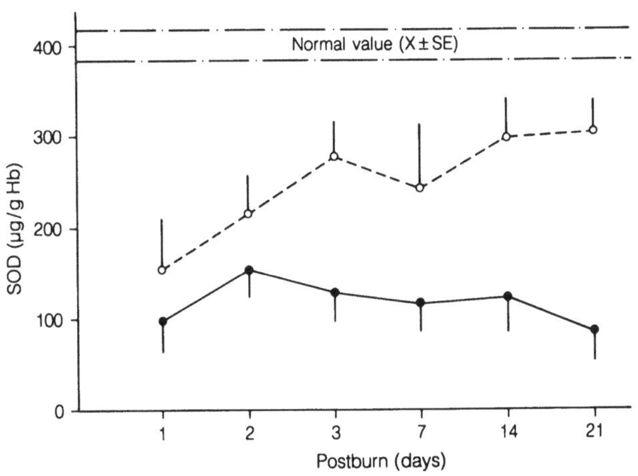

Fig. 11.18. Changes in superoxide dismutase (*SOD*) content in blood of burned patients with MOF. ●———●, nonsurvivors; ○---○, survivors

and the level of MDA in urine were all significantly higher than in those who showed no signs of organ failure.

The role of free oxygen radicals in causing organ failure has also been demonstrated in our animal experiments with partial occlusion of the superior mesenteric artery (see below). A marked decrease in SOD and elevation of MDA were identified in both the liver and the lungs, in collaboration with marked impairment of their functions and decisive histopathological changes simulating MOF in clinical cases.

It has repeatedly been proved that organisms from the intestinal tract of a burned subject with compromised immunity and disturbed microecology of the intestinal flora, owing to prolonged use of broad-spectrum antibiotics, can translocate through the mucosa into the portal circulation and mesenteric lymphatics [25–33]. This was again proved by our experiment [19].

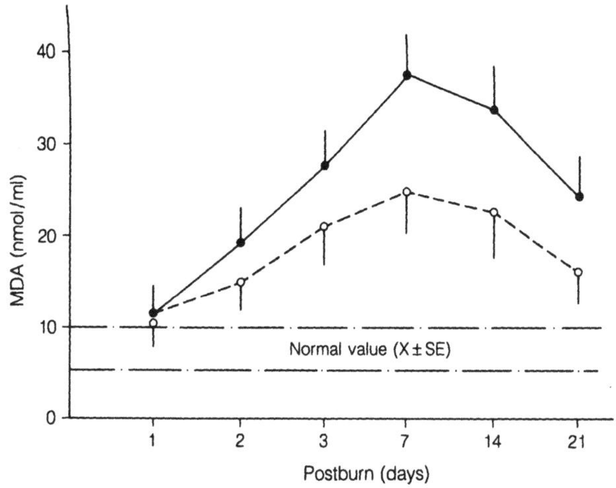

Fig. 11.19. Changes in malondialdehyde (*MDA*) content in plasma of burned patients with MOF. ●——●, nonsurvivors; ○---○, survivors

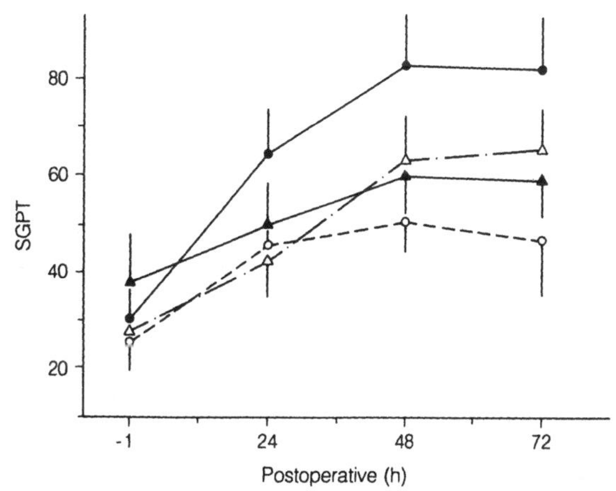

Fig. 11.20. Changes in serum glutamic pyruvic transaminase (*SGPT*) in plasma of each group. Group I (——○——), sham operation control; group II (——●——), partial occlusion of the superior mesenteric artery for 1 h; group III (——▲——), partial occlusion of the superior mesenteric artery + vitamin E; group IV (——△——), partial occlusion of the superior mesenteric artery + rubiside

Our experiment started with the premise that there would be a sharp reduction in blood supply to the gastrointestinal tract after the onset of hypovolemic shock. Consequently, the portal flow would be reduced. As the portal vein supplies about 70% of the blood supply to the liver, the latter would then suffer from ischemia. The animals, including both rabbits and dogs, were first fed neomycin for 3 days to eliminate a high proportion of the intestinal flora. Fourteen hours before the experiment, they were fed with *E. coli*. The superior

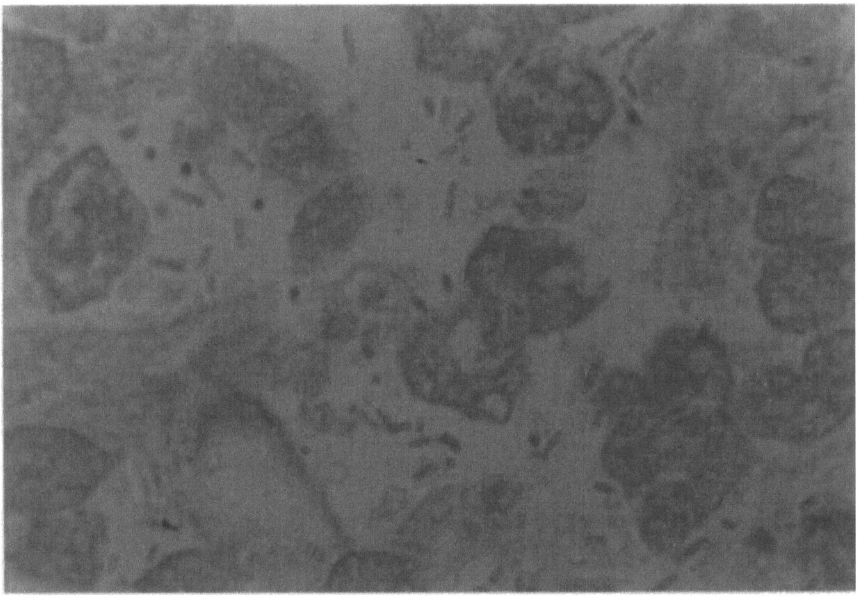

Fig. 11.21. Group II: numerous gram-negative bacilli in liver sinuses. Modified gram stain, × 1000

Fig. 11.22. Group II, showing immunofluorescence-marked *E. coli* $O_{111}B_4$ in liver sinuses

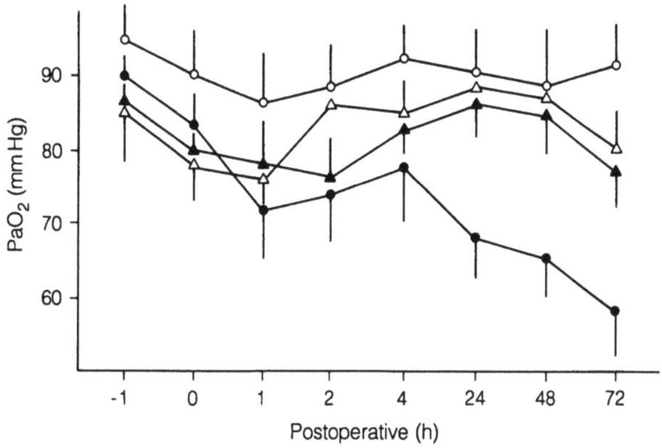

Fig. 11.23. Changes in PaO_2 in each group. Group I (——○——), sham operation control; group II (——●——), partial occlusion of the superior mesenteric artery for 1 h; group III (——▲——), partial occlusion of the superior mesenteric artery + vitamine E; group IV (——△——), partial occlusion of the superior mesenteric artery + rubiside

mesenteric artery was then partially occluded until the portal blood flow was reduced by 55%. This was maintained for 1 h. Serum glutamic pyruvic transaminase (SGPT), serum glutamic oxaloacetic transaminase (SGOT), alkaline phosphatase, SOD, and MDA of blood, and liver biopsies were sequentially examined, and lung SOD, MDA, and pathological changes were determined immediately after death or euthanasia. It was shown that the liver consistently exhibited marked changes, both functional and pathological, soon after the release of superior mesentery artery occlusion (Fig. 11.20, p. 203). Pathological changes in the liver were essentially sinusoid congestion, granulocyte infiltration, hyperplasia of Kupffer's cells, liver cell degeneration, and focal necrosis of the liver perenchyma. Transmission electron microscopy confirmed the live cell degeneration. Bacilli could be seen in the liver sinusoids (Figs. 11.21, 11.22). The liver pathology was progressive until the animals developed respiratory symptoms, which were fatal in 80% of the animals. Respiratory symptoms included hyperpnea, and lowering of the PaO_2 and SaO_2 (Fig. 11.23). Pathological examination revealed focal hemorrhage, proteinaceous exudation into the alveoli, marked thickening of the alveolar septa with marked neutrophilic infiltration, hyaline membrane formation in the alveoli, congestion in small vessels, and the presence of hyaline thrombi in the arterioles. These changes were less conspicuous with the administration of antioxidants, e.g., vitamin E, rubiside, tanshinone, or *Rubia yunnanensis* [24] (Table 11.5). Demonstration of the microorganism, which was fed before the experiment, in the liver sinusoids, and partial protection afforded by amikacin after the release of the artery implied that the intestinal flora related infection also contributed to the pathogenesis of MOF in the experimental animals (Figs. 11.24–11.29).

In brief, the pathogenesis of MOF is probably a biological summation of numerous humoral mediators, and it may actually be a biphasic disease. The

Table 11.5. Pathological changes in lung, heart, liver, and small intestine in each animal group

Groups	I	II	III	IV
No. of animals	10	10	10	10
Lung				
PMN aggregation	1	9	5	2
Alveolar hemorrhage	2	8	3	1
Interstitial or alveolar edema	1	8	3	2
Formation of microthrombus	0	7	2	1
Hyaline membrane	0	7	1	0
Bronchopneumonia	0	6	3	1
Detection of G-bacillus	0	6	3	0
Heart				
PMN aggregation and infiltration	0	7	1	0
Interstitial congestion	2	10	5	5
Interstitial hemorrhage	0	5	2	1
Interstitial edema	1	9	2	1
Myocardial myofibril degeneration	0	9	2	1
Focal necrosis	0	5	0	0
Liver				
PMN aggregation and infiltration	2	8	5	3
Fatty degeneration	2	9	4	2
Focal necrosis	0	8	1	0
Activation phagocytosis of Kupffer's cells	0	8	1	2
Detection of G-bacillus	0	5	3	0
Small intestine				
Mucosal and submucosal PMN infiltration	2	10	5	3
Mucosal congestion	6	10	5	4
Mucosal edema	1	9	5	4
Mucosal necrosis	0	8	2	0
Mucosal microthrombus	0	8	2	1
Detection of G-bacillus	0	9	5	1

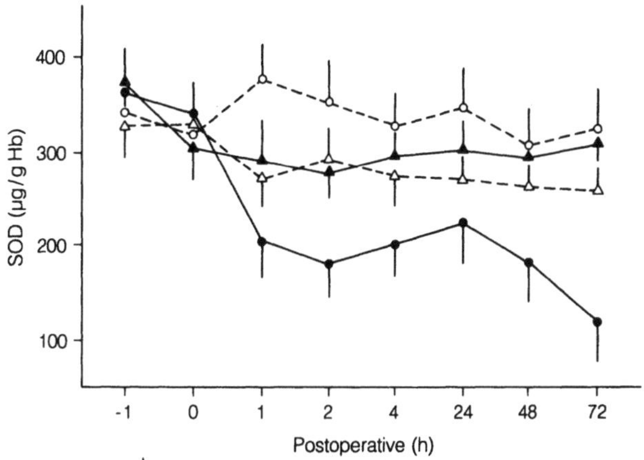

Fig. 11.24. Changes in superoxide dismutase (*SOD*) in the blood of each group. See Fig. 11.23 for key

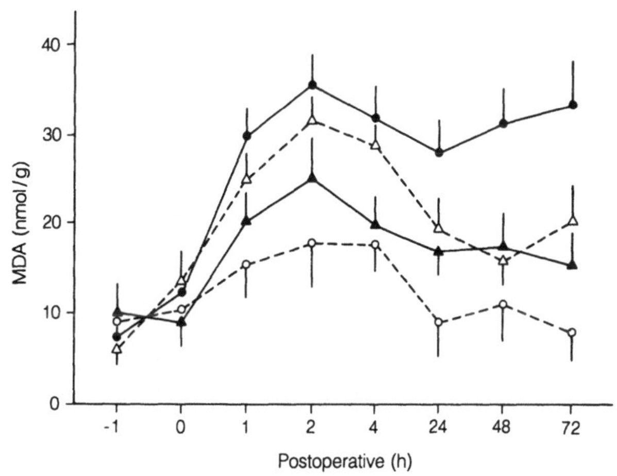

Fig. 11.25. Changes in malondialdehyde (*MDA*) content in the plasma of each group. See Fig. 11.23 for key

trigger of these mediators in early failure may possibly be lipid peroxidation, initiated by reperfusion after prolonged hypovolemia and activation of complement cascade and the multiple organ system, accompanied by translocation of the intestinal flora (or bacterial products) to berpetuate the septic response. Late failure probably represents the sequelae of protein-calorie malnutrition, an exhausted, failing host defense, following a sustained course of strong stress, and also failure of the barrier function of the intestinal mucosa.

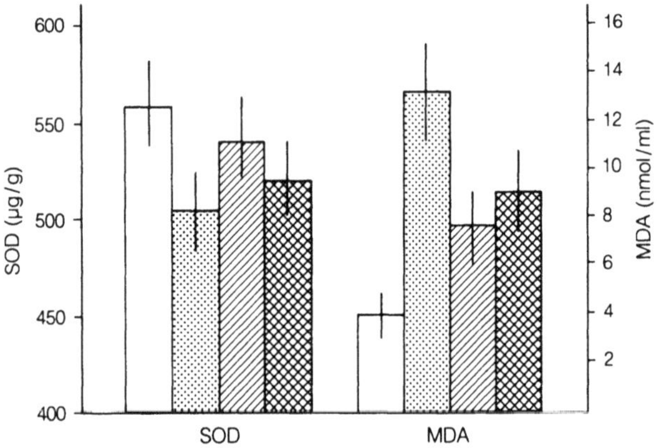

Fig. 11.26. Changes in superoxide dismutase (*SOD*) and Malondialdehyde (*MDA*) content in hepatic tissue. Group I (□), sham operation control; group II (▦), partial occlusion of the superior mesenteric artery for 1 h; group III (▨), partial occlusion of the superior mesentric artery + vitamin E; group IV (▩), partial occlusion of the superior mesenteric artery + rubiside

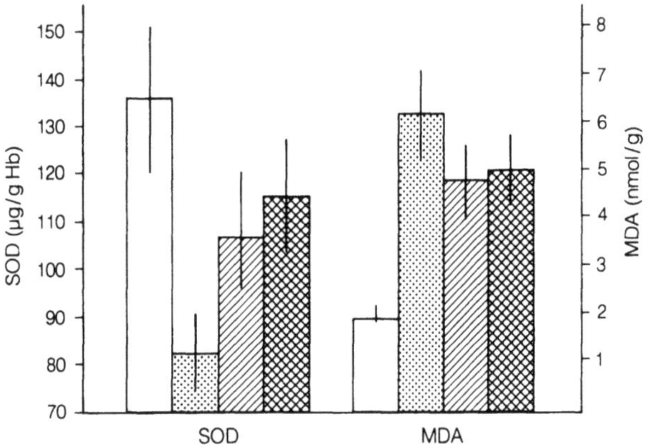

Fig. 11.27. Changes in superoxide dismutase (*SOD*) and malondialdehyde (*MDA*) contents in lung tissue. See Fig. 11.26 for key

11.6 Prevention and Treatment of MOF

11.6.1 Combating Burn Shock as Early as Possible

With all the deleterious effects of hypovolemic shock in mind, one should never hesitate to resuscitate a patient with an excessive amount of deep burns immediately after the injury, or before full-blown shock develops. The problem occurs with the patient suffering from burn shock for some time before being

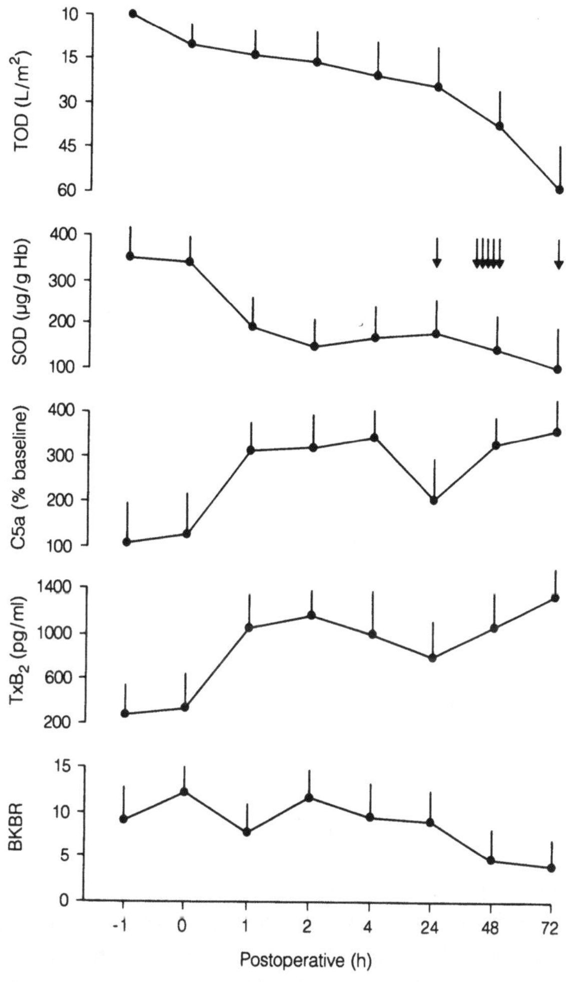

Fig. 11.28. Changes in superoxide dismutase (*SOD*), C5a, TxB_2, blood ketone body ratio (*BKBR*), and tissue oxygen debt (*TOD*) in blood in group II: partial occlusion of the superior mesenteric artery for 1 h (dog). *arrows*, bacteremia

brought to a burn institute for treatment. At least in China, we sometimes see patients to whom resuscitation fluid has been inadequately given and they are transported in a rough way. They usually receive an adequate amount of resuscitation fluids as soon as they reach a burn institute, and their hemodynamic status is quickly stabilized. In such cases, the fluid replacement restores the circulating volume as expected, but, on the other hand, it may create a reperfusion state, engendering free oxygen radicals. We preliminarily demonstrated in our experimental burn model that there is more intensive lipid peroxidation after 4 h of burn shock than after 1/2 h [34]. We postulate that the use of several free radical scavengers such as vitamin E, dimethylthiouria, superoxide dismutase, catalase,

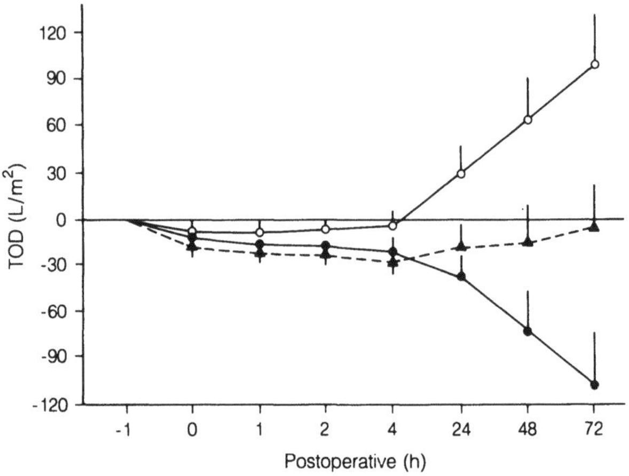

Fig. 11.29. Changes in cumulative tissue oxygen debt (*TOD*) in group I (○——○), survivors in group II (▲---▲), and nonsurvivors in group II (●——●). Group I, sham operation control; group II, partial occlusion of the superior mesenteric artery for 1 h

and others simultaneously with replacement fluids will be beneficial in the prevention of postburn MOF. Some Chinese herbs, such as *Salvia miltiorrhiza*, *Ganoderma lucidum*, rubiside, and *Rubia yunnanensis*, are also promising, but they are still in the experimental stage.

11.6.2 Sound Primary Wound Care

The burn wounds should not be cleansed before the patient is hemodynamically stabilized or until a venous line is installed. The wounds are washed gently with a standard detergent. Loose skin is debrided. A topical antibiotic is used to minimize bacterial growth. Theoretically exposure to dry air increases the depth of damage to the skin. In practice, it makes little difference for deep burn wounds, while infection seems to be delayed when the wounds are allowed to dry. Thus, for circumferential burns of the trunk, the patient is best kept on a air flotation bed in the first 48 h, and then turned over every 2–4 h on a Stryker frame.

11.6.3 Maintenance of the Airway Patency

A patient airway should be carefully maintained, especially in those patients who show signs of respiratory burn. Close observation is essential when the patient is in the prone position, as acute edema of the glottis is prone to occur. It should always be remembered that even a transient hypoxia is devastating to an already highly stressed patient.

11.6.4 Accurate Definitive Surgery with Zero Deficit

It is mandatory that the best part of the deep wounds be excised in stages as early as possible. Necrotic tissue and toxins orginating from the burn wounds are known to possess the effect of activating complements, thus inciting a systemic inflammatory process which, when uncontrolled, may lead to conditions favorable for the development of MOF. Furthermore, necrotic tissue will readily be colonized by bacteria, and extensive infection will ensue. Careful planning is important so that macerated or infected wounds, or anything which impedes respiration, is given priority. No nonviable tissue should be left in place where skin grafting is to be performed. No unexcised superficial wound should remain amid the excised wound, as often the superficial wound becomes the nidus of infection, leading to failure of skin grafting. It has to be emphasized that the best prevention of wound infection is complete closure of the wound.

11.6.5 Good Coverage of the Wounds

All excision wounds should be securely covered with viable skin autograft or allograft. Complete hemostasis should be achieved before the skin grafts are applied. An elastic dressing should be applied to prevent accumulation of blood underneath the skin graft, which is a frequent reason for graft failure and secondary infection. The elastic dressing also assures firm contact of the skin grafts with the raw wound surface, which is absolutely necessary for the take. Failure of skin grafting is often disastrous, and we have had the painful experience of several deaths from MOF as a result of graft failure and subsequent fulminating secondary infection.

11.6.6 Avoidance of Iatrogenic Errors

Our data show that in several instances an iatrogenic error can be blamed for initiating the development of MOF, for example, suppurative thrombophlebitis as a consequence of an inadvertently infected venous line. Most iatrogenic causes should be preventable.

11.6.7 Early Oral Feeding

Recent progress in research on nutrition after extensive burn injury has stressed the importance of early oral feeding. Saito et al. [35] demonstrated that a protein diet was necessary to maintain a healthy state of the intestinal mucosa. Alverdy et al. [36, 37] showed that translocation of the intestinal flora occurred after total parenteral nutrition. O'Dwyer et al. [38] found that glutamine was essential for the integrity of the intestinal mucosa, and glutamine was absent from current parenteral nutritional formulas. Since translocation of the intestinal bacteria may play an important role in precipitating MOF, early oral feeding should be considered a preventive measure against MOF.

As much as 5000–6000 calories of food should be supplied to a patient of average weight with an extensive deep burn. Within this calorie value, the ratio between nonprotein calories and nitrogen in grams should be 100–150:1. As there is usually an intolerance of sugar, as shown by the appearance of persistent hyperglycemia despite ample exogenous insulin, fat can be given to supplement glucose, constituting as much as 60% of the total calorie value. When parenteral nutrition is instituted, it is advisable to restrict the amount of aromatic amino acids, especially phenylalanine.

11.6.8 Appropriate Use of Antibiotics

Improper use of antibiotics may not only produce strains of bacteria resistant to most antibiotics currently used clinically, but also a disturbance of the intestinal flora. Resistant bacteria contribute to a continuation or aggravation of local or systemic infection, while a disturbance of the intestinal flora is one of the major factors which augments bacterial translocation. On the other hand, antibiotics are essential for the prevention of systemic infection, especially in the perioperative periods of wound excision and skin-grafting.

11.6.9 Prevention of Pulmonary Failure

Prevention of pulmonary failure is important because it is usually the first in a sequential failure of organs. It can best be achieved by early support of the lungs using nasotracheal intubation or tracheostomy, assisted ventilation frequently with intermittent mandatory ventilation, or less preferably with positive end expiratory pressure (PEEP), as soon as there are signs of inadequate oxygenation with more or less labored voluntary respiration. When there is circulatory overload jeopardizing the lungs, as evidenced by an excessive rise in central venous pressure, diuresis is necessary. Humidification of the respiratory tract is important, especially if there is a tracheostomy. FiO_2 should be kept as low as possible to avert oxygen toxicity, provided an adequate arterial oxygen tension is maintained. Frequent reevaluation of the PaO_2/FiO_2 ratio is required. Careful monitoring of the colonizing bacteria in the airway greatly helps to combat infection. Needless to say, any restriction of chest wall movement due to the presence of circumferential third-degree burns of the chest or abdomen should be released promptly with escharotomies, followed by excision in a few days when the general condition allows. The administration of systemic steroids should be avoided in view of its questionable therapeutic value and adverse immunodepressive effect.

11.6.10 Hepatic Support

It is difficult to measure early abnormalities in hepatic function. To date, there have been few definitive ways of supporting the liver. Adequate blood flow, prevention of bacterial translocation from the bowel, and nutritional support may be helpful. Indiscriminate use of hepatotoxic antibiotics should be guarded against.

11.6.11 Gastrointestinal Tract Support

The stomach and duodenum are protected mainly by constant emptying of the stomach by suctioning if there is hypotonicity of the stomach. The administration of antacids and H_2 receptor blocking agents to maintain the pH of the gastric contents at or above 4 seems to be useful to a certain extent to eliminate stress ulceration and bleeding. Though the use of allopurinol has been shown to be partially effective in preventing stress ulceration in animal experiments [39], it has not yet been put to clinical trial. It is advisable to use the gastrointestinal tract for early feeding to maintain mucosal activity and the barrier function of the gut.

11.6.12 Kidney

In the early stage, prevention of acute renal failure requires maintenance of adequate circulation and blood flow to the kidneys, and good diuresis. When sepsis sets in, it is important to recognize that a normal or increased urinary output may not necessarily indicate normal renal function as the kidneys may not be able to hold water due to juxtaglomerular tubular injury. The possible methods of supporting the kidneys are removal of necrotic tissues and effective control of systemic infection. Generally, nephrotoxic antibiotics should be avoided. However, when there is an infection by gram-negative bacilli giving rise to a strong indication for the use of an aminoglycoside, its use should be duely considered, because renal impairment is often the result of the infection. Azotemia may diminish with the control of the infection.

References

1. Skillman JJ, Bushnell LS, Goldman H et al. (1969) Respiratory failure, hypotension, sepsis, and jaundice: a clinical syndrome associated with lethal hemorrhage from acute stress ulceration of the stomach. Am J Surg 117: 523–530
2. Tilney NI, Bailey GL, Morgan AP (1973) Sequential system failure after rupture of abdominal aortic aneurynsms: an unsolved problem in postoperative care. Ann Surg 178: 117–122
3. Baue AE (1975) Multiple, progressive, and sequential systems failure: a syndrome of the 1970s. Arch Surg 110: 779–781

4. Fry DE, Pearlstein B, Fulton RL et al. (1980) Multiple systems organ failure: the role of uncontrolled infection. Arch Surg 115: 136–140
5. Cerra FB (1989) The hypermetabolism organ failure complex. World J Surg 11: 173–181
6. Sheng CY, Liu SH (1982) Multiple system organ failure complicating major burns. Presented before the 9th army conference on burn injuries, 1982
7. Liu SH, Sheng CY et al. (1983) Multiple system organ failure complicating major burn injuries. Chin Med J 63(8): 518
8. Dong YL, Sheng CY et al. (1989) Clinical analysis of 68 cases of multiple system organ failure after burns. Gen Surg Clin 4: 246
9. Ozawa K, Aoyama H, Yasuda K et al. (1983) Metabolic abnormalities associated with postoperative organ failure: a redox theory. Arch Surg 118: 1245
10. Hassett J, Cerra FB, Siegel J et al. (1982) Multiple systems organ failure—a very brief summary. Injury. J Accident Surg 14: 93
11. Xu SH, Sheng CY, Zhu YN et al. (1989) Changes of insulin receptors on monocytes in severe burn patients. Presented before 2nd Sino-American conference on burn injury and trauma, May 22–25, 1989, Beijing
12. Cerra FB, Siegel JH, Colman B et al. (1980) Autocannibalism, a failure of exogenous nutritional support. Ann Surg 192: 570
13. Fry D (1986) Multiple-organ-failure syndrome. Arch Surg 121: 201
14. Dong YL, Sheng CY, Li JY et al. (1989) Postburn multiple system organ failure. The characteristics of plasma amino acids profiles. Chin J Surg 27: 541–545
15. Goris RJA, Boekholtz WKF, van Bebber IPT et al. (1986) Multiple organ failure and 'sepsis' without bacteria. Arch Surg 121: 897–901
16. Schirmer WJ, Schirmer JM, Naff GB et al. (1988) Systemic complement activation produces hemodynamic changes characteristic of sepsis. Arch Surg 123: 316
17. Steinberg S, Flynn W, Kelly K et al. (1989) Development of a bacteria-independent experimental model which faithfully simulates the pathophysiology and histopathology of the multiple organ failure syndrome. Presented before the 2nd Sino-American conference on burn injury and trauma, May 22–25, 1989, Beijing
18. Lu JY, Liang YJ (1990) A morpho-pathological study of zymosan induced multiple organ failure in rat (to be published)
19. Dong YL (1990) Clinical and experimental studies on postburn multiple system organ failure. Doctoral thesis
20. Fry DE, Polk HC (1987) Host defense and organ system failure. In: Richardson JD, Polk HC, Flint LM (eds) Trauma: clinical care and pathophysiology. Year Book Medical Publishers, Chicago, p 41
21. Dong YL, Sheng CY, Zhu ZM et al. (1989) Prostaglandin release and multiple system organ failure in severe trauma patients. Chin Med 69: 655
22. Maier RV (1986) Multiple-organ-failure syndrome. Arch Surg 121: 204
23. Zhao ZD, Li A, Yang ZC (1989) The role of lipid peroxidation in the pathogenesis of MOF after burn injury. Presented before the 2nd Sino-American conference on burn injury and trauma, May 22–25, 1989, Beijing
24. Dong YL, Sheng CY, Ban FS et al. (1989) The release of oxygen free radicals and multiple system organ failure in bowel ischemia and reperfusion. Presented before the 2nd Sino-American conference on burn injury and trauma, May 22–25, 1989, Beijing
25. Berg RD (1983) Bacterial translocation from the gastrointestinal tracts of mice receiving immunosuppressive chemotherapeutic agents. Curr Microbiol 8: 285–292
26. Berg RD et al. (1988) Immunosuppression and intestinal bacterial overgrowth synergistically promote bacterial translocation. Arch Surg 123: 1359
27. Deitch EA, Maejima R, Berg R (1985) Effect of oral antibiotics and bacterial overgrowth on the translocation of the gastrointestinal tract microflora in burned rats. J Trauma 25: 385–392

28. Deitch EA et al. (1987) Endotoxin promotes the translocation of bacteria from the gut. Arch Surg 122: 185–190
29. Deitch EA et al. (1987) The gut as a portal of entry for bacteremia. Ann Surg 205: 681–692
30. Maejima R, Deitch EA, Berg R (1984) Promotion by burn stress of the translocation of bacteria from the gastrointestinal tracts of mice. Arch Surg 119: 166–172
31. Lan FS, Shi ZG, Yu Y et al. (1989) Immunosuppression promotes bacterial translocation from intestinal tract and sepsis after burn injury: a pathological study. Chin J Micro Ecol 1(2): 22–27
32. Shi ZG, Yu Y, Lan FS et al. (1989) Penicillin promotes bacterial translocation from intestinal tract in burned SPF rats. Chin J Micro Ecol 1: 53–56
33. Shi ZG, Yu Y, Lan FS et al. (1989) Changes in intestinal flora and their translocation in rat after burn injury. Chin J Micro Ecol 1: 30–33
34. Yang P, Zhu AM, Sheng CY (1990) Changes in oxygen free radical release in relation to duration of burn shock in rabbit
35. Saito H, Trocki O, Alexander JW et al. (1987) The effect of route of nutrient administration on the nutritional state, catabolic hormone secretion and gut mucosa integrity after burn injury. JPEN 11: 1–7
36. Alverdy JC, Aoys E, Moss GS (1988) Total parenteral nutrition promotes bacterial translocation from the gut. Surgery 104: 185–190
37. Alverdy JC, Chi HS, Sheldon GF (1985) The effect of parenteral nutrition on gastrointestinal immunity. The importance of enteral stimulation. Ann Surg 202: 681–684
38. O'Dwyer ST et al. (1987) Glutamine-enriched nutrition decreases intestinal injury and increases nitrogen retention. Br J Surg 74: 1162
39. Gao WY, Sheng CY (1987) The preventive effect of allopurinol on stress ulcer following burns. Chin J Exp Surg 4(3): 114

12 Skin Preservation

Zhu Zhao-ming

12.1 Importance of Skin Preservation

In the case of extensive deep burns, owing to the lack of available donor sites for autografting, or if the patient's general condition is too poor for surgery, wound-covering materials are used to enable the patient to survive the critical period.

There are a number of wound-covering materials of different types. In our experience and that of our Chinese colleagues, homologous skin has proved to be the most effective material. Homograft is not used as a biological dressing; it is changed every 2–3 days as is practised outside China, but if necessary is left on the wound until rejection takes place.

In our clinical practice, it is very difficult to obtain adequate fresh homograft to meet requirements. Often there is no suitable patient requiring skin graft when a fresh homograft is available, and valuable material is thus wasted. Therefore, for a burn unit with regular admissions of patients with extensive burns, it is necessary to install equipment to preserve viable skin in good condition.

Our skin bank for deep-frozen storage of skin (modified from Bondoc [1]) was established in 1973. Since then more than 20 skin banks have been successfully established in China and the survival rate of patients with major deep burns has improved.

With skin storage facilities, not only cadaver skin can be preserved, but autograft left over after skin grafting and the skin from amputated limbs can also be preserved for future use.

As the antigenicity of homologous skin may be attenuated after cryopreservation, the transplanted skin may be able to survive for a longer period.

12.2 Relationship Between Skin Preservation and Structure

Skin consists of epidermis, dermis, and subcutaneous tissue. The stored skin is usually prepared in split thickness devoid of subcutaneous tissue. The quality, viability, and regenerative ability of the skin depend mainly on the basal layer cells of the epidermis. Superficial to the basal cells, there are spinous, granular, clear, and keratin layers as well as a lipid membrane. These layers prevent noxious agents from entering the body, but as far as skin storage is concerned they hinder the penetration of cryoprotective agents through the superficial layers to the basal cells. Unlike the vascularized organs, such as kidney, cryoprotective agents can be perfused via the arteriovenous system. The cryoprotective agent reaches the basal layer of the skin mainly by means of penetration through the dermis. So the skin for storage should not be too thick.

For patients with extensive burns, the area of skin grafting is usually rather large. Accordingly, the size of the stored homograft should not be too small, certainly not smaller than 400–500 cm^2. When the homograft is stored in very large sizes, not only the nonuniform permeation of the cryoprotective agent but also the uneven conductivity of heat due to the thermoinsulating effect of skin itself during cooling and thawing will have an unfavorable effect on the viability of the stored skin.

Embryologically, the epidermis derives from the ectoderm, while the dermis, a connective tissue, originates from the mesoderm. Tissues developed from different origins may react divergently to cooling, i.e., the effects of the same freezing technique on the viability of the cells in these two skin structures are not necessarily identical.

12.3 Skin Preservation in a Refrigerator

The method of storing skin in a common refrigerator at 4°C for future grafting has been widely employed by surgeons. It has the merit of simplicity and convenience and no complicated equipment is necessary, but the preservation time is relatively short.

12.3.1 Storage in Normal Saline

Pieces of skin are immersed in normal saline containing penicillin (400 000 U/500 ml) or gentamicin (80 000 U/500 ml). The amount of skin stored should not exceed 2 cm^2/ml. Skin may be stored in a sterile closed bottle after being wrapped up in a gauze wet with normal saline. The temperature must be kept at 4°C, and in order to minimize variations in temperature every effort should be taken to reduce the number of times the refrigerator door is opened. Our experimental work shows that succinate dehydrogenase (modified Hershey's method [2]) and oxygen consumption (microelectrode method) in the stored skin decrease to 60%–70% of the prestorage values after 3 days of storage, and to 34%–48% after 1 week of preservation. It is likely that transplantation of this type of skin would be unsuccessful. Therefore, when the skin is stored in normal saline at 4°C, it should be used within 3 days.

12.3.2 Skin Preservation with Nutrient Medium

In this technique, cell culture media such as minimum essential medium (MEM), Dulbecco's modified Eagle's medium (DMEM), or RPMI-1640 medium are used as the preservation solutions. These media are balanced solutions containing

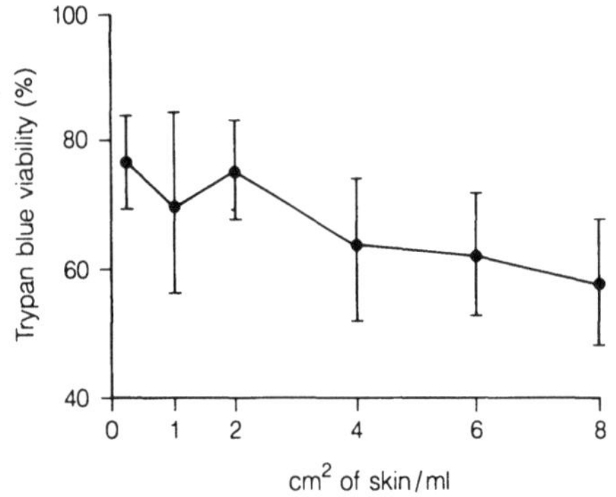

Fig. 12.1. Trypan blue viabilities (fresh skin as 100%) of different ratios of skin and RPMI-1640 (cm^2/ml) stored at 4°C for 1 week

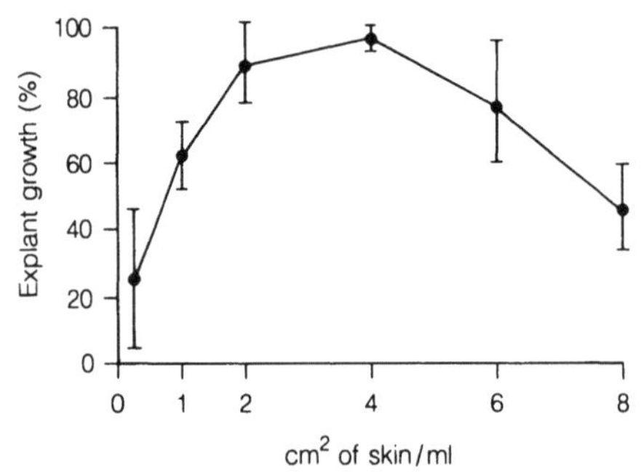

Fig. 12.2. Values of in vitro skin explant (fresh skin as 100%) of different ratios of skin and RPMI-1640 (cm^2/ml) stored at 4°C for 1 week

various amounts of amino acids, vitamins, trace elements, and a buffer system necessary for cell growth and metabolism. The powdered ingredients are dissolved in distilled water according to the prescription and the adjusted to pH 7.3–7.4. The solution is then filtered with a Millipore filter for sterilization. Of the media mentioned above, RPMI-1640 is the best, and is even better if 10% bovine serum is added. In order to find out the best ratio of the amount of skin to that of the stored medium, homologous skin pieces were immersed in RPMI-1640 medium in the following proportions: 0.2, 1, 2, 4, and 6.8 cm^2/ml, and stored at 4°C for 7 days. The viability of the tested skin pieces was assayed by means of trypan blue dye exclusion, [^{14}C]leucine incorporation, and the in vitro skin explant method. It was shown that 2–4 cm^2 to every milliliter of medium was the best for maintaining the viability of the skin (Figs. 12.1–12.3). Too small an amount of stored medium is inadequate to meet the needs of skin nutrients, leading to metabolite accumulation, resulting in a decrease in pH and adverse effects on the viability of the skin. If too much medium is added, it will be more

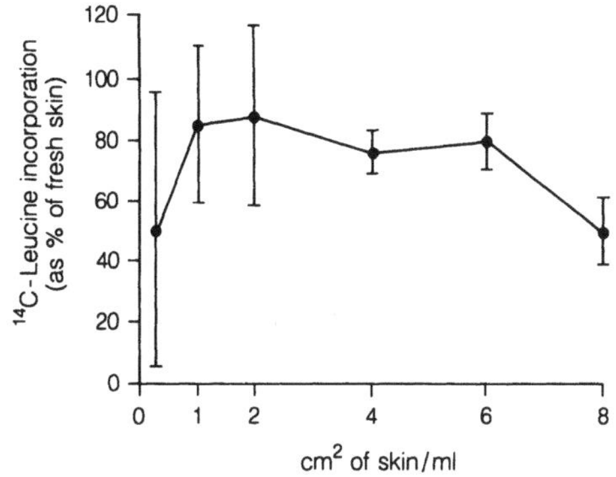

Fig. 12.3. [^{14}C]Leucine incorporation into protein value (fresh skin as 100%) of different ratios of skin and RPMI-1640 (cm^2/ml) stored at 4°C for 1 week

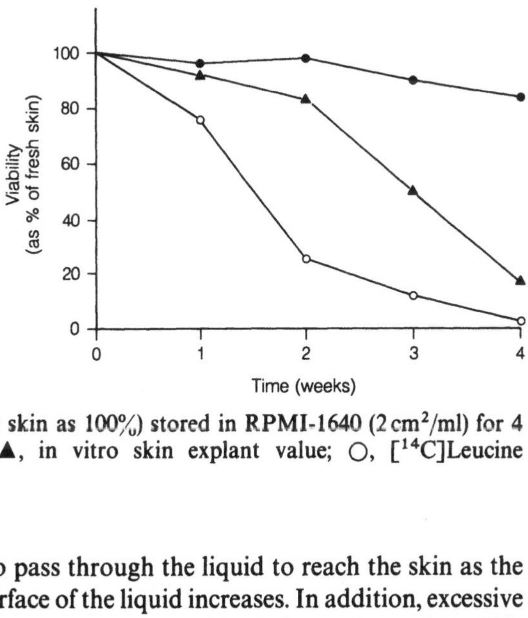

Fig. 12.4. Viabilities of skin (fresh skin as 100%) stored in RPMI-1640 (2 cm^2/ml) for 4 weeks. ●, trypan blue value; ▲, in vitro skin explant value; ○, [^{14}C]Leucine incorporation into protein value

difficult for oxygen in the air to pass through the liquid to reach the skin as the distance from the skin to the surface of the liquid increases. In addition, excessive liquid causes an increase in hydraulic pressure, which also exerts an unfavorable influence on skin viability. Stored at 4°C by this method, on average, the skin would retain 95% the viability of normal skin after 1 week, 50% after 2 weeks, 30% after 3 weeks, and 20% after 4 weeks (Fig. 12.4). Electron microscopy after 1 week of preservation showed intact fine ultrastructures of the organelles, with only scanty vacuole formation (Fig. 12.5).

According to the above-mentioned results, skin kept in the refrigerator at 4°C with RPMI-1640 should be used within 2 weeks. Within the 1 week there is little difference between the viability of the preserved skin and fresh skin. A preservation period of 2 weeks will reduce the viability down to 50% and considerably reduce the therapeutic effect of skin grafting.

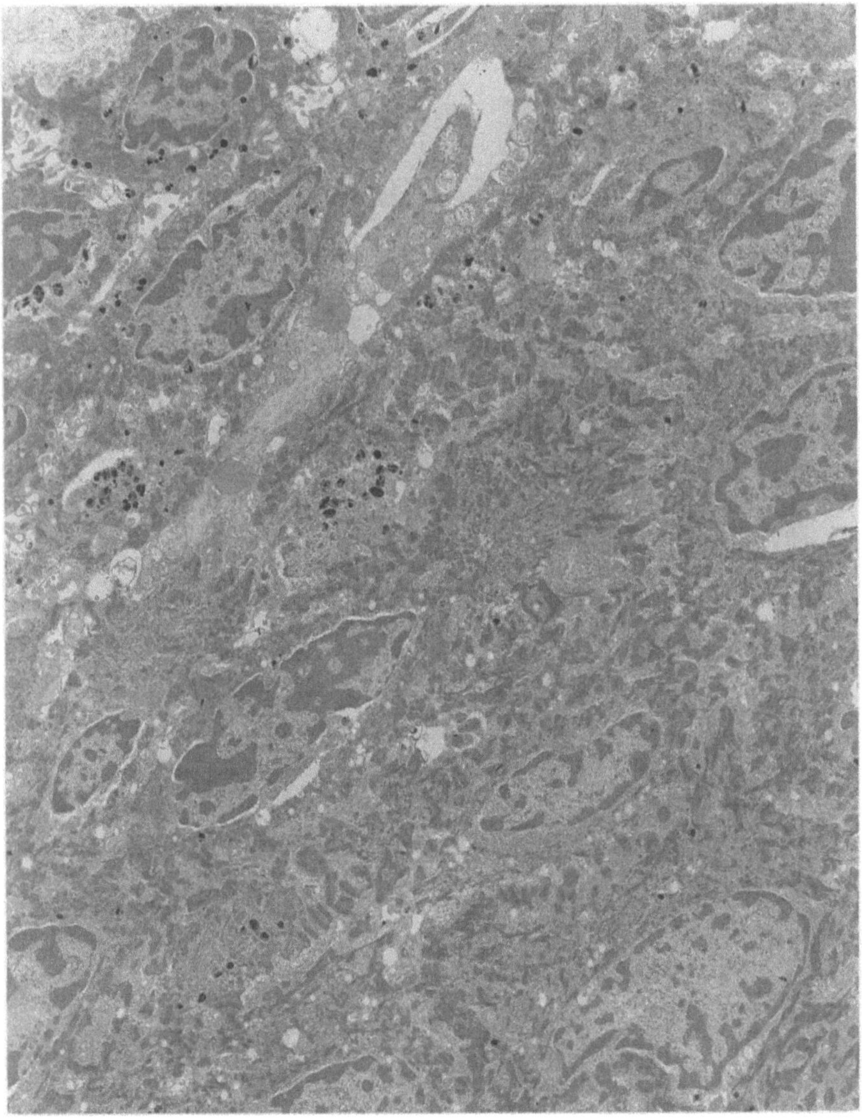

Fig. 12.5. Electron microscopy of skin stored in RPMI-1640 ($4\,cm^2/ml$) for 1 week showed an intact ultrastructure of organelles with only scanty vacuole formation, × 7800

12.4 Cryopreservation of Skin by Deep Freezing

12.4.1 Importance of Deep Freezing

The skin stored at 4°C will lose its viability substantially by the end of the 2 week, and cannot therefore fulfill the clinical requirements. During deep freezing (usually at −80°C or −196°C), especially at −196°C in liquid nitrogen, the metabolism of the cells is decreased to a very low level, being nearly completely inhibited, and the cells are kept in a so-called life suspension state. Theoretically, cells or tissue could be preserved under this condition for an indefinite period. It has been shown in our clinic, the 304th Hospital of the People's Liberation Army, that skin is still intact and suitable for grafting after preservation in liquid nitrogen for 15 years. Hence, when deep-freezing facilities are available to supply homografts whenever the need arises, surgeons will no longer have to worry about the source of skin.

12.4.2 Mechanism of Freezing Injury to Skin

When the ambient temperature decreases to 0°C, the water in tissue will form ice crystals and induce a series of changes. When the temperature is less than 0°C, extracellular water begins to crystallize first. The crystal grows from a droplet form to a tubular structure, then assumes a reticular configuration, and eventually forms a large piece of ice. The extracellular ice crystals can injure cells by direct crushing, but this is not the main cause of cellular injury.

When extracellular water begins to crystallize, the remaining unfrozen part of the extracellular fluid will become hypertonic, and the cell will be surrounded by a hyperosmotic environment. It has been reported that the concentration of extracellular fluid of mammalian tissue will increase tenfold when the ambient temperature is decreased to −5°C. The hypertonic extracellular fluid will induce cell shrinkage and injury to the membranous structure and internal structures of the cell. This constitutes the major cause of cellular damage at low temperatures.

As the extracellular water crystallizes, the buffer system of the acid-base balance will be disturbed. As a result, partial pressure of toxic gas and toxic substances such as urea will elevate. All these will aggravate cellular injuries.

In nature, the spores of some bacteria and the eggs of certain animals such as frogs and silkworms can tolerate temperatures down to −24°C. In contrast, ordinary tissues and cells will lose their viability after freezing if no special preventive measure is undertaken. The lowest temperature which mammalian cells can tolerate is −5°C.

12.4.3 Measures to Reduce Skin Injury During Freezing

12.4.3.1 Use of Cryoprotective Agents

Cryoprotective agents are divided into two groups: penetrating and non-penetrating. The most-used agents of the former group are dimethylsulfoxide (DMSO), propylene glycol, and glycerine. The latter group consists of polyethylene, polyvinylpyrolidone (PVP), albumin, hydroxy starch, mannitol, etc.

The mechanism of cryoprotective action is not yet very clear. The probable beneficial effects of the cryoprotective agent are: (a) to decrease the speed of ice crystal formation so as to diminish the crystal size and reduce the pressure exerted on the cells, thereby mitigating cell damage; (b) after passing through the membrane and entering the cell, to attract and pull the intracellular water molecules so that crystallization is markedly retarded; and (c) to smoothen the course of thawing and protect the cell from injury induced by abrupt diminution of pressure. Nonpenetrating cryoprotective agents should be used at higher concentrations than penetrating ones and with a longer treatment period; otherwise the cryoprotective effect is not achieved.

The cryoprotective agent itself, especially at high concentrations, has a certain toxic effect on cells. The viability of skin will be decreased markedly when it is immersed in a protective agent for too long a period. Therefore, every effort should be taken to minimize the toxic effect, with the prerequisite that the cryoprotective action has been brought into play.

There are several methods of decreasing the toxicity of cryoprotective agents: (a) reduce the concentration of the agent; (b) shorten the immersion time in the agent; (c) use several cryoprotective agents in combination and; (d) raise the atmospheric pressure during treatment of the skin with the cryoprotective agent. Under high pressure, the toxic effect of the protective agent is lessened somewhat because the temperature at which the fluid produces crystals declines. It is a pity that this method is scarcely practical due to the complicated equipment and processes required.

12.4.3.2 Control of Cooling Rate

There are two ways to transfer skin from 4°C after being treated with a cryoprotective agent to deep-frozen environment.

Slow Cooling Method. The temperature is usually decreased by 1°–3°C/min to – 60°C or – 80°C, and after being kept at that temperature for 4–12 h the skin is finally placed directly into liquid nitrogen. Although the slow cooling method is favorable in reducing freezing injury of cells, it is unable to prevent completely the hyperosmotic dehydration effect induced by freezing.

The ideal equipment for the slow cooling process is the microcomputerized controlled-rate cooling apparatus, in which liquid nitrogen is used as the cooling source. Liquid nitrogen is sprayed into the cooling vessel at defined intervals controlled by a microcomputer, so that the temperature in the vessel decreases at a preset rate. Another method is to place the skin in a deep freezer (– 80°C) with the pieces of skin separated from one another. Measurements show that a cooling rate of around 1°–3°C/min can also be achieved by this method (Fig. 12.6). Thirdly, a gradual cooling effect can also be achieved by hanging the skin in a liquid nitrogen container high above the liquid surface, and then lowering it step by step until the skin is finally immersed in liquid nitrogen.

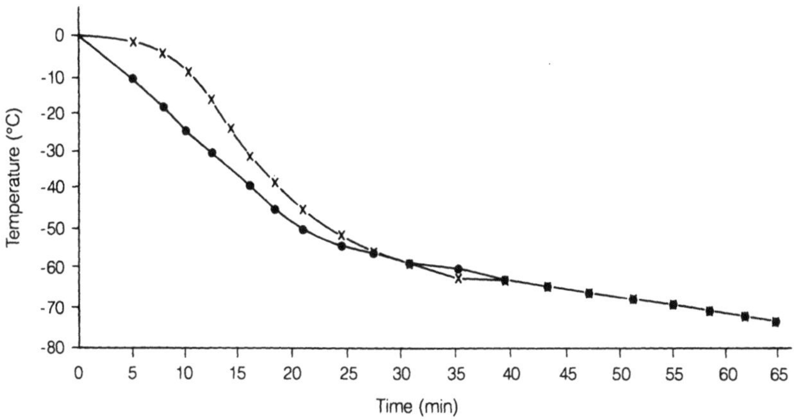

Fig. 12.6. Cooling rate of skin in a −80°C deep freezer. —×—, thermocouple placed between two layers of skin; —●—, thermocouple placed between a plastic bag and the skin

Since 1973, we have preserved homografts by the slow cooling method, and this skin has been used in more than 400 cases of major deep burns. The viability of the preserved skin processed by this method is only 50%–60% that of fresh skin as assayed with the trypan blue dye exclusion test, succinate dehydrogenase determination, and oxygen consumption measured with the microelectrode method. When transplanted onto burn wounds, this preserved skin can act as a wound coverage, but sometimes blisters are formed under the epidermis and the take is not as satisfactory on heavily colonized granulation wounds. Therefore, the quality of the skin stored by this method needs further improvement.

Rapid Cooling Method. This is also called the vitrification method. The skin temperature after being treated with cryoprotective agents is quickly reduced to − 196°C. Under such rapid cooling conditions, the water both inside and outside the cells is not allowed to form crystals but only to increase in viscosity. The water inside the skin approaches a homogeneous state like glass, and the cellular damage caused by ice crystals and the hyperosmotic state during freezing is thus reduced. In order to obtain a satisfactory result, the type and concentration of cryoprotective agent should be reconsidered for vitrification.

No reports on skin stored by the rapid cooling process have been published in China or elsewhere up to the present. We investigated this area with different types of cryoprotective agent for vitrification and different sizes of guinea pig skin as test samples. The viability of stored guinea pig skin was determined. A solution (H solution) composed mainly of a combination of DMSO and propylene glycol was selected, and was found to have a lower toxicity and a higher cryoprotective effect during vitrification. The viability of skin stored by this method was about 20% higher than that of skin subjected to the slow cooling method used previously. The results with homograft stored by this method used previously.

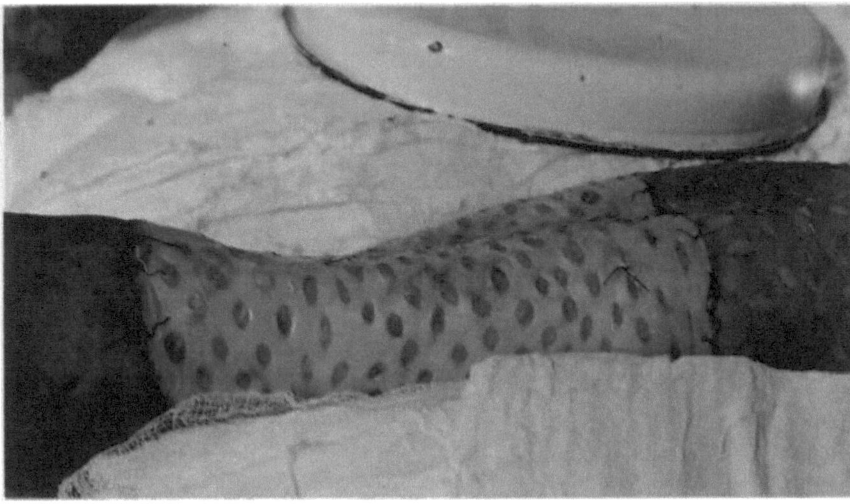

Fig. 12.7. A 45-year-old man sustained third-degree burn of 90% TBSA. Escharectomy of the left leg was performed on the tenth postburn day. The wound was covered by homograft stored by slow cooling (*upper part of leg*) and by rapid cooling (*middle part of leg*). The photograph was taken on the fifth postoperative day. The color of the homograft stored by rapid cooling (*bright red*) is better than that stored by slow cooling (*brown*)

Table 12.1. Comparison of viability of skin ($500\,cm^2$) stored by vitrification and slow cooling

Groups	Oxygen consumption (%)	Succinate dehydrogenase (%)	Mean viability (%)
Vitrification ($N = 70$)	85.5 ± 9.4	72.8 ± 2.6	$79.2 \pm 5.4^*$
Slow cooling ($N = 70$)	61.4 ± 3.8	58.1 ± 5.5	$59.7 \pm 4.7^*$

$^*p < 0.05$.

The results with homograft stored by this method were the same as with guinea pig skin (Table 12.1).

A quantity of $100\,000\,cm^2$ homograft was stored with the rapid cooling method and transplanted onto the wounds after escharectomy in 30 patients with major deep burns, and a take of over 91% of the transplanted homograft was observed. The color of transplanted homografts turns reddish very quickly, with occasional blister formation. Satisfactory take has been seen even when homograft is transplanted onto infected granulation wounds. These clinical results indicate that the quality of skin stored by rapid cooling is better than that preserved by slow cooling (Fig. 12.7).

12.4.4 Control of the Thawing Rate

The stored skin can be used clinically only after being thawed to above 0°C when it is removed from liquid nitrogen. During the course of thawing, the pressure exerted on the skin cells changes rather rapidly, especially when the temperature rises to the range of – 30°C–0°C, in which ice crystals both inside and outside the cells undergo a course of repeated crystallization and recrystallization; which in turn will damage the cells. Therefore, the thawing rate should be as rapid as possible, in order to shorten the course of recrystallization of ice. Skin should be thawed in a water bath with a relatively large volume of water, the temperature of which is maintained at 40°C with a stirrer.

12.5 Procedure for Skin Storage by Deep Freezing

1. Selection of cadaver: The cadaver should not remain at room temperature for longer than 6 h or in a refrigerator after death for longer than 24 h. Infectious disease, tumor, jaundice, or dermatological disease should not be present at the time of death.
2. Large sheets of skin with subcutaneous tissue are flayed from the cadaver under nonaseptic conditions and transported to the skin bank in an ice box for further processing.
3. Large sheets of skin with subcutaneous tissue are shaved, washed thoroughly with soap and water, and rinsed with tap water. After beng rinsed with 1/1000 bromogeramine solution for 15 min, the skin is washed with sterile normal saline. From this point on, further processing is done with the aseptic technique. The subcutaneous tissue is removed with a dermatome; thus the skin thickness is reduced to 0.3–0.4 mm. The skin is finally trimmed into sheets 500–1000 cm^2 in area.
4. The skin is placed in a sterile container, and 10% DMSO balanced solution or 20% glycerol balanced solution is added for slow cooling storage. The skin should not be left in DMSO for longer than 15 min, while 2 h are required for glycerol solution. If the vitrification method is used, the skin should be treated with a specific cryoprotective solution (H solution) for 30 min. The whole process is performed under 4°C.
5. Skin sheets should be removed from the cryoprotective solution in time, and they are then transferred into plastic bags. Large sheets can be folded once, but wrinkles should be smoothed. The bags are labeled, securely sealed, and put directly into a liquid nitrogen container for vitrification storage.
6. In the slowing cooling method, the plastic bags are kept in a deep freeze (– 80°C) or a container with dry ice (– 79°C) for 4–12 h. Then the bags are quickly transfered into a liquid nitrogen container.
7. Whenever homograft transplantation is to be performed, the plastic bags are rapidly taken out of the container and thawed immediately in a 40°C water bath until the skin becomes soft. The thawing time is usually not longer than 3 min.

8. The bag is sterilized with 75% alcohol and the sealed edge of the bag cut open. Then the skin is taken out from the plastic bags with the aseptic technique and washed with normal saline to remove the remnants of the cryoprotective agent. Then the skin is ready for transplantation. In order to obtain better results, the skin should be used immediately after thawing. The skin should not be left of room temperatures for too long. The remainder of the skin should be discarded and should not be refrozen for storage again.

12.6 Determination of Skin Viability

The outward appearances such as color, flexibility, and elasticity of the preserved skin do not differ from those of fresh skin. Therefore, the quality of skin cannot be judged by gross inspection. Methods for appraisal of the viability and quality of the stored skin should be carried out to judge whether the skin should be transplanted to the patients, and these methods form the essential constituents of the research work into skin storage.

12.6.1 Trypan Blue Dye Exclusion Method

A quantity of 0.25% trypsin is used to digest the test skin in a 37°C water bath for 1 h and in 4°C overnight. A suspension of 0.1 ml epidermal cells is removed and 0.4 ml 0.1% trypan blue solution is added to it. After mixing, one drop of the cell suspension is placed in the bloodcell-counting chamber and 100 cells examined under the light microscope. The blue-stained cells are dead ones and the unstained cells are viable cells. The percentage of unstained cells counted is regarded as the viability percentage. This method is simple and quick to perform and no specific apparatus is required. The result can be obtained in 1–2 h. However, false results can sometimes be encountered, which can be caused by the adhesion of a rather large quantity of protein-like substance to the surface of the dead cells, thus preventing the dye from entering the interior of the dead cells. Besides, errors in the digestion process of the skin could also influence the result of the determination.

12.6.2 Quantitative Determination of Succinate Dehydrogenase in Epidermal Cells

The mitochondria of basal layer epidermal cells contain succinate dehydrogenase, the main function of which is to catalyze succinic acid by dehydrogenation to form fumaric acid. This biochemical process is an important link in the Kreb's cycle of energy metabolism. Quantitative determination of this enzyme reflects skin viability.

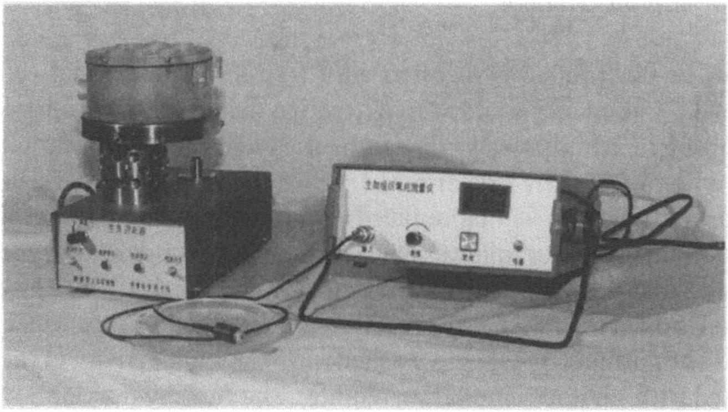

Fig. 12.8. Apparatus for determination of oxygen consumption of skin

$$\text{Sodium succinate} + \text{red tetrazoline} \xrightarrow[\text{dehydrogenase}]{\text{Succinate}} \text{fumaric acid} + \underset{\text{(red precipitate)}}{\text{formazan}}$$

The determination procedure is as follows: After weighing the skin sample to be determined, it is cut into small pieces and placed in the bottom of a Thunberg's tube containing sodium succinate and red tetrazoline. Air is removed and the tube filled with nitrogen. Then the test solution is poured to the bottom of the tube and incubated at 37°C for 1 h. The skin pieces, which are now stained red with formazan, are taken out and the red color extracted with ethylene glycol ether for 4 h. The extract is subjected to colorimetric determination with a wavelength of 490 μm in a spectrophotometer. The result is expressed as OD/mg weight of skin.

12.6.3 Determination of the Oxygen Consumption of Skin with Microelectrodes

The main principle of this method is that the viable tissue undergoes metabolism and thus consumes oxygen. In a nutrient medium at constant temperature, the partial pressure of oxygen on the surface of the microelectrode (platinum and silver electrodes) in contact with the viable skin is reduced. The degree of reduction of the partial pressure of oxygen can be recorded with a magnifier; thus the viability of the skin can be recorded. The entire determination can be completed within 1 h (Fig. 12.8).

12.6.4 Isotope Incorporation Method

The skin sample to be determined is digested with trypsin, an epidermal cell suspension is made. [^{14}C]Leucine is added to determine the percentage isotope incorporated with protein. Alternatively, ^{3}H can be used and the incorporation rate of the isotope with nuclear DNA determined. When the viability of the cells decreases, the incorporation rate will be reduced accordingly. A simple way of performing this determination is as follows: The isotope solution is added to the epidermal suspension and incubated for a certain length of time at 37°C. Then trichloroacetic acid is added to interrupt the reaction. The residual isotope which is not incorporated with protein or DNA is washed out. The radioactivity of the sample is determined with a liquid scintillation counter, and thereby the viability of the skin can be calculated. The unit used is decay per minute per milligram of protein in cell suspension.

12.6.5 In Vitro Skin Explant

Using a sharp knife, the skin sample is cut into small pieces each 0.2–0.3 mm in size. They are put into a culture plate with 24 small wells together with culture medium, and incubated in a CO_2 incubator at 37°C. At the end of 7 days, outgrowth of cells from the periphery of the skin specimens in any one well indicates that the test skin is viable. Percentage viability is calculated according to the number of wells with proliferation of cells.

12.6.6 Animal Transplantation Test

The skin to be determined is cut into small pieces and transplanted onto the back of mouse, rabbit, or nude mouse without thymus. The transplant is examined 5–7 days later. If the skin graft is soft with adequate blood circulation, it indicates that the graft is in good viable state.

12.6.7 Electron Microscopy of Skin

The skin sample is regarded as having satisfactory viability when the ultrastructures of the epidermal cells are intact and no abnormalities are seen, especially when there are no vacuoles and edema in the intercellular space or inside the cells. This method is not as sensitive as others and the result is only conjectural. In brief, there are a number of methods to determine the viability of skin, each of them reflecting one aspect of the biological function of the skin. Therefore, they are all biological assays and a number of factors can influence the results of each determination. Thus, it would be more reliable if more than two methods were used concomitantly, and the average percentage viability (as compared with that of the fresh skin) obtained. Of the above-mentioned methods, trypan blue dye exclusion, succinate dehydrogenase determination, and oxygen consumption determination are comparatively simple, speedy, and reliable, and generally only 1–2 h are needed to obtain the results. Usually several days are required for other methods to give results; therefore, they can only be used in research work in the field of skin storage.

References

1. Bondoc CC, Burke JF (1971) Clinical experience with frozen human skin and a frozen skin bank. Ann Surg 174: 371
2. Hershey FB, Cruickshank CND, Mullins LI et al. (1958) The quantitative reduction of 2,3,5,tri-phenyl tetrazoline chloride by skin in vitro. J Histochem 6: 191

13 Epithelial Cell Culture and Its Clinical Application in the Treatment of Burns

Wang Wen-zheng

13.1 Introduction

The human skin is a complex organ in structure and function. There are at least four types of cell present in the epidermis. The skin keratinocytes are the major epidermal cells. This cell or a related stem cell has the capacity to form both the stratified epithelium of the epidermis and the epidermal appendages found largely in the dermis.

The melanocytes are the second type of cell found in the epidermis, and provide pigment for the keratinocytes. The third type of cell present in the epidermis is the Langerhans cell, which is found in the mid-epidermis with cytoplasmic processes. These dendritic cells extend between the keratinocytes down to the junction of the dermis and epidermis. They appear to belong to the reticuloendothelial system and are involved in immunological reactions of the skin. The fourth type of cell in the epidermis is called Merkel's cell.

The complex system of immune response-associated cells present in normal skin is defined as the skin immune system (SIS). B lymphocytes are absent from normal human skin; lymphocytes of the SIS are exclusively T cells. Lymphocytes are relatively rare in the dermis, and account for less than 2% of the total number of T cells in the normal skin. Most of the intradermal T cells belong to the $CD8^+$ suppressor-cytotoxic T-cell subset.

The human epidermis, because of its availability and well-characterized pattern of growth and differentiation, is particularly suitable for adaptation to cell culture and facilitates a variety of experimental studies. Several culture systems for better growth of adult human keratinocytes in vitro have been established [1].

The epidermal cell culture discussed in this chapter takes into account the cultivation of keratinocytes only. Isolation and cultivation of other kinds of epidermal cells are found elsewhere.

Owing to the rapid progress in the field of cell culture, rapid growth of confluent sheets of epidermal cells suitable for grafting a large surface area can be obtained, and a viable graft sufficient to cover extensive deep burn wound can be grown a few weeks after injury. This provides new prospects for improvements in burn care [2].

13.2 Basic Methodology

13.2.1 Types of Epidermal Culture

Different types of epidermal cell culture have been established for the investigation of various problems [3].

Organ Culture. These cultures are often used to maintain full-thickness skin, the skin blocks usually being attached to the bottom of the culture vessels and submerged in the culture medium.

Explant Culture. This is established primarily to obtain an outgrowth of a stratifed sheet of epithelial cells from split-thickness skin explants. Skin blocks are attached to the bottom of the culture vessels.

Cell Culture. Epidermal cells are dispersed and plated in a substrate. The inoculated cells may be epidermal cells, including keratinocytes, and some melanocytes and Langerhans cells; pure keratinocytes; or cocultured with fibroblasts.

Suspension Culture. Dispersed epidermal cells or explants attached to the surface of microcapsules (Cytotex), which float in a methycellulose solution.

Air-Exposed Culture. The epidermal cells or explants are plated onto a substrate (collagen film, dermal equivalent, or artificial skin), which is raised to the air-liquid interface during cultivation [4].

Combination Cultures. Cells are grown in one type of culture at first, and then transferred to a second or even third type of culture.

Selection of culture system depends on the specific question to be explored and the experience and equipment available.

13.2.2 Media and Supplements

13.2.2.1 Basic Medium

Dulbecco's modified Eagle's medium (DMEM), TC199 medium, McCoy's 5A medium, and Ham's F-12 medium have been recommended, but these were originally designed for the culture of cells other than keratinocytes; therefore they are not suitable for keratinocytes culture, especially in serum-free cultures. An improved serum-free culture system has been developed by Boyce and Ham, which is specifically designed for normal human epidermal keratinocytes. The basic nutrient medium adapted in the system is MCDB 153 [5].

13.2.2.2 Serum

Epidermal cell culture is rarely successful unless chemically defined media are supplemented with serum. A concentration of 10%–20% by volume is commonly used, although a lower concentration of appropriately selected batches of serum is often satisfactory. Recent reports shows that keratinocyte cultures have been performed in serum-free medium with some success [6, 7].

Investigations have shown that serum can be substituted by bovine or human serum albumin (1%) to provide the necessary factors for the cultivation of epidermal cells in a serum-free culture system.

13.2.2.3 Growth Factors

Epidermal Growth Factor. Epidermal growth factor (EGF) is a single-chain polypeptide consisting of 53 amino acid residues and exhibiting potent mitogen activity for a variety of cell types in vivo and in vitro. EGF was first described by Cohen, and it was isolated from submaxillary glands of adult male mice. The gross effects of EGF are to prevent differentiation, increase mitosis, and especially increase the motility of the epidermal cell. In tissue culture, EGF stimulates the net accumulation of RNA and protein, increases the activity of isolated ribosome for cell-free protein synthesis, induces a rapid conversion of ribosomal monomers into functional polymers, and increases ornithine decarboxylase activity.

Cyclic AMP. Cyclic AMP stimulates both growth and maturation. The end effect depends on the proportion of cells in each stage, which may be activated in either growth or maturation.

Insulin and Transferrin. Insulin and transferrin are cell growth factors, which are necessary components of the culture medium for most cell strains. Insulin is a weak mitogen but a type of anabolic stimulating agent for maintaining a healthy growth of cells, and for improving the mitogenic activity of other growth factors.

Steroids. Steroids (hydrocortisone, dexamethasone) increase the proliferation of keratinocytes in both the presence and absence of serum.

Whole Bovine Pituitary Extract [5]. Boyce and Ham reported that the growth of epidermal keratinocytes in serum-free culture was improved by whole bovine pituitary extract (WBPE), which was the only undefined supplement in his culture system. WBPE is stored at $-20°C$ for at least 6 months. The concentration of WBPE used in culture is 70 μg/ml and 700 μg/ml for frozen storage of epidermal cells.

Others. Triiodothyronine ($2 \times 10^{-9}\,M$), ethanolamine (0.1 mM), and phosphoethanolamine (0.1 mM) have been recommended for the culture of human keratinocytes.

13.2.2.4 Metal Ions

Many types of metal ion have obvious effects on the growth of epidermal cells in vitro, of which calcium and selenium are notable. The reduction in calcium ion concentration shifts the balance between cell growth and maturation to one of growth. The increase in concentration of calcium ion shifts the balance to maturation.

A marked effect of selenium in promoting clonal growth of keratinocytes has been reported.

13.2.2.5 Vitamin A

It has been reported that vitamin A regulates differentiation, increases proliferation, and decreases keratinization. The lowered serum levels permit expression of in vivo like traits and high-molecular weight keratins, more keratohyalin granules, and increased nuclear destruction [7].

13.2.2.6 pH

Growth studies of keratinocytes in vitro show optimal growth and maturation at pH 7.2–7.4. But reduction of the culture medium pH to 5.8 has been reported to facilitate growth of the epidermal cells.

13.2.3 Substrate [8]

Human epidermal cells are anchorage dependent and require substrate to attach to, grow, and function. Proliferation capacity and growth requirements of keratinocytes can be markedly influenced by the type of substrate on which they are plated and maintained. The growth of keratinocytes is facilitated by collagen and/or fibronectin. Type IV collagen shows increased attachment of keratinocytes when compared with other collagen types. The substrate has been noted to have major effects on the morphology and growth characteristics of keratinocytes with chemical modification of collagen or changes in the content of the extracellular matrix.

Acid-soluble collagen is extracted and purified from various tissue sources according to the types of collagen to be used, or it is purchased. Laminin, fibronectin, and other components of the extracellular matrix, and the coating agents (polylycine, protamine) can also be purchased.

13.2.4 Examination of Cultured Epidermal Cells

13.2.4.1 Routine Observation

The growth pattern of the cultured epidermal cells can be closely observed daily under the inverted-phase contrast microscope, and recorded by photography. Contamination from fibroblast, bacteria, or fungus, and fibroblast overgrowth should be monitored and treated carefully and properly.

13.2.4.2 Staining of Keratinocyte Colonies [9]

Rhodanile Blue Method. Rhodanile blue is an aqueous solution of 1% rhodamine B and 2% Nile blue A, prepared by mixing equal volumes of filtered 2% solution of the two compounds. The cultures are rinsed briefly with tap water and fixed for at least 20 min with 10% formalin in neutral phosphate-buffered saline. The fixed cultures are stained for 30 min with rhodanile blue, and then rinsed under running tap water for 30 s to 2 min to remove excess stain and achieve differential staining of the feeder layer and the keratinocyte colonies.

Acid Fuchsin-Aniline Blue-Orange G Method. A modification of the Mallory connective tissue stain has been found to be useful for cultured keratinocytes.

The fixed cultures are stained for 3 min with 5% acid fuchsin solution (w/v) in distilled water, rinsed briefly with running tap water, stained for 45 min in aniline blue-orange G solution (a distilled water solution 0.5% water-soluble aniline blue, 2% orange G, and 1% phosphotungstic acid), rinsed quickely three times with 95% ethanol and once with absolute ethanol, and then drained and air dried in an inverted position.

Giemsa Stain. The cultured epidermal cells can be fixed and stained with Giemsa stain as recommended for general histology.

13.2.4.3 Quantitative Methods for Measuring Cell Growth

Cell Count. Cell number is most commonly obtained by counting well-dispersed cells or nucleus suspensions in a standard hemocytometer chamber or counter.

The dye exclusion test for cell viability depends upon the fact that viable cells do not take up certain dyes whereas nonviable cells do. A 0.4% aqueous solution of either trypan blue or erythrosine B can be used.

Measurement of Surface Area. A more convenient method is the use of a calibrated ocular micrometer. The diameter of a colony or explant may be measured in two or more directions in one plane, then the surface area of a monolayer of the epidermal cell sheet can be roughly calculated by the formula for the area of a circle.

NAG Colorimetric Method [10]. A rapid colorimetric assay for human epidermal keratinocyte growth in culture is based on the color reaction of NAG (ρ-nitrophenol-N-acetyl-β-D-glucosaminide), and the result is recorded by spectrophotometer. The result of this method correlates well with cell count.

Other Methods. Determination of cell protein concentration of the cultured cells and determination of the DNA-synthesizing cells by autoradiography after a [^{3}H]TdR pulse are two other methods.

Kinetic Parameters of Epidermal Cell Growth. This is based on the data from measurement of cell number or surface area. The growth curve, expected doubling time, mitotic index, and mitotic time can be calculated.

13.2.4.4 Histological Examination

Light Microscopy. The cultured epithelium is fixed in 10% buffered formalin and embedded in paraffin, and sections are stained with hematoxylin and eosin, argentaffin, or periodic acid-Schiff stain.

Electron Microscopy. The specimens are fixed in 3% glutaraldehyde, postfixed in osmium tetroxide, dehydrated in alcohol, and embedded in epoxy resin. Ultrathin sections are contrast stained with uranyl acetate and lead citrate, and examined under the electron microscope.

Immunofluorescent Examination. The specimens are frozen in liquid nitrogen, stored at $-80°C$, and examined by immunofluorescence using conventional methods for the presence of various markers of human epidermal differentiation.

13.2 Current Culture Systems

Three standard culture systems used for the culture of human epidermal keratinocytes for autologous or allologous grafts are available.

13.3.1 Cell Culture System [1, 2, 11, 12]

13.3.1.1 Procedure

Preparation of Skin Specimens. For autologous graft the split-thickness skin samples are obtained from unburned area (axilla or scalp), usually within the first few days after admission. For allograft the skin samples can be obtained from skin removed at surgery. The skin blocks are placed aseptically into bottles containing sterile DMEM medium plus 5% fetal calf serum (FCS) for transport to cell culture laboratory, and are processed within 2 h.

The skin samples are rinsed with serum-free medium in a culture dish three times. The skin blocks are fixed on a wooden block with the dermal side upward. The subcutaneous fat and deeper portion of the dermis are removed, and then cut into pieces about 3 × 3–8 mm in size.

Preparation of Dispersed Cell Suspension. Separation of the epidermis proceeds by either floating skin fragments in a solution of 0.25%–0.3% trypsin at 4 °C for 12–16 h, or placing the skin fragments in a flask equipped with a magnetic stirring bar and stirring at 37 °C in a trypsin solution for 30–45 min. A 0.2% trypsin solution plus 0.2% collagenase or Dispase (1.2 U/ml) may also be used. After enzymatic digestion, the epidermis is removed easily from the dermis by gentle blowing with a pipette in DMEM solution, filtered through nylon cloth, and counted. The cell suspension is diluted with complete DMEM growth medium to the desired cell density.

Medium and Supplements. The basic medium of DMEM is supplemented with 10%–15% FCS or NCS (new born calf serum), penicillin 100 U/ml, streptomycin 100 μg/ml, amphotericin B 2.5 μg/ml, bovine insulin 5 μg/ml, hydrocortisone 0.4 μg/ml, EGF (epidermal growth factor) 5–10 ng/ml, and cholera toxin 10^{-9} *M*. Several authors have also used 3:1 DMEM and F12 medium as the basic medium with success.

Preparation of a Substrate. Collagen coating of the culture dishes is performed by adding sufficient solubilized collagen in 0.1 *M* acetic acid to yield 10 μg protein/cm^2 dish surface. The growth surface substrate is ammonium hydroxide fume cross-linked, or cross-linked by adjusting the collagen suspension to physiological pH and ionic strength and jelly at 37 °C.

Fibronectin is diluted in the medium to a concentration of 10 μg/ml and dispensed into a culture dish precoated with collagen. The dishes are incubated at 37 °C for 20–30 min, washed with warm D-Hank solution, and are then used immediately for cultivation.

Primary Culture. Dispersed epidermal cell is suspended in complete culture medium containing 10% FCS, antibiotics, and other supplements. The cell number is counted, the percentage of viable cells is estimated, and plating is performed using a cell density of $4 \times 10^4/cm^2$. The dishes are incubated at 37 °C in an atmosphere of 5% CO_2 in air saturated with water vapor. The medium is changed after 24 h and twice weekly thereafter.

Subculture. Once the cells have reached confluence, passage can be attempted by withdrawing the medium and adding a solution of 0.25% trypsin in calcium-free and magnesium-free Hank's solution. The separation is monitored under an inverted microscope. Approximately one-half of the cells at the free edge of the cell sheet which have floated free from the surface cells are withdrawn and centrifuged for 5 min at 500 rpm, and resuspended in the medium.

The cells are then replated in new flasks. The original flasks are again kept in the incubator if the parent cultures are to be continued.

Cryopreservation and Thawing. Exponentially growing keratinocyte cultures are dispersed to single cells and resuspended at a concentration of 2×10^5 to 10^6 cells/ml in the medium supplemented with serum. Sterile glycerol is added to a strength of 10%, and the suspension is introduced into 2-ml glass or plastic ampules with a pasteur pipette. The temperature of the ampules is slowly brought down to −190 °C by placing them within a Styrofoam container, exposing them to the vapors of liquid nitrogen for at least 2 h, before storing them in the freezer.

Ampules are thawed by placing them in a 37 °C water bath. The thawed suspension is transferred to a plastic centrifuge tube with a pasteur pipette, 10 volumes warm medium plus serum are slowly added in drops, and the suspension is then pelleted, resuspended in the culture medium, and plated at the desired density.

13.3.1.2 Growth Characteristics of Keratinocyte Cultured in the Cell Culture System

The dissociated epidermal cells attach either individually or in clumps within a few hours of seeding, the time and efficiency of cell attachment being dependent on the substrate type, medium ion concentration, and state of differentiation of the inoculated cells. Attached cells spread, proliferate, and form cell colonies within 25–48 h after seeding. By continuous proliferation they become confluent and form a monolayer. This may occur in a few days, or in weeks, depending on cell density and supplements (Figs. 13.1, 13.2).

Once the cells are confluent, they begin to stratify into layers that differ from one another morphologically and correlate with the state of differentiation.

Basal cells organize themselves into a single layer of loosely associated squamoid or cuboid cells that attach to the substrate. The cytoplasm of the cultured basal cells contains abundant mitochondria, a well-developed Golgi zone, a few cisternae of rough endoplasmic reticulum and vesicles of smooth endoplasmic reticulum, melanosomes, and abundant free ribosomes and polyribosomes. The nucleus contains one or more large nucleoli. Cytoskeletal elements present in cultured basal cells include microtubules, microfilaments, and small bundles of keratin filaments. Structurally complete hemidesmosomes have been recognized in cultured epidermal cells.

Bullous pemphigoid antigen is synthesized by basal cells (Figs. 13.3, 13.4).

The basal cells join together and with cells of the first intermediate layer by desmosome and gap junction, and in some places by intercellular spaces.

Basal cells in long-term stratified cell cultures often contain lipid, multivesicular bodies, and other secondary lysosomes. Basal cells in culture, as in vivo, synthesize DNA, proliferate, migrate upward, and undergo differentiation. Intermediate layer cells are flat and have an elongated nucleus oriented with

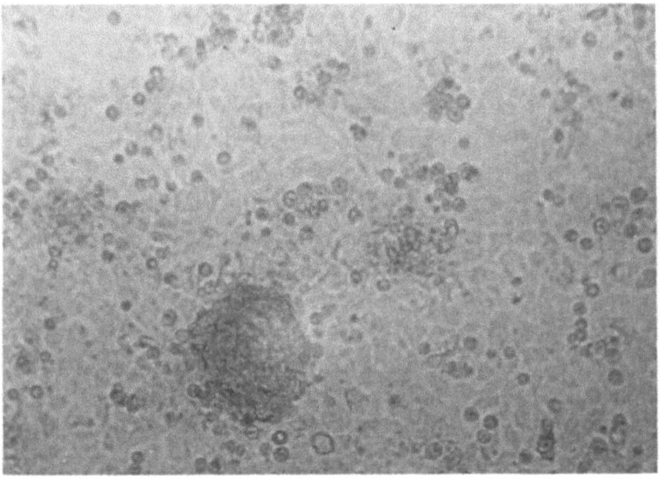

Fig. 13.1. Pattern of attachment, spread, and growth of human epidermal cells on the surface of extracellular matrix substrate in a cell culture system (2-day culture). Inverted microscopy, × 160

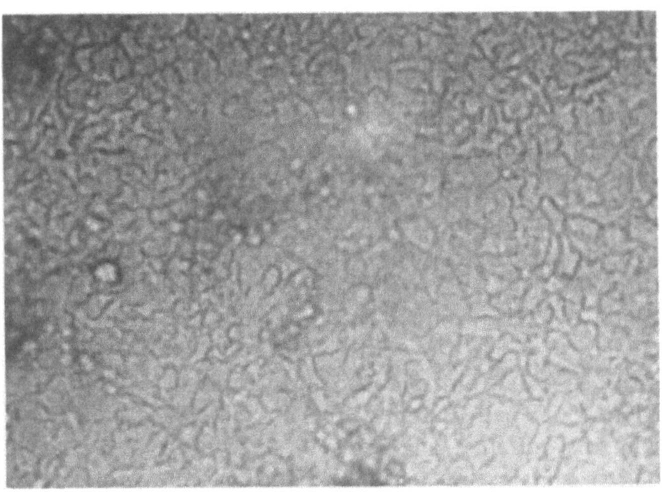

Fig. 13.2. Confluent culture of human keratinocytes in a cell culture system 2 weeks after plating. Note the typical closely packed polygonal cells with a cobblestone appearance. Inverted microscopy, × 160

the long axis of the cell. They join with one another by desmosomes, but cells from each layer are usually widely separated and have microvilli on the upper and lower surfaces. Keratin filaments are more abundant in intermediate cells than basal cells and have more prominent associations with desmosomes. Intermediate cells contain the organelles that are associated with cellular

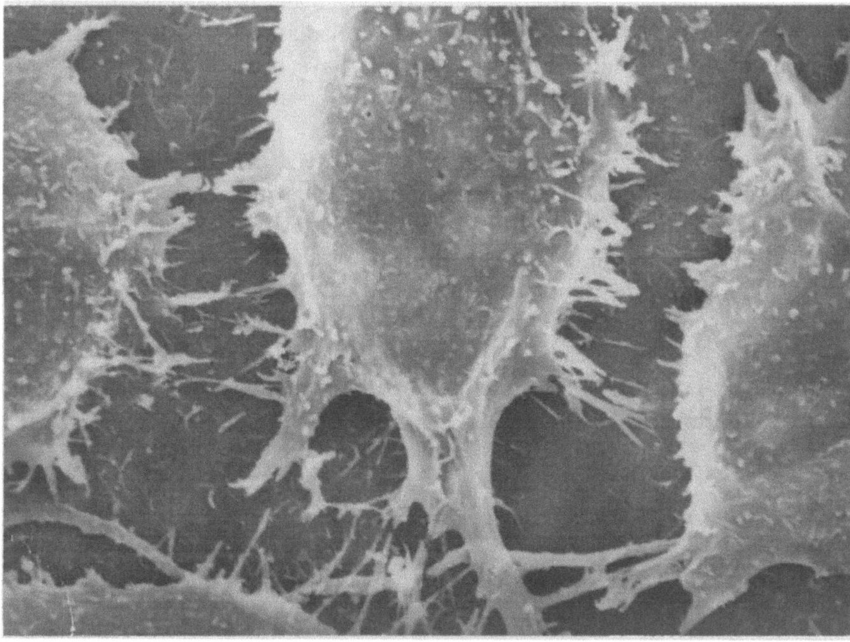

Fig. 13.3. Scanning electron micrograph of a few keratinocytes cultured for 6 days in a cell culture system. Note the pseudopodia extending from the cell body, × 3000

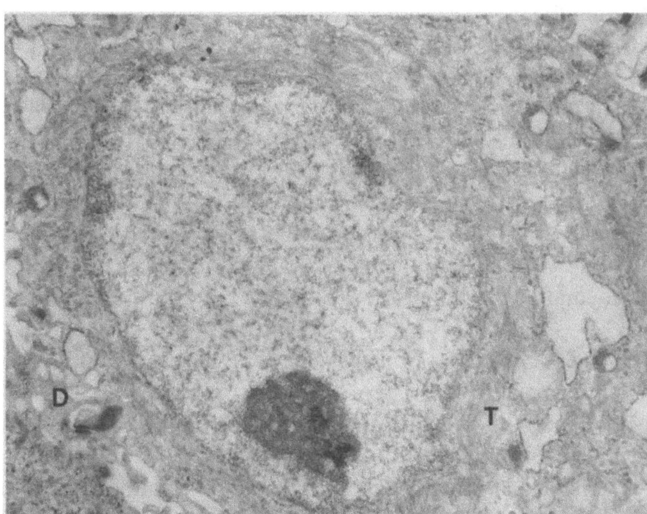

Fig. 13.4. Electron microscopic appearance of cultured human epidermal keratinocytes in a 30-day culture. Note the abundant tonofilament (*T*) and typical desmosomes (*D*), × 17 000

metabolism, and degenerative vacuoles and glycogen. Pemphigus antigen and upper-cytoplasmic antigens are present in intermediate cells. Histocompatibility antigens of the *H-2* locus and weak *H* loci have been detected in cultured epidermal cells. The numbers of cell layers in the intermediate zone depends on the culture system and the age of the culture.

The upper layer zone includes only two cell layers. All the cells in the upper zone have a cornified cell envelope, and many cells retain the nucleus in some stage of degeneration, some cells lacking a nucleus. Most are filled with keratin filaments, and some still contain keratohyalin granules.

The life span of a primary epidermal cell culture depends on the ability of the culture conditions to support cellular proliferation. Culture can be terminated in 2–3 weeks or can survive up to 6–10 weeks. When culture conditions limit differentiation, the epidermal cells can be maintained in a monolayer for up to 1 month.

13.3.2 Feeder Layer Culture System [1, 7, 9, 13]

Application of the 3T3 feeder layer to the cultivation of human epidermal keratinocytes has been successfully established by Rheinwald and Green (1975).

13.3.2.1 Procedure

Skin Source and Preparation of Cell Suspension. These are similar to those in the cell culture system.

Preparation of 3T3 Feeder Layer. The established fibroblast line 3T3, developed from random-bred Swiss mouse embryo cells, is used as the feeder cells. Confluent 3T3 culture is rendered reproductively dead by irradiating with 6000 rads of γ-rays from a cobalt source, or by incubating with 4 μg/ml mitomycin C for hours. Treated 3T3 culture is trypsinized and replated as a feeder layer at slightly more than one-third of its confluent density (approximately 2×10^4 cells/cm^2) 1 day before the seeding of the keratinocyte suspension.

Culture Medium and Supplements. The basal medium used is DMEM, and it is supplemented with 15%–20% FCS (selected lots), hydrocortisone 0.4 μg/ml, penicillin 100 U/ml, streptomycin 100 U/ml, and amphotericin B 2.5 μg/ml for primary keratinocyte culture growing with 3T3 feeder cells.

Epidermal growth factor 10–20 ng/ml is added to the medium in the first refeeding of the primary keratinocyte cultures 4 days after plating and at subsequent refeedings until subculture. DMEM is supplemented with 10% FCS, penicillin 100 μ/ml, and streptomycin 100 mg/ml for the growth of 3T3 cells.

Primary Culture of Keratinocytes in the 3T3 Feeder Layer. Dispersed epidermal cell suspension is plated in complete DMEM plus 10%–20% FCS at 10^4–10^5 cells/100-mm dish containing 3T3 cell feeder cells.

Five to seven days after plating, dishes yielding 100 and 1000 keratinocyte colonies are purified by incubating at room temperature for 30 s in 0.2% ethylenediaminetetra-acetic acid (EDTA) solution, followed by vigorous pipetting to dislodge dermal fibroblasts and the 3T3 feeder layer, while the keratinocytes remain firmly adhered to the dishes.

Fresh 3T3 feeder cells are then added back to the culture medium, and the keratinocyte colonies are allowed to continue their growth until subculture, EGF is included at 10 ng/ml in the first refeeding of the primary keratinocyte cultures 4 days after plating and at subsequent refeedings.

Subcultivation. The subconfluent cultures of growing keratinocytes are first taken from their feeder layer as described above. The keratinocyte colonies are then dispersed to single cells by incubating with 0.05% trypsin plus 0.01% EDTA at 37 °C for 15–30 min. An equal volume of DMEM plus 20% FCS is added to the suspension to stop the enzyme action. The cells are counted with a hemocytometer, pelleted by low-speed centrifugation, resuspended in an appropriate volume of complete DMEM medium, and seeded in densities ranging from 10^3 to 10^5 cells/60-mm culture dish with a standard number of 3T3 feeder cells.

Cryopreservation and Thawing. These are similar to the techniques described for the cell culture system.

13.3.2.2 Growth Characteristics of Keratinocyte Culture on 3T3 Feeder Cells

The keratinocytes attach directly to the culture flask surfaces in the first few hours, and then spread by migration and proliferation to form colonies. As the colonies expand, they push away the reproductively dead 3T3 feeder cells.

The displaced feeder layer cells often appear as a rolled-up cuff at the periphery of the colonies. The keratinocytes are closely packed in a polygonal epithelioid arrangement (Fig. 13.5). After 1 week, the feeder layer density begins to decrease through cell detachment, resulting in rapid expansion of large colonies, centrally located cells become slightly more flattened after the feeder layer is removed, and exponential growth of the colonies continues until the culture is confluent.

The majority of the cells in a growing colony are basal cells with an intermitotic time of about 24 h. The expanding keratinocyte sheet tends to stratify and undergo terminal differentiation. The growing colonies, enlarge, di-sulfide-link their keratins, and eventually form a cornified envelope. The morphological characteristics of stratified epithelium are similar to those described for the cell culture system.

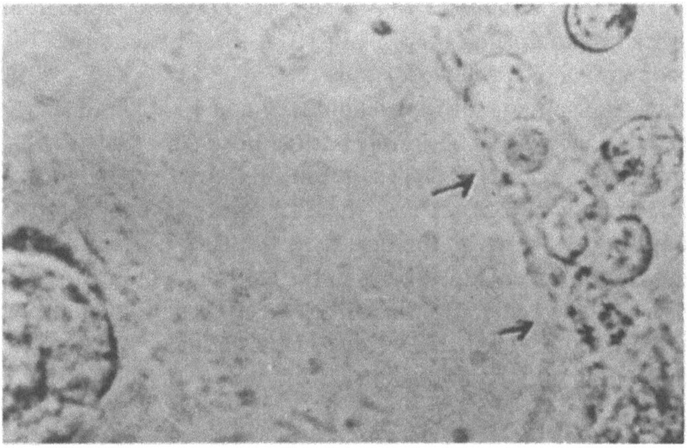

Fig. 13.5. A typical keratinocyte colony grown in a 3T3 feeder layer culture system 6 days after coculturing. Note the 3T3 cells are pushed away by rapid expansion of the keratinocyte colony. Inverted microscopy, × 160

In preparaton for cell suspension, a number of fibroblasts with colony-forming potential are also released from the skin, but they grow very slowly when surrounded by a dense monolayer of 3T3 feeder cells. Selective removal of fibroblasts with EDTA 1 week after plating and the addition of fresh feeder layer cells for the remainder of the culture period eliminates all or nearly all the dermal fibroblasts. If necessary this operation is repeated 1 week after plating the secondary culture.

13.3.3 Explant Culture System

Explant culture of the human skin is one of the oldest tissue culture techniques. Specific media have been developed and tissue culture ware and controlled environments have improved along with the efficiency of the method.

Since the explant culture is simple, it is suitable for all sources of skin. There is no need to disperse tissues with enzymes, and no requirement for a feeder layer. The explant culture system has been adopted by some laboratories to obtain keratinocyte growth for burn wound coverage. However, proliferation of epidermal cells using this method is insufficient to produce the large amounts of epidermis required for grafting extensive burns, and fibroblast overgrowth in the culture is a troublesome problem.

13.3.3.1 Procedure

Tissue Source and Preparation. These are similar to those of the cell culture system.

Medium and Supplements. The basal medium used is DMEM, which is supplemented with 10% FCS, penicillin 100 U/ml, streptomycin 100 mg/ml, amphotericin B 2.5 μg/ml, hydrocortisone 0.4 μg/ml, insulin 5 μg/ml, and EGF 10 ng/ml.

Primary Culture. The skin sample is stretched and fixed after being rinsed in PBS. If possible, the subcutaneous tissue and dermis are removed with scissors, and cut into blocks (1 × 1 mm) with a scalpel or razor blade.

The blocks are transferred to a tissue culture dish, are equally spaced, and are allowed to stand in the incubator to let the fluid decrease by evaporation. Just before they are completely dried out, complete medium is added and incubated at 37°C and 5% CO_2. The medium is changed every 3–4 days.

Subcultures. The use of 0.25% trypsin in 0.04% EDTA for 5 min at 37 °C has been found effective in dissociating the epidermal cell sheet into a monocellular suspension. With slow centrifugation much of the horny material remains suspended; plating of the pellet results in more than 90% cell attachment.

13.3.3.2 Growth Characteristics of Keratinocytes in Explant Culture

The epithelial cells begin to grow out from the tissue block within a few days after explantation. This occurs by a process known as epiboly, during which the epidermal cells grow down from the side of the block onto the dish.

After a lag period of about 24 h, epithelial cells in the explant extend outward onto the surface of the culture dish like a circular apron of cells. This outgrowth appears to be function of cell migration rather than proliferation. The radial outgrowth of the epithelial cells progresses, with the leading edge of the cells giving a slight scalloped appearance (Fig. 13.6). The outgrowth is made up of cells approximately 50 μm in diameter with distinctive oval nuclei and one to six prominent nucleoli. These cells synthesize bullous pemphigoid antigen (BPA) and secrete type AB_2 collagen. Basal laminin becomes evident by day 7.

After the outgrowth reaches several millimeters in length, stratification occurs, beginning immediately around the explant and expanding outward with the growing cultures, so that a monolayer exists only near the leading edge. A confluent culture is formed by the extension of the outgrowth from the adjacent explant.

During the first 48 h BMA appears beneath all the migrating cell surfaces, and the appearance of type IV collagen and laminin lag behind.

Epithelial cell outgrowth occurs more rapidly than that of the fibroblasts, although ultimately it is restrained and the fibroblasts overtake the culture. If fibroblast outgrowth is troublesome, it can be controlled by careful trypsinization or by other measures.

A series of degenerative changes followed by regeneration characterizes the survival of the original skin blocks in explanted cultures. In the first few days,

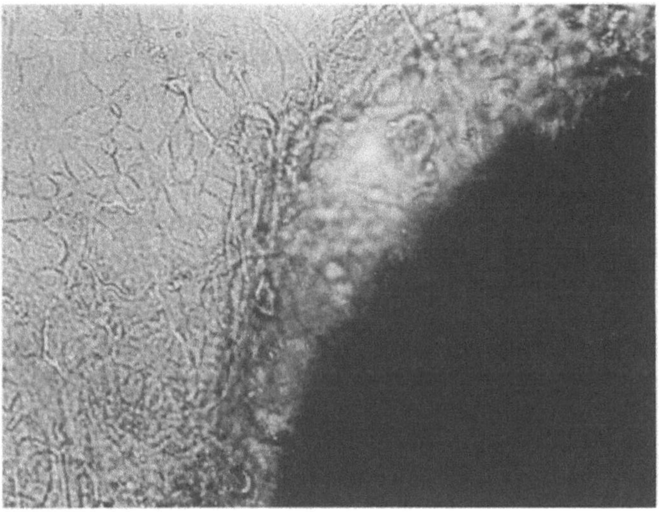

Fig. 13.6. Pattern of outgrowth of human epidermal keratinocytes from the edge of a skin block in an explant culture system 14 days after plating. Inverted microscopy, × 160

the tissue appears hyperproliferating, and parakeratotic and orthokeratotic cells may form. Cells of the basal layer begin to pull apart from one another. The original stratum corneum usually separates from the newly formed epidermis. Subsequently, the hyperplastic epidermis layer degenerates and detaches. The secondary epidermis regenerates from the remaining foci of basal cells. This tissue also stratifies but in fewer layers, keratinization is incomplete, and the tissue architecture is disorganized.

The dermis, like the epidermis, initially appears hyperplastic, and then fragments and degenerates, followed by incomplete regeneration.

13.4 Clinical Application of Cultured Epidermis in the Treatment of Burns

There are three types of clinical application of cultured epitheliun in the treatment of burns.

13.4.1 Cultured Autograft [2, 11, 14–17]

Cultured autograft, which is grown from a small skin biopsy specimen from the burned patient, is grafted to full-thickness burn wound. The graft grows to cover the burn wound. This method has been successfully used in the treatment of extensive burn wound and has proved to be lifesaving. Ten patients treated with cultured autologous epidermis have been reported by Gallico and O'Connor.

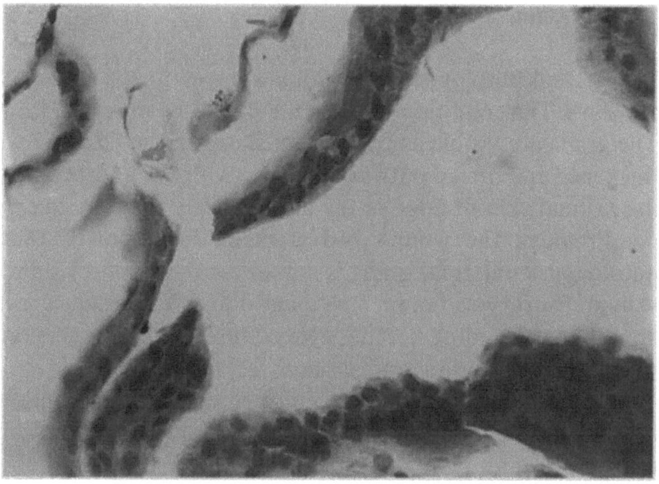

Fig. 13.7. Section of a cultured human epidermal sheet in a 30-day culture, H&E × 60

13.4.1.1 Preparation and Grafting of Cultured Epidermis

The thickness of the epidermis formed after cultivation for 2–3 weeks ranges from two to seven or more cell layers. It can be detached as a coherent sheet from the culture flask with the aid of enzyme Dispase II, which is neutral protease. The use of this enzyme facilitates easy handling and minimizes contracture and fragmentation of the cell sheet (1.2 U/ml medium, GODO Shusel, Tokyo, Japan) (Fig. 13.7).

The epithelial sheet is washed with serum-free culture medium, and it is then attached basal side up to a piece of petrolatum (Vaseline) gauze with hemoclips. The gauze together with the epithelial sheet is transported to the operating room in cooled culture medium.

The burn wounds which have been excised and covered with allografts or other types of skin substitute during the early postburn period should be prepared by peeling off the allografts or skin substitutes, careful hemostasis, and washing the wound bed with normal saline-containing antibiotics.

The cultured epidermis is placed onto the prepared site with the basal cell layer against the recipient bed. It should be sutured to the wound edge, or held in place by a single layer of petrolatum gauze and covered with several layers of sterilized gauze. The outer layers of the dressing are changed daily, and the petrolatum gauze is removed 5–8 days after grafting. The dressing is changed when necessary for 10 days. Thereafter, the graft is left exposed.

13.4.1.2 Clinical Follow-up

The grafted autologous epithelium adheres to the underlying tissue within a few days. The condition of the graft should be observed from the first dressing. The grafts are visible as translucent sheets in the first 1–2 weeks; they are then thickened and spread outward to merge with one another, meeting the surrounding normal skin or edge of the autograft during subsequent weeks.

Provided the wound bed is clean, the reported take rate of cultured autologous epidermal grafts is still lower than that of standard split-thickness skin grafts, varying between 80% and 100%. The results are influenced by many conditions, including keratinocyte culture technique, general patient condition, wound bed condition, and surgical tcchniqucs.

Wound contraction of the cultured epidermal autografts is similar to that in split-thickness skin grafts, depending more on anatomical body site than on the type of grafting employed. Usually there is a contraction to 60%–70% of its original size.

The cultured grafts appear similar to split-thickness skin grafts in thickness, durability, and texture after $\frac{1}{2}$ year. The cosmetic appearance of the cultured grafts appears to be superior to that of split-thickness skin graft after 5 years.

Identification of the growth of cultured cell sheet in the grafted area should be established by serial skin biopsies, using conventional microscopy and electron microscopy.

13.4.1.3 Morphological Maturation of Grafted Epidermis

After adhering to the wound bed, the epithelium thickens uniformly within 1 week and develops both granular and cornified layers above the basal layer.

The ultrastructural features are those of an epidermis with keratinocytes at different stages of their terminal differentiation.

The dermoepidermal junction is linear (Fig. 13.8); the rete ridges are lacking at first, but form slowly over a minimum of $\frac{1}{2}$ year. A delicate basement membrane can be seen 1 week after grafting, and an increase in thickness is noted progressively.

Collagen type IV, laminin, and basement membrane zone (BMZ) antigen can be identified. Melanocytes with dendritic processes can also be identified, but Merkel's cells are never found.

Langerhans cells and class II antigen are absent in the cultured epithelium, but Langerhans cells with Birbeck granules can be found 1 month following grafting, indicating their recipient origin. These changes suggest that the cultured epithelium, although not fully differentiated, may successfully regenerate a permanent epidermis after grafting.

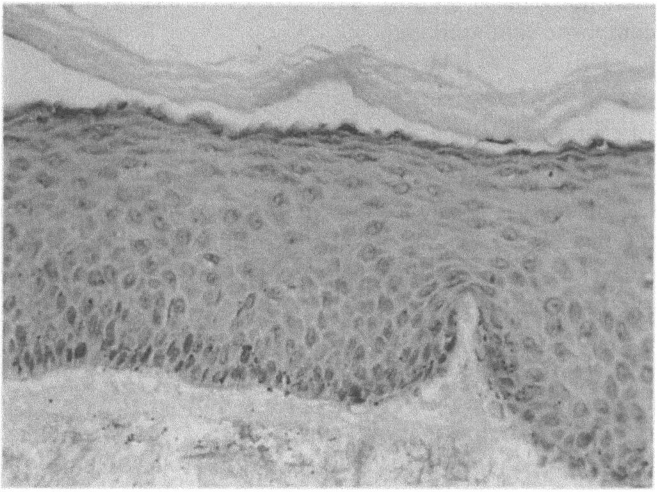

Fig. 13.8. Section of a cultured human epidermal autograft 1 month after grafting on a third-degree burn wound. Note the well developed epidermis with orthokeratosis on the surface and absence of skin appendages. H&E ×400

13.4.1.4 Progress and Problems

The availability of sheets of cultured epidermal cells for the treatment of large surface area wounds can provide a virtually unlimited source of graftable autologous skin for permanent wound coverage. Therefore cultured epidermal graft is a major advance in the treatment of extensive burns.

However, despite the successful results obtained, several problems remain to be solved: The use of cultured autologous grafts necessitates an interval of 2–3 weeks for the growth of a sufficient quantity of epidermis; they are initially more vulnerable than split-thickness skin grafts; the lack of dermal structure in the cultured epidermis leads to less take and more contraction. Skin fragility in the healed epidermal autograft and spontaneous blistering within the sites of the graft have been reported, and discontinuous lamina densa and sparse anchoring fibrils in the reconstituted basement membrane beneath the grafts may be the causative factors. The lack of formation of epidermal rete ridges and dermal papillae in the reconstitution of the grafted wound may contribute to poor epidermal-dermal adherence in the autografted sites. The search for the ideal skin substitute, which will take less time to produce and give better cosmetic results with no blistering, wound contraction, or scarring, continues.

13.4.2 Composite Skin Graft

Since wound contraction and scarring following skin graft are inversely proportional to the dermal thickness, and the use of cultured epidermal autograft does not replace the lost dermis, research has been carried out to develop a composite skin graft.

13.4.2.1 Composite Autologous-Allogeneic Skin Graft [18]

Cuono reports a composite skin grafting method for the management of the severe burn. The graft is composed of allogeneic dermis and autologous epidermis. The allograft skin is grafted immediately on the excised burn wounds and functions as a true graft. After the "take," the allograft is abraded, leaving a dermal base which supports the grafting of the keratinocyte sheets, and integration of the duplex into a permanent skin coverage ensues. Hence the composite skin graft.

The allograft skin is obtained from a skin bank, and the cryopreserved skin is viable at the time of application. Keratinocyte cultures are initiated with split-thickness skin harvested from unburned areas. They are cultured on 3T3 feeder layer in a serum-free medium.

The allogeneic dermis promotes rapid stratification, maturation, and synthesis of anchoring fibrils. There was no evidence of rejection of allogeneic dermis in a patient who was followed up for 11 months.

The author hypothesizes that removal of the epidermis from the grafted allogeneic skin eliminates the majority of cells which constitute expressing class II antigens, leaving behind a viable allogeneic bed that serves as an ideal substrate for grafting and integration of keratinocyte cultures but does not initiate rejection. Composite autologous-allogenic skin grafts have shown promising results with burn patients.

13.4.2.2 Living Skin Equivalent [19, 20]

A living skin equivalent used as a skin prosthesis has been developed by Bell. It consists of two components: a dermal equivalent made up of fibroblasts in a collagen matrix that is contracted and modified by the resident cells, and an epidermis that develops from tissue culture is plated on the dermal equivalent.

This skin equivalent provides the barrier property of an epidermis as well as the contraction-reducing property and structural integrity of a dermis.

From initial skin specimens, one needs to obtain fibroblasts and basal cells. The fibroblasts are grown to confluence and recultured when necessary to obtain nearly 5×10 cells/cm^2. The cells are removed, suspended in acid-swollen collagen and serum, and the lot is coprecipitated by neutralization. This loose collagen and fibroblast mat is then contracted by the fibroblasts, resulting in a thin, firm matrix. The matrix is washed and seeded with an epidermal cell suspension, and maintained in culture, until it grows to become confluent. Then it can be used for grafting.

In experimental studies, the rate of take of these grafts is reported to be 80%. Autografts and allografts of skin equivalents are rapidly vascularized. The graft grows in thickness with remodeling of the collagen. The graft appears scaly and dry due to lack of sweat and sebaceous glands. By 10 weeks a normal dermal collagen pattern can be seen, and the dermis of the graft is about one-half the thickness of normal dermis. It lasts essentially for the life span of the host. The graft remains free from hair and sebaceous glands. Contraction of the wound is limited to 50% or less in most grafts.

One distinct problem in translating this work to human grafting is that it requires 20–26 days to effect only a 100-fold increase in the area of wound that can be covered.

Recently a preliminary clinical study of the skin equivalent in burn patients was reported by Wassermann. Eight patients with full-thickness burn wounds covering 15% TBSA were partially grafted with skin equivalents. In every patient extensive lysis (60%–90%) of the skin equivalent graft was observed at first dressing. In only one patient was a significant percentage of take (40%) observed 14 days after grafting. These disappointing results were probably related to the presence of collagenases or proteases produced on the wound bed either by bacteria or by surrounding tissue cells. It appeared that the dermal component must be biochemically modified before routine clinical application.

13.4.2.3 Bilayered Synthetic Membrane and Autologous Epidermis [21]

Yannas and Burke developed a synthetic membrane to act as a temporary barrier and a permanent framework. The synthetic skin is composed of covalently linked bovine collagen, glycosaminoglycan, and chondroitin 6-sulfate, expanded into a sponge with a pore size of approximately 150 μm. The glycosaminoglycan is understood to render the collagen nonantigenic, and the cross-linking, which is achieved with glutaraldehyde and/or dehydrothemeryl, controls the rate of breakdown and resorption at the wound site. A nonporous silastic surface is vulcanized onto the matrix to form the temporary epidermal layer.

When the bilayered synthetic skin is placed on the prepared wound, it adheres and is invaded by fibroblasts from the recipient. Two to seven weeks after the application, the silastic outer layer is stripped away and replaced by thin meshed autograft or/and autologous epidermal cells. In animal trials, epidermal cells are found to grow within the membrane.

13.4.3 Cultured Allograft [22–26]

The use of cultured graft from autologous epidermal cells may be limited not only by the availability of the suitable donor sites but also by the time required for the growth of the cells in vitro.

Prolongation of nonsyngenetic graft survival of pancreatic, thyroid, ovarian tissue and skin that had been cultured in vitro prior to transplantation have been reported. Hefton used epidermal allografts, which were grafted after in vitro epidermal cell culture, resulting in rapid healing of the wound. As Langerhans cells and other class II antigen expression cells degenerate when epidermal cells are cultured in vitro, it is suggested that cultured allogeneic epidermis might be used as a permanent skin substitute. This possibility has stimulated tremendous interest and controversy in the field of tissue transplantation.

This approach offers several advantages over autologous epidermis, including the ready availability of cultured grafts, a nearly unlimited source of supply, and elimination of the painful donor site, if skin transplants are obtained from cadavers.

Grafting of cultured allogeneic epidermis on second- and third-degree burn wounds in 26 patients has been reported by Madden. Deep second-degree burn wounds in 11 out of 12 patients healed rapidly within a mean time of 10 days, after being covered with cultured allogeneic epidermal cells. The BSA grafted with cultured cells varied from 1% to 12%. Nine patients with third-degree burns were grafted with cultured allografts after excision or on a bed of granulation tissue. This cultured graft was not able to survive on the wound bed and on granulation tissue, even after repeated application and reepithelialization from the wound edges.

Some authors have claimed that the survival time of cultured allografts was markedly prolonged or immunologically tolerated. However, these studies were performed on partial-thickness wounds and the possibiliy of epithelialization from the remaining dermal element could not be excluded.

Attempts have been made to determine the extent of survival of the cultured cells in the healed wound. However, data suggested that these cells survive only temporarily after grafting, and are eventually replaced by host epithelium [26].

However, the cultured epidermal allografts seem to provide a potent stimulation to wound healing. Th technique has been found to be beneficial in covering small skin wounds, such as small burns, leg ulcers, and split-thickness skin donor sites.

References

1. Wang WZ, Wang W, Liu JL et al. (1985) Studies on the cultivation and transplantation of epidermal cells: growth of cultured human epidermal keratinocytes in three culture models. J 2nd Milit Med Coll 6: 399–403
2. Phillips TJ (1988) Cultured skin grafts. Arch Dermatol 124: 1035–1038
3. Holbrock KA, Henning H (1983) Phenotype expression of epidermal cells in vitro: a Review. J Invest Dermatol 81: 11s–23s
4. Prunirrs M, Regnier M, Woodley D (1983) Methods for cultivation of keratinocytes with an air-liquid interface. J Invest Dermatol 81: 28s–33s
5. Boyce ST, Ham RG (1985) Cultivation, frozen storage and clonal growth of normal epidermal keratinocytes in serum-free media. J Tissue Cult Methods 9: 83–94

6. Wang WZ, Dai FP, Zhang SC (1988) Studies on cultivation of adult human epidermal keratinocytes in serum-free media. Proc Milit Med Symp Burns Plast Surg 12: 162
7. Gilchrest BA (1982) Attachment and growth of human keratinocytes in a serum-free environment. J cell physiol 112: 197–204
8. Tong GW (1988) Subculture of human epidermal cells. Proc Milit Med Symp Burns Plastic Surg 12: 161
9. Rheiwald JC (1980) Serial culture of normal human epidermal keratinocytes. Methods Cell Biol 21A: 230–254
10. Dai FP, Wang WZ (1988) Comparative studies on the effect of different culture media on the growth of human epidermal cells in vitro. Proc Pan China Symp Surg 11: 178
11. Wang WZ, Wang W, Liu JL (1988) Cultivation of human epidermal keratinocytes with fibronectin coated substrate and its clinical application. J 2nd Milit Med Coll 9: 120–124
12. Liu JL, Pan YL, Yu LY (1988) Studies on subculture of human epidermal cells. Proc Milit Med Symp Burns Plast Surg 12: 159
13. Green H, Kehinde O, Thomas J (1979) Growth of cultured human epidermal cells into multiple epithelia suitable for grafting. Proc Natl Acad Sci USA 76: 5665–5666
14. Le YY, Shi JX (1988) Culture of epidermal cells and application. Proc Pan China Symp Surg 11: 177
15. Gallico GG, Compton CC, O'Connor NE (1984) Permanent coverage of large burn wounds with autologous cultured human epithelium. N Engl J Med 31: 448–451
16. Cheng B, Tong CW, Cheng MD (1986) Cultivation and grafting of human epidermal cells. Proc Milit Med Symp Burn Plastic Surg 11: 165–166
17. Gallico GG, O'Connor NE (1985) Cultured epithelium as a skin substitute. Clin Plast Surg 12: 149–157
18. Cuono DCB, Langdon R, Birchall N et al. (1987) Composite autologous allogenic skin replacement: development and clinical application. Plast Reconstr Surg 80: 626–635
19. Bell E, Ehrlish HP, Butter DJ et al. (1981) Development and use of living skin equivalent. Plast Reconstr Surg 67: 356–392
20. Wassermann D, Schlotterer M, Cazalet C et al. (1988) Preliminary clinical studies of a biological skin equivalent in burned patients. Burns 14: 326–330
21. Burke JF, Yannas IV Wuinby MC et al. (1982) Successful use of a physiologically acceptable artificial skin in the treatment of extensive burn injury. Ann Surg 194: 413–420
22. Hefton JM, Madden MR, Finkelsein JL et al. (1983) Grafting of burn patient with allografts of cultured epidermal cells. Lancet 1: 428–430
23. Madden MR, Finkelstein JT, Stino-Coco et al. (1986) Grafting of cultured allogenic epidermis of second and third degree burn wounds on 26 patients. J Trauma 26: 955–960
24. Thivolet J, Faure M, Dmidem A et al. (1986) Long-term survival and immunological tolerance of human epidermal allografts produced in culture. Transplantation 42: 274–280
25. Zhao ZF, Hu JN, Lu SC (1985) Cultivation of human epithelial cells and its preliminary application for wound coverage. Chin J Surg 23: 247–250
26. Celen V, Faure M, Mauduit G et al. (1987) Progressive replacement of human cultured epithelial allografts as evidences by HLA class I antigen expression. Dermatologica 175: 166–170

14 Skin Substitutes

Ge Sheng-de

It is well known that burns may be associated with many local and systemic problems due to the loss of the skin barrier and function. Local burn management to promote wound healing of course is of great importance, because it not only treats local wounds but also resolves systemic problems. In extensive deep burns, wound coverage is achieved by skin grafting. When there is an inadequate amount of intact skin, i.e., shortage of skin donor sites, alternative material is applied. Skin substitutes have been developed for the conversion of an open wound to a closed wound.

Different types of material have been used in local burn treatment. Most are commercially available and some are promising products still under clinical trial. Many have been developed abroad and several are available in China. The purpose of their clinical application is to establish permanent or temporary wound coverage which helps or leads to wound healing. This chapter will focus mainly on the skin substitutes used in China with a mention of the products developed abroad.

Although many products are frequently used in burn treatment and their beneficial effects have made them useful, none has proved totally effcacious. Indeed, they are far from ideal.

14.1 Ideal Skin Substitute

To provide temporary wound covering, an ideal skin substitute should possess certain properties, which are thought to be critical for its clinical application. The commercially available skin substitutes possess most of these properties in order to meet clinical requirements. The following are the critical properties of an ideal skin substitute.

1. It adheres to the wound surface and serves as a temporary covering.
2. It is easily applied and removed.
3. It minimizes local pain.
4. It protects the wound and provides a bacterial barrier.
5. It is elastic and durable and conforms to the body contours.
6. It maintains body fluid and transports water vapor.
7. It is antiseptic and hemostatic
8. It is nontoxic and nonantigenic.

9. It is easily produced, preserved, and stocked and has a relatively long shelf life.
10. It is inexpensive.

Actually, the skin substitutes available possess not only merits but also demerits. New products are being developed for further improvement with more beneficial effects and less drawbacks relative to the alternatives.

14.2 Skin Substitutes

Skin substitutes may be classified into biological, synthetic and biosynthetic substitutes. The products used in China and some products available abroad will be described individually according to their preparation, properties, indications, procedures, and application results.

14.2.1 Biological Skin Substitute

14.2.1.1 Skin Allograft

Skin allograft is the skin graft obtained from an individual and is transferred to another individual of the same species. Clinically it is obtained from a donor, a patient's relative, or a normal individual, and transplanted to the patient to provide temporary coverage for partial- or full-thickness wounds. When a large amount of skin allograft is needed to treat extensive deep burns, skin allograft is obtained from a fresh cadaver without premortal hepatitis, septicemia, dermopathy or skin cancer. Skin allograft is therefore not always available. It is usually preserved in a 4°C refrigerator for a period of less than 1 week. The period for which skin allograft at 4°C can be preserved may be prolonged by using nutrient medium [1, 2, 3]. Skin allograft preserved with nutrient medium will maintain its viability above 90% after being preserved for 1 week. Most burn centers use a cryopreservation technique with a $-80°C$ refrigerator or liquid nitrogen at $-190°C$. We have found that cryopreserved skin allograft has a relatively normal configuration under gross and microscopic observation. Recently, the technique has been improved using vitrification [4].

Skin allograft may be used in large sheets or small pieces. It will be rejected 2 weeks after its transplantation due to its antigenicity. The rejection reaction could be inhibited by using an immunosuppressant such as azathiopurine, cyclosporin A, antilymphocytic serum (ALS), or antilymphocytic globulin (ALG). However, the rejection reaction may follow if immunosuppression is discontinued, since establishment of immunotolerance has not been observed.

The survival time of skin allograft may be prolonged after its transplantation if the graft is pretreated in vitro with fluocinolone acetonide, triamcinolone acetonide, azathiopurine, or a combination of these. Fluocinolone acetonide treated skin allograft take was prolonged probably by decreasing infiltration monocytes in the graft and the recipient bed [5].

14.2.1.2 Skin Xenograft

Skin xenograft is the skin graft transferred between two individuals from different species. Clinically skin xenograft is usually obtained from mammals such as pig and sheep. Pig skin is more frequently used because its configuration resembles that of human skin much more and it is readily available, while sheep skin is used because of the religious regulations in autonomous moslems regions.

The preserving and transplanting techniques are quite similar to those for skin allograft. However, cryopreservation is not often used, since skin xenograft is more readily available in fresh form. Nonviable forms of xenograft such as glutaraldehyde-treated or further lyophilized product [6] have been introduced, since they are readily available.

Xenograft can also be preserved by using some other techniques such as alcohol. Cryopreserved skin xenograft using liquid nitrogen has proved effective. The technique has been modified by using H solution, a mixture of DMSO and propylene glycol. H solution is highly effective in cryopreservation, having a low toxicity. The new technique can save much time, with the sealed plastic bag of the skin xenograft being placed directly into liquid nitrogen. The results of a study of cryopreservation technique using vitrification show the preserved skin xenograft has a better viability. A study using guinea pig skin showed that the viability of skin stored by vitrification was 20% higher than that stored by slow cooling. Clinical application of vitrified autografts on granulation wounds showed 60% permanent take. No autografts or allografts stored by slow cooling were found to take on granulation wounds. Vitrified allografts for covering excised deep burn wounds showed a 91% overall take rate [5].

Xenograft can also be treated in vitro for prolonged take. Take of fluocinolone acetonide treated skin allograft was prolonged probably by decreasing monocyte infiltration in the graft and recipient bed [7].

14.2.1.3 Radiation Skin Graft

Radiation skin xenograft is a type of biological dressing prepared by radiation of split-thickness porcine skin [8]. It is completely sterilized and totally nonantigenic. A comparative study of the antigenicity of porcine skin sterilized by radiation and by the conventional method showed that the titer of antibody derived from porcine skin sterilized by the conventional method was 1:128 while that of radiation-sterilized porcine skin was 1:8. A significant correlation was observed between the lymphocyte transformation potency and the cAMP/cGMP ratio; the lower the ratio, the lower the potency [9].

Radiation skin xenograft is indicated in the treatment of superficial and deep second-degree burns. It is also used in third-degree burns for covering on either early postburn wound or granulation wound, or even after skin grafting. It is well accepted probably due to its texture being similar to that of fresh xenograft, having a better conformation to the body contours. Limited experience has shown that radiation skin can serve as a good wound covering or protector in clinical application. However, it is far from being popular, although it has shown promise in some clinical trials.

14.2.1.4 Amniotic Membrane

Human amniotic membrane has been used in clinical burn practice with some success. It can be used in freshly prepared form or may be available in forms preserved by new geramine, chlorhexidine, alcohol, or glutaraldehyde. It can also be prepared in dried form simply by exposure.

Bovine amniotic membrane has been used in local burn treatment. Microscopic examination of bovine amniotic membrane showed that there was interdigitation in between cells. The intracellular gaps measured about 20–50 nm and were too narrow for pathogenic bacteria to pass through. Clinical practice has shown that bovine amniotic membrane has the following characteristics: It stops bacteria from invading the wounds; it prevents further fluid loss from the wound surface, its refrigerated form can offer immediate relief of local pain; its therapeutic effects seem to have nothing to do with its viability; and its clinical application reduces the frequency of dressing change, saves dressing material, and lessens the work load of nursing care. The healing time of superficial and deep second-degree burn was 6–9 days and 12–16 days [8]. It is larger than human amniotic membrane; hence, it is better accepted in clinical practice.

Glutaraldehyde-treated bovine amniotic membrane has been used in local burn care with good results. It can reduce dressing changes, save dressings, simplify nursing care, and reduce healing time. Since bovine amniotic membrane is larger, thicker, and more pliable than human amniotic membrane, it is therefore preferable [10].

14.2.1.5 Peritoneum

Fresh porcine peritoneum used as a biological dressing in local burn management has been introduced by Liu Bing-Shen [11]. The technical procedure of obtaining fresh porcine peritoneum is very simple; hence it is easily prepared. Its clinical trial provide to be effective. More clinical trials and further laboratory study are required to demonstrate its effectiveness in burn treatment. Since it has an abundant source, it may show promise if it could be accepted as a biological material.

14.2.2 Synthetic Skin Substitute

Skin substitute made from synthetic material is referred to as artificial skin. It is usually prepared using high molecular weight polymers as its material.

Several types of synthetic skin substitute have been used in China. Some are home products and others are from other countries.

14.2.2.1 Number 2 Artificial Skin

A yellowish-brown semitransparent soft velour membrane was introduced as No. 2 artificial skin in 1973 [12]. It is composed of a base membrane made from polyurethane as the outer layer and a collagen velour inner layer. It is nontoxic, nonantigenic, and nonirritant and has a soft and pliable texture. It is slightly acidic but does not produce obvious local stimulation, inflammation, or foreign body reaction. The acid velour has a positive electric charge, while that of the fibroblast is negative. The difference in electric charge is, therefore, beneficial to the adhesion of the artificial skin to the wound surface where it is applied. The adherent effect of No. 2 artificial skin keeps it in close contact with the wound surface on the basis of affinity between its collagen velour and the collagen fiber of the wound. The collagen velour is very short, which allows elimination of dead space after its application on the burn wound. Its permeability and vapor transport effect are able to minimize fluid accumulation. Bacterial proliferation could be limited due to the limited opportunity for fluid accumulation in the dead space and nutrient supply, as well as elimination of bacterial growth by the immune effect. Moreover, bacterial infection is effectively prevented, since herbal medicine with its bacteriostatic and bactericidal effects is an additional component in the production of No. 2 artificial skin [13].

Number 2 artificial skin has been used in local burn treatment as a synthetic skin substitute for temporary coverage of the wound with some success [14–17], which helps the establishment of epithelialization and reestablishment of a body surface barrier.

14.2.2.2 Number 204 Artificial Skin

Number 204 artificial skin is a type of synthesized skin prosthesis similar to No. 2 artificial skin but with an additional Silastic membrane. It has been used in the treatment of superficial burns with some success.

14.2.2.3 T_{41} Artificial Skin

T_{41} artificial skin is a bilayer skin prosthesis which is composed of an inner layer velour of Nylon 6 polyethylene propanamide and an outer layer membrane of Silastic membrane treated by polysorbate 60 (Tween 60). It meets the clinical requirements of burn wound treatment, with no space-occupying effect when applied to deep burns and a satisfactory result without influencing epithelial growth.

14.2.2.4 Polyurethane Film

A polyurethane film developed recently by the cooperation of our Burn Center and the Textile University of China has been used in our burn ward [18]. Polyurethane has been well accepted as a nontoxic and nonantigenic high polymer. It adheres readily to the wound surface and has proved effective in the management of burn wound and skin donor sites. It helps minimize local pain soon after its application. It is elastic and durable, and is a temporary skin barrier effective in preventing fluid loss and bacterial contamination. Loss of water vapor is reduced to 27% in second-degree burn wound and 69% in excised third-degree burn wound. The amount of fluid loss controlled depends on the diameter of the porous structure. We have formed the initial impression after clinical use that it helps to promote wound healing and reduce pigmentation compared with controls.

14.2.2.5 Hydron Wound Dressing

Hydron Wound Dressing (HWD) is a commercially available dressing. The Hydron Kit is a well-prepared sterilized complete set of Hydron power, poly(2-hydroxyethyl methacrylate, with polyethylene glycol 400/H_2O as its solvent and an applicator). It has been used as a material in local burn care. It has the beneficial effect of reducing local pain when a film is formed soon after its application. The barrier it forms has the benefit of preventing excessive fluid loss and bacterial contamination. The film is demonstrated to promote wound healing in the treatment of superficial second-degree burns and skin donor sites [19]. Fluid accumulation and cracks or fissures have been observed. Reapplication of HWD is required during dressing changes.

14.2.2.6 Lyoform

Lyoform is a type of synthetic dressing which can be used as a skin substitute. It is made from polyurethane with a double-layered foamy structure. Its inner layer is more dense, flatter, smoother, and hydrophilic. When it is applied to the wound it adheres. Water at the wound surface is readily absorbed, transferred, and evaporated from the outer hydrophobic layer. Its special configuration makes it a bacterial barrier after being applied to an open wound. It is indicated for the treatment of burn wounds.

Lyoform C modifiers Lyoform when a layer of active carbon-treated nonfabric viscose staple is added to cover the hydrophobic layer. The active carbon helps to eliminate bad odor from the wound. It is commercially available and is more frequently used in Europe. Lyoform is available in various products such as sterile dressing, carbonaceous dressing, tracheostomy dressing, and burn sheet to meet clinical requirements.

14.2.3 Biosynthetic Skin Prosthesis

14.2.3.1 Chimeherb

Chimeherb is a recently developed biosynthetic skin. It is made from chitosan and keratin acetate with some trace elements and a Chinese herbal medicine component [20]. It possesses spiracles and holes, and is, therefore, good for water and vapor transport. It is nontoxic and nonantigenic, has no adverse effects, and can adhere to the wound surface with properties of elasticity and durability. It protects local wound by preventing stimulation and alleviating local discomfort and pain. It is commercially available and can be stored with a relatively long shelf-life. The product should be stored at a temperature of less than 30°C , should be kept dry, and direct sunlight must be avoided. It has been used in burn clinics with some success. However, it is not yet widely popularized. Evaluation of its efficacy requires further study.

14.2.3.2 Biobrane

Biobrane is a biosynthetic skin substitute or dressing. It is a temporary skin substitute for excised deep burn wounds and compares favorably with fresh cadaver allograft. It consists of a custom-knit nylon fabric bonded to a silicone rubber membrane. Following the provision of the silicone membrane with the appropriate functional groups, collagenous peptides of porcine skin origin are covalently bonded to both the nylon and silicone with 2,4,6-trichloro-*S*-triazine.

The elastic properties of Biobrane have been demonstrated. It is significantly more adherent than biological dressing, allograft, or xenograft 72 h after use. There is an immediate decrease in evaporative water loss with mean values less than 90% that of open wound. Biobrane is thought to be safe for clinical application because of its lack of irritation, toxicity, antigenicity, and pyrogenicity. When Biobrane was kept on the wound it markedly reduced wound contraction. However, contraction proceeded rapidly once Biobrane was removed [21].

Bacterial study using quantitative cultures showed that colony counts were lowest on wounds subjacent to dressings, with counts for Biobrane-covered wounds being ten times less than those of xenograft- or allograft-covered wounds. Colonies derived from open wounds had counts 100 times more than those of Biobrane-covered wounds. Biobrane is permeable to antimicrobial agents. The efficacy of silver sulfadiazine topically applied to Biobrane to control bacterially contaminated wounds has been demonstrated.

Biobrane is thought to be useful for treatment of outpatients for its efficacy and efficiency in treating partial-thickness burns. It is an effective wound covering for clean superficial partial-thickness burns [22, 23].

14.2.3.3 Burke's Artificial Dermis

Burke introduced an artificial dermis in 1981 [24], which is composed of a bilaminar membrane with a bovine collagen matrix and a Silastic cover, in between which is placed chondroitin-6-sulfate from shark cartilage, making it similar to a sandwich. It is indicated for the treatment of extensive deep burns where an adequate skin donor site is not readily available. It may be used as a permanent dermal graft for excised burn wounds, and epidermal grafts are applied after removal of the Silastic cover at the second operation. The artificial dermis offers a material superior in texture, function, and appearance, with satisfactory short- and long-term results. It may also be applied to the skin donor site, having an average healing time 5 days shorter than that of the control [21]. Although it has proved quite efficacious, it is still far from being popular, probably due to its high cost.

References

1. Zhu ZM (1989) The best condition for skin preservation at 4°C. Proceedings of the 1st national conference on burns, Shanghai, p 106
2. May SR (1980) Integrated study of the structural and metabolic degeneration of skin during 4°C storage in nutrient medium. Cryobiology 17: 125–129
3. Zhu ZM, Wu ZG, Zhou YQ et al. (1989) Study on several problems in skin preservation at 4°C. Chin J Plast Surg Burns 5: 139–140
4. Zhu ZM, Jia XM, Gao WY et al. (1989) Cryopreservation of skin by vitrification. Proceedings of the 2nd Sino-American conference on burn injury and trauma, Beijing, p 159
5. Zhu ZM, Jia XM, Gao WY et al. (1979) Study of vitrification in skin preservation. IV. Clinical effect of auto- and allo-graft preservation. Proceedings of the 2nd national conference on burns, Nanchang, Chinese Burn Association, p 82
6. Sully L, Bailey BN (1978) Lyophilized pig skin in the treatment of superficial and deep dermal burns. Burns 4: 271–276
7. Zhao XF, Huang WH, Zhong LH et al. (1985) Histological evaluation of fluocinolone acetonide effect on prolonged take of xenograft transplantation. Chin J Plast Surg Burns 1: 206–208
8. Liu R, Wang TY, Sun BT (1989) The use of bovine amnion in the management of burn wounds. Proceedings of the 2nd Sino-American conference on burn injury and trauma, Beijing p 100
9. Tang ZY, Lu XA, Lin W et al. (1989) Antigenicity of porcine skin sterilized by radiation and by conventional method. Proceedings of the 2nd Sino-American conference on burn injury and trauma, Beijing, p 116

10. Mu XX, Xu FX, Liu YL et al. (1987) Use of glutaraldehyde treated bovine amniotic membrane on burn wound. Chin J Plast Surg Burns 3: 265–267
11. Liu BS (1989) Laboratory study and application of animal peritoneum on burn wound. Proceedings of the 2nd national conference on burns, Nanchang, Chinese Burn Association, p 57–58
12. General Hospital of Nanjing Area Command (1976) A brief introduction to no. 2 artificial skin. In: Clinical data on no. 2 artificial skin. Nanjing, pp 2–7
13. General Hospital of Nanjing Area Command (1976) Preliminary evaluation of biphysical problems of no. 2 artificial skin. In: Clinical data on no. 2 artificial skin. Nanjing, pp 107–116
14. General Hospital of Nanjing Area Command (1976) Experience of clinical application of no. 2 artificial skin. In: Clinical data on no. 2 artificial skin. Nanjing, pp 32–35
15. Shanghai Changhai Hospital (1976) Conclusion of clinical use of no. 2 artificial skin. In: Clinical data on no. 2 artificial skin. Nanjing, p 65
16. Shanghai Ruijin Hospital (1976) Conclusion of clinical application of artificial skin. In: Clinical data on no. 2 artificial skin. Nanjing, p 41–42
17. Beijing Jishuitan Hospital (1976) Experience of no. 2 artificial skin in treating deep burn wound. Nanjing pp 63–64
18. Ge Sheng-De, Hua Zheng-Lu, Xia Zhao-Fan et al. (1985) Insensible water loss of local burn wound – clinical observation and laboratory study. Chin J Plast Surg Burns 1: 10–13
19. Ge SD, Huo ZL, Liu YL et al. (1987) Use of Hydron® wound dressing in minor and moderate burns. Acad J 2nd Milit Med Univ 8: 211–213
20. Wu HC, Xui GS, Qiu MX et al. (1989) Use of 864-artificial skin in burn treatment. Proceedings of the 2nd national conference on burns, Nanchang, Chinese Burn Association, p 58
21. Robson MC (1989) Fresh cadaver allograft vs a biosynthetic dressing (Biobrane) on excised burn wound. Proceedings of the 2nd Sino-American conference on burn injury and trauma, Beijing, p 94
22. Warder G, Heimbach D, Luterman A et al. (1989) Artificial dermis for major burns: a multi-center randomized clinical trial. Proceedings of the 2nd Sino-American conference on burn injury and trauma, Beijing, p 37
23. Hansbrough JF, Zapata-Sirvent R, Carroll WJ et al. (1984) Clinical experience with Biobrane® biosynthetic dressing in the treatment of partial-thickness burns. Burns 10: 415–419
25. Burk JF, Yannas IV, Quiby WC et al. (1981) Successful use of a physiologically acceptable artificial skin in the treatment of extensive burn injury. Ann Surg 194: 413–428

15 Nutritional Support in Burns

Wang Shi-liang and Li Ngao

After a short duration of ebb phase or shock phase, the burn patient enters a hypermetabolic state, characterized by an elevated metabolic rate, increased protein catabolism and gluconeogenesis, and loss of body weight. Energy requirements are often high, up to 4000 kcal (16 736 kJ) or more per day. Thus vigorous nutritional support is needed in order to prevent complications precipitated by catabolism, and to promote early anabolism and wound healing.

15.1 Hypermetabolism in Burns [1, 2, 3, 4, 5]

Basal energy expenditure (BEE) increases curvilinearly with an increase in burn size up to 50% of the total body surface area (TBSA), and it reaches a maximum at about twofold that of normal BEE. The postburn hypermetabolism is the result of many stimuli, such as pain, hypotension, hypoxia, and tremendous water and heat loss. For many years the explanation for hypermetabolism has been controversial. The elevated metabolic rate can be lowered to a certain extent when the burn patient is placed in a warm environment or the burn wound is covered with a water-impermeable membrane or/and bulky dressings, but would still not return to normal levels. Thus it seems that the prime stimulator of the hypermetabolism is not "externally cold," but rather "internally warm." The current explanation for this postburn hypermetabolic response has concentrated on hormonal changes, mediators such as catecholamines, insulin, glucagon, cortisol, growth hormone, interleukin I, endorphins, prostaglandins, possibly thyroid hormone, and many others which are thought to be responsible.

Catecholamine released after burning seems to be the primary mediator. It is well known that increased catecholamines (increased adrenergic activity) are the major calorigenic mediators responsible for the hypermetabolic response following injury. Fang et al. [6] found that the urine catecholamine content of the group of patients who survived showed an initial increase followed by a gradual return to normal, while that of the group who died was constantly and slightly below normal. In the survivors, elevation of the epinephrine level was more obvious than that of norepinephrine (Table 15.1). Catecholamine levels also increased during escharectomy, skin grafting, and sepsis following burn injury. In sepsis, the urine catecholamine level can reach a value of 74.3–124.5 $\mu g/24\,h$ (normal value, $28.7 \pm 9.1\ \mu g/24\,h$), which will return to

Table 15.1. Changes in urine levels of catecholamines, epinephrine, and norepinephrine in severely burned patients ($\bar{x} \pm SE$ μg/24 h)

Postburn	Catecholamines		Epinephrine		Norepinephrine	
	Group A ($n = 17$)	Group B ($n = 3$)	Group A ($n = 17$)	Group B ($n = 3$)	Group A ($n = 17$)	Group B ($n = 3$)
Within 2 days	57.77 ± 19.07	–	18.22 ± 5.82	–	39.47 ± 13.70	–
2 weeks	38.57 ± 8.83	20.33 ± 1.59	20.88 ± 6.42	8.57 ± 1.47	23.60 ± 5.32	11.76 ± 2.60
3 weeks	32.46 ± 8.21	26.68	8.74 ± 1.21	3.84	22.46 ± 7.22	23.04
4 weeks	39.85 ± 8.64	8.60	12.69 ± 3.56	4.30	25.09 ± 7.00	4.30
5 weeks	20.71 ± 3.99	–	15.42 ± 5.77	–	22.18 ± 6.22	–
Normal values	28.70 ± 9.10		7.60 ± 5.30		20.50 ± 7.10	

Group A, patients that survived; group B, patients that died.

Table 15.2. Changes in plasma cortisol levels in severely burned patients ($\bar{x} \pm SE\ \mu g/ml$)

Postburn	Group that survived ($n = 17$)	Group that died ($n = 3$)
Within 2 days	40.82 ± 7.67	66.25 ± 11.93
2 weeks	40.57 ± 6.86	39.75 ± 9.81
3 weeks	42.87 ± 5.36	51.75 ± 1.14
4 weeks	20.33 ± 4.55	24.45 ± 8.15
5 weeks	31.33 ± 9.36	87.50
Normal value	12.00 ± 2.00	

Table 15.3. Plasma levels of insulin and glucagon in rabbits with 30% third-degree burns

	Preburn	Postburn day			
		1	3	6	10
Insulin (mU/l)	6.29 ± 2.44	8.88 ± 2.42	9.20 ± 2.67	11.30 ± 5.13	16.80 ± 5.31
Glucagon (ng/l)	19.70 ± 9.24	86.4 ± 14.2	64.5 ± 9.26	54.70 ± 14.52	33.30 ± 9.18
I/G	0.32	0.10	0.14	0.21	0.50

approaching normal levels as the sepsis is controlled, or will increase further up to 354 $\mu g/24\,h$ in the nonsurvivors.

The elevation in plasma level of corticosteroids after burning is not only pronounced but also sustained. In burn rats, the plasma level of corticosterone was kept high, at up to 257.72 ± 22.51 nmol/l (154.40 ± 12.41 nmol/l in controls) on PBD (postburn day) 12 [7]. In a group of severely burned patients, even 3–4 weeks postburn, the level of plasma cortisol was about three times higher than normal [6] (Table 15.2). After 4 weeks, it gradually decreased in the survival group, but remained higher in the group of nonsurvivors.

Generally during the early resuscitation phase, at first, 1–2 PBD, the plasma insulin level is decreased, and increased shortly after the resuscitation stage. These changes are related to the circulating plasma glucose level and are proportional to the degree of elevation of the metabolic rate. The plasma glucagon level stimulated by catecholamines is also increased after burn injury. The insulin to glucagon ratio (I/G) is an important index for the prediction of the metabolic state of the victim. A decrease means that the metabolism is changing from the anabolic to the catabolic state as is usually seen during the early postburn stage, and the ratio will increase if anabolism occurs as in the convalescence stage. However, in our severely burned rabbit experiment, it was

Table 15.4. Plasma levels of insulin in severely burned patients ($\bar{x} \pm$ SE mU/l)

Postburn	Group that survived ($n = 17$)	Group that died ($n = 3$)
Within 2 days	33.00 ± 9.51	33.00 ± 2.47
2 weeks	27.73 ± 6.23	14.00 ± 0.25
3 weeks	43.42 ± 11.69	71.00 ± 25.10
4 weeks	33.22 ± 12.63	–
5 weeks	17.22 ± 6.28	–
Normal value	10–30	

found that the plasma insulin level was not lowered on PBD 1 [8] (Table 15.3). And similar trends could be seen in severely burned patients [6] (Table 15.4).

Growth hormone (GH), because of its ability to promote protein synthesis and wound healing, and decrease nitrogen excretion, has been used to reduce postburn catabolism. But there have been quite different reports concerning its plasma level postburn, and studies on the postburn pathological changes of GH cells are rare. Wu and Shi [9] showed that after burn injury: (a) the synthetic activity in GH cells was enhanced, the process of secretion was more rapid, and the rate of granule maturation was increased; (b) the nude GH granules were found in both sinusoids and endothelial cells; (c) the newly formed mitochondria may originate from the Golgi complex and divide by themselves; and (d) some endothelial cells manifested degenerative changes and others were in the active stage. According to these findings, variations in GH cells were divided into stress, modulation, and functional recovery stages. Some reports claimed that GH could promote anabolism in burn patients; however, further study is needed concerning its clinical application.

In a group of 57 severely burned patients with average $61.2\% \pm 22.1\%$ TBSA burns, it was demonstrated that the plasma levels of both thromboxane A_2 (TXA_2) and prostacyclin (PGI_2) shoswed significant changes following burns. The TXA_2/PGI_2 ratio increased markedly and correlated positively with burn size and the severity of the patient's general condition [10]. It was also stated [4] that the administration of prostaglandin inhibitors to hypermetabolic burned animal models resulted in a marked decrease of the hypermetabolic response to injury. But it seems that more studies are needed to clarify the relationship between prostaglandin secretion and the metabolic rate in burns.

It is generally considered that thyroid function is inhibited after burns, although some differences have been observed. Jin et al. [11] reported that thyroid glands play an important role in burn stress, finding that the mean serum thyroxine levels in 21 burn patients were higher than those in normal subjects ($p < 0.01$), and that thyroxine levels increased gradually after the shock stage. But others have found that thyroxine is lowered postburn. Tian et al.

[12] reported that the T_4 level was lower in most burns ($p < 0.05$), but became significantly higher than normal ($p < 0.01$) in those complicated by systemic sepsis. Chen et al. [13], Gao et al. [14], and Jin and Chen [15] all reported diverging serum levels between T_3 and T_4. The T_4 concentration ranged from normal to slightly below normal, whereas that of T_3 was found to be obviously decreased and that of T_3 increased significantly ($p < 0.05$) in either burn patients or burn animal models. Besides, the serum levels of T_4 were different for various burn sizes [12]. They were normal or slightly increased in patients whit burns less than 30% TBSA, or decreased in those with burns more than 30% TBSA. The larger the burn size the lower the concentration of T_4. Moreover, the serum levels of T_4 were also different in various burn stages. In a severe burn rat model, Jin and Chen [15] concluded that: (a) in the early stage (within 2 days postburn), there was a marked damage to the follicular cells of the thyroid, and synthesis function and thyroid hormone release were significantly inhibited, this being referred to as the inhibition phase; (b) around 1 week or so postburn, damage to the follicular cells of the thyroid was attenuated, and synthesis function and thyroid hormone release were restored to normal levels, this being referred to as the recovery phase; and (c) about 2 weeks later, thyroid function became active, and organelles reflecting synthesis and release function of the thyroid hormone were well developed, this being the active phase. Jin et al. also showed a considerable decrease in T_3 serum levels during the first 2–3 weeks postburn [13, 15], and considered that the inhibition of T_3 was related to the lower serum concentration of T_4, the metabolic disturbance of T_4 deiodination, and the inhibition of thyroid secretion.

To summarize, mediators concerned with hypermetabolism after burn injury are complicated. Catecholamines, glucagon, insulin, cortisol, and interleukin I are considered to be the primary ones. With regard to the growth hormone, prostaglandins, thyroxine, and others might play a role in postburn metabolic rate.

15.2 Glucose Metabolism and Its Requirement

Usually, hyperglycemia, increased gluconeogenesis, insulin resistance, and lactacidemia occur following burn injury. Increased gluconeogenesis and insulin resistance have been considered to be the main factors inducing hyperglycemia.

For a long period most investigators studying burn gluconeogenesis focussed their attention on hepatic and rarely on renal function. Zhai et al. in 1986 [16] demonstrated the gluconeogenic capacity of kidney in a severe burn rat model. They found that on PBD 3 and PBD 7 the ability of renal cortex to convert glutamic acid, aspartic acid, lactic acid, and glycerol into glucose was markedly increases ($p < 0.05$), but the renal cell could not properly utilize alanine to produce glucose. On PBD 1–PBD 7, the activities of glucose-6-phosphatase, fructose-1,6-diphosphatase, and phosphoenolpyruvate carboxykinase in both renal and hepatic cytoplasm were significantly elevated. In both renal and hepatic cytoplasm, no overt change in glutamic oxaloacetic transaminase (GOT) was found, whereas glutamic pyruvic transaminase (GPT) activity was exaggerated in hepatic but not in renal cytoplasm. These findings suggested that gluconeogenesis in the renal cortex plays an important role in maintaining the blood glucose level during the "flow phase" of burn injury. At present, most authors [3, 4, 5] emphasize the importance of liver in burn gluconeogenesis. After burn, a large proportion of the endogenous glucose production appears to be converted from the three carbon precursors provided by the alanine-glucose cycle and anaerobic glycolysis – pyruvate and lactate – which depend on skeletal and visceral protein as a major energy source. A small fraction of endogenous glucose originates from the glycerol.

Another important factor inducing hyperglycemia is insulin resistance, which is characterized by elevated plasma levels of glucose and insulin and glucose intolerance. There are also defects in both insulin receptors and postreceptors. Xu et al. [17, 18, 19] carried out a series of studies on insulin resistance in different burn animal models. They found that insulin resistance occurred not only in the burned or injured area or tissue, but also in the uninjured area or tissue. This phenomenon may last from the shock phase to the flow phase. After investigating the insulin receptors on cell membranes of erythrocytes as well as isolated hepatic and skeletal muscle cells, they also showed that the highest binding rates (B/T%) of the cells with [^{125}I] insulin in burn animals showed no significant difference from those of normal animals. However, the maximal binding capacities (R_0) and the number of receptors were obviously reduced, and the average affinity was significantly increased in burn animals.

Results of glucose consumption studies in the burned limb were quite controversial. Thrinsky (1983) reported that glucose consumption in skeletal muscle of the burned limb was significantly greater than that of the opposite unburned limb, whereas Thomas et al. (1979) indicated that in the burned limb there was obvious reduction of glucose consumption in skeletal muscle and decrease in insulin sensitivity, which was apparently normal in unburned limb. Xu et al. [19] found that postburn glucose consumption in skeletal muscle was decreased but showed no significant difference between the burned and unburned limb of rat. Further exploration is needed to explain this phenomenon.

Hyperglycemia, whether induced by gluconeogenesis or by insulin resistance, was considered to be the result of increased release of catecholamine, glucagon, cortisol, and other mediators. Infusion of epinephrine, glucagon, and cortisol for 3 days would induce changes in both glucose and protein metabolism, closely resembling the changed pattern after burn injury [20]. When combined α- and β-adrenergic blockades were administered to burned guinea pigs, glucose production increased. Thus the stimulation of glucose production after burn injury cannot be explained by the increased catecholamine activity. On the other hand, if somatostatin is infused, glucagon will lowered, and glucose production decreases, indicating that glucagon is a prominent stimulator of glucose production in burn pateients [21]. Nevertheless, Qin and Xu [22]

Table 15.5. Changes in serum glucose, insulin, and glucagon levels

	Tolbutamide-treated group ($n = 8$) postburn day					Control group ($n = 8$) postburn day				
	0	1	3	6	10	0	1	3	6	10
Glucose (mmol/l)	6.44 ±0.97	6.69*** ±1.39	5.83** ±1.17	5.44** ±0.78	5.05** ±0.82	6.11 ±0.60	10.47 ±1.29	7.99 ±1.23	7.44 ±1.17	7.05 ±1.33
Insulin (mU/l)	6.13 ±2.25	19.8*** ±3.21	23.4*** ±0.60	26.7*** ±8.38	24.3* ±4.22	6.29 ±2.44	8.88 ±2.42	9.20 ±2.67	11.3 ±5.13	16.8 ±5.31
Glucagon (ng/l)	17.7 ±8.75	64.7* ±10.57	52.9 ±11.4	42.9 ±8.86	27.6 ±7.89	19.7 ±9.24	86.4 ±14.2	64.5 ±9.26	54.7 ±14.52	33.3 ±9.18
I/G $\left(\frac{\text{insulin}}{\text{glucagon}}\right)$	0.35	0.31***	0.44**	0.63***	0.88*	0.32	0.10	0.14	0.21	0.50
I/Gs $\left(\frac{\text{insulin}}{\text{glucose}}\right)$	0.95	2.96***	4.01**	4.91**	4.81*	1.03	0.85	1.15	1.52	2.38

* $p < 0.05$.
** $p < 0.01$.
*** $p < 0.001$.

showed that hyperglycemia was blocked in burned rats after injection of α-blockade phentolamine (10 mg/kg) or β-blockade propranolol (50 μg/g), or after adrenalectomy. These findings were consistent with the study by Wilmore [3], who also demonstrated a significant reduction in the metabolic rate after administration of phentolamine and propranolol in burn patients, but did not define the relationship between the α-, β-blockade, and hyperglycemia. However, the clinical usefulness of blockade still appears limited.

Up to present, hyperglycemia induced by insulin resistance after burn cannot be completely eliminated clinically, but its severity can be reduced by several measures. Besides infusion of somatostatin [21] and insulin, we found that tolbutamide could combat burn hyperglycemia to a certain degree due to comparatively low levels of serum insulin and tissue insulin resistance [8]. The serum glucose level was obviously lowered, and the insulin level and I/G (insulin/glucagon) ratio were significantly higher than those of the control group (Table 15.5). The cumulative nitrogen balance, oxygen expenditure, and serum albumin in the tolbutamide-treated group were better than those of the controls. It was proposed that the mechanism of tolbutamide in reducing burn hyperglycemia and hypermetabolism was probably stimulation of insulin secretion, enhancement of insulin effect, inhibition of glucagon secretion, improvement in tissue insulin resistance, and promotion of glucose utilization of skeletal muscles. Its initial dosage used in burn adult patients is about 3 g/day (1 g tid). Several days later, the dosage is reduced to 1–2 g/day, as adjusted according to the serum levels of glucose, insulin, glucagon, and the I/G ratio after treatment with tolbutamide (90 mg/kg per day) in burn rabbit.

Besides I/G (insulin/glucagon), insulin/glucose (I/Gs) is also a simple and reliable index of glucose metabolism as shown in Table 15.5. Tian et al. [12], after analyzing the variation in I/Gs in 68 burn adults, found that the higher the burn TBSA, the lower the I/Gs ratio. The I/Gs ratio was slightly higher only in the group with burns less than 30% TBSA. The I/Gs ratio in the groups with burns above 30% TBSA gradually increased only after PBD 3, reaching a peak on PBD 7, and then reduced. Usually, the lower the I/Gs ratio, the poorer the prognosis of the burn patient.

In addition to hyperglycemia, hypoglycemia may sometimes occur in severely burned patients [1, 23], especially those in a state of malnutrition and those with sepsis and septicemia. In view of the fact that both hyperglycemia and hypoglycemia may occur in burns, it is better to maintain serum glucose levels in the range of 150–250 mg/dl. The rate of glucose infusion should be maintained at about 5 mg/kg per minute or 500 g/day in burned adults. It is harmful to liver and lung function if excessive quantities of glucose are given [4, 5].

15.3 Protein Metabolism and Its Requirement

During the flow phase, the negative nitrogen balance of burn victims was rapidly established in a catabolic state. The negative nitrogen balance increased in proportion to the extent and depth of the burn. Zhang and Shi [24] reported that the negative nitrogen balance was around 7–12 g/day in adults with burns of about 54% TBSA during the catabolic stage. According to our data, during the catabolic state, the negative nitrogen balance was in the range of 10–20 g/day in patients with burns of 40%–50% TBSA, of which more than one-third were third degree, and in the range of 5–10 g/day in patients with burns of 60%–70% TBSA without third-degree burns. Nitrogen loss originates not only from the skeletal muscle proteins in patients with a greater mass and slower turnover rate, but also from the proteins of visceral organs and others, which have a smaller mass and faster turnover rate.

Another index, 3-methylhistidine, is used for determining the degree of protein catabolism. As released from the degradation of muscle protein, it would not take part in recycling of protein metabolism; therefore the urinary output of 3-methylhistidine can be used as a quantitative measure of the catabolic state of protein. Zhang and Shi [24] reported that in a group of severely burned patients (mean burns about 54% TBSA), the urinary output of endogenous 3 methylhistidine was about 3.4 μmol/kg per day, which is consistent with other reports. Calculating from the output of 3 methylhistidine, the average decomposition rate of muscle protein is 2.3 times that of the normal controls.

In a study of a group of 19 patients with severe burns 56% mean TBSA, it was found that the mean protein supplied was 1.69 g/kg per day. Usually the protein supply was lower, within the range of 1.01–1.94 g/kg per day (mean, 1.19 g/kg per day) during the early stage, especially 1–2 week postburn, and/or severe conditions such as serious toxemia and septicemia were present. Protein administration reached a mean of 2.4 g/kg per day (range, 2.35–2.64 g/kg per day) during the stable and/or convalescent stage.

Excessive protein administration seems to be useless or even harmful especially in patients with impaired renal and hepatic function. Nevertheless, the protein dosage considered excessive still needs further study. Wolfe et al. [25] claimed that excessive protein supply did not increase the net protein synthesis, and they found no increase in protein synthesis beyond 1.4 g protein/kg per day. There is no effective clinical treatment so far to eliminate the protein catabolism, although measures to reduce hypermetabolism have been reported. It was found [7] that oxygen free radicals (OFR) and lipoperoxide (LPO) could have some effect on protein catabolism in a severe burn rat model. Superoxide dismutase (SOD) and catalase (CAT), the oxygen radical scavengers, could reduce protein catabolism to some extent. It is possible that OFR–LPO mediates catabolism postburn by affecting catabolic and anabolic hormones, directly modifying the protein structure, enhancing its degradation through the intracellular proteolytic system, and influencing the metabolism of arachidonic acid to increase PGE_2 production more than that of PGF_2 [26].

The free amino-acid levels in serum determined in burn patients are quite different [2, 27, 28]. The variables influencing their serum levels might be many, such as timing of determination, extent and depth of burn injury, nutritional state, and supply. Protein supplementation enriched with branched-chain amino acids (BCAA) to 50% of total amino acids was often recommended to promote anabolism in trauma patients. However, there was no definite information about the effectiveness of BCAA-enriched diets in nutritional support for burns. Orrawin et al. [29] found that supplementation of BCAA-enriched diets had no beneficial effect on postburn enteral nutritional management. Furthermore, when protein intake was either very low or very high, BCAA supplementation might instigate an adverse effect. It has been suggested that supplemental dietary arginine could lessen protein catabolism and enhance immune responses after trauma. Saito et al. [30] demonstrated that 1% and 2% arginine supplementation could improve metabolism and enhance immunity, and reported that the 2% arginine-supplemented group showed the best response, while there were no beneficial effects in the 4% arginine-supplemented group. It thus seems probable that aggressive amino acid supply is essential, but the adverse effect of excess amino acid supplementation should be avoided.

The serum levels of phenylalanine at various burn phases are found to be obviously high, which not only reflects the degree of protein decomposition in skeletal muscles, but also indicates the severity of impairment of hepatic function.

15.4 Lipid Metabolism and Its Requirement

According to the respiratory quotient, a rough indicator of fuel utilization, lipid is the major fuel source for energy production after burn.

Lipolysis and lipid mobilization from adipose tissue are increased after burn. Triglyceride is decomposed into glycerol and free fatty acids (FFA). In liver, glycerol can be converted to glucose, which is essential for brain and kidney tissue, and burn wound repair. There are two major pathways of FFA transformation which take place in the liver, i.e., reesterification of FFA to triglycerides and/or phospholipids, and the carnitine-dependent transfer of the FFAs into energy, acetyl-coenzyme A, and ketone bodies. After burn injury, the latter is usually inhibited [4], and is probably the result of the lack of carnitine, mitochondria dysfunction due to ischemia and anoxia, and the inhibition effect of catecholamine on this metabolic pathway.

The production of ketone body is decreased and peripheral use of ketone body is obviously increased after burn injury. Usually, the serum level of ketone body is not higher than normal but in fact lower than normal. There has been controversy as to whether the exogenous ketone body decreases protein consumption. Yang and Dong [31] showed that, before the use of exogenous Na-DL-3 hydroxybutyrate (3-HOBNa) and insulin in a burn rat model, the FFA decreased markedly and the urinary 3-methylhistidine excretion and the protein degradation rate of the soleus muscle of the injured hind limb increased markedly. Infusion of 3-HOBNa for three consecutive days following burns reduced the urinary 3-methylhistidine excretion and the protein degradation rate of the soleus muscle with no significant influence on the skeletal muscle protein anabolism. Moreover, there was no synergistic effect of the insulin-ketone body combination on anticatabolic capacity in burned rats. However, the clinical use of exogenous ketone body in burn patients has not yet been attempted and needs further exploration.

There are three main functions of dietary fat: to provide calories and minimize catabolism, fat is a more concentrated source of calories; to act as a carrier for the soluble vitamins; and to prevent essential fatty acid deficiency [32].

As to the lipid provision and its type in the diet of burn patients, Alexander et al. suggested that only 10%–15% of nonprotein calories should be derived from a lipid source and approximately 5% of nonprotein calories should come from linoleic acid. Using fish oil to provide about 50% of lipid calories appeared to be beneficial [32]. According to our clinical data in patients with burns of about 50% TBSA, the energy supply was lower and the lipid percentage of the total calories was also lower, usually below 15%, during the first 10 days postburn. Thereafter, the energy supply and lipid percentage gradually increased. The latter was usually about 20%–30% of the lipid in the total calorie supply. Of course, from these limited data, it can not be concluded that this lipid percentage is the optimal one.

15.5 Methods of Nutritional Support for Reduction of Hypermetabolism

So far, there have been no effective clinical measures to eliminate hypermetabolism. Many methods have been attempted for the reduction of catabolism. It was found [7] that SOD and CAT and the other oxygen radical scavengers reduced hypercatabolism and protein catabolism to some extent. It was also found [8] that tolbutamide reduced burn hypermetabolism probably through the stimulation of insulin secretion, improvement of tissue insulin resistance, and inhibition of glucagon secretion. Besides, the antagonist thromboxane(TXA_2), naloxone, somatostatin (reducing glucagon and growth hormone), insulin, etc. have been recommended as being able to reduce postburn hypermetabolism. But none have shown conclusive results, and further study is required especially in clinical practice.

15.5.1 Calorie and Protein Requirements

Various formulas have been devised for calculating daily energy and protein requirements for burned patients [5], such as 2000 cal/m^2 body surface, 20 cal/kg + 70 cal/% TBSA burned, and 2 × BMR. The most popular one is Curreri's formula, but the energy requirement calculated from this formula seems too

Table 15.6. Formula for estimating the calorie and protein requirements of burn patients

% TBSA burned	Calories/ day	Protein g (g/day)	Protein % of total calories	Calories to nitrogen ratio
< 30	40/kg	1.5–2.0/kg	15–20	
30–70	50/kg	2.0–2.5/kg	15–20	166:1–125:1
70–100	60/kg	2.5–3.0/kg	15–20	

Table 15.7. Nutritional requirements of burn patients

	Glucose	Lipid	Protein
% of total calories	60–70	15–20	15–20

high for the needs of Chinese burn patients. In our clinical practice, the following formula has been used for determining calorie and protein administration for burn adults (Table 15.6). Using this formula, which is by no means the best, but which is practicable and simple, of the total calories provided, 15%–20% are from lipids and 60%–70% are from glucose, as shown in Table 15.7.

15.5.2 Parenteral Nutrition

Because of the high incidence of sepsis caused by indwelling central venous catheters in burn patients, the application of parenteral nutrition by the central venous route is often limited. In a group of our patients with burns of 70% mean TBSA, the positive culture rate of central venous catheter tip was as high as 47.8%. Therefore, in clinical burn practice the first choice would be enteral and/or peripheral parenteral nutrition. Central parenteral nutrition is only selective, unless the above-mentioned route of nutritional support can not meet the calorie requirement.

Peripheral parenteral nutrition can be used immediately after the resuscitation stage. The osmolarity of amino acid infusion, fat emulsion, and a glucose concentration below 13% (722 mOsm/l) can be tolerated by the peripheral veins. The peripheral venous route is much safer than the central one, but is often limited by the tolerance of the peripheral veins to hyperosmolar infusions.

15.5.3 Enteral Nutrition

Dysfunction of the gastrointestinal tract is often seen in the first several days of severe burns. However, in most cases only gastric emptying is impaired, and small bowel functions may still be maintained or only slightly impaired. Enteral nutrition may become possible and can be started earlier, if the feeding tube is delivered through the pylorus and enters the small bowel. Our transnasal enteral feeding tube [33] can pass through the pylorus within 6 h with the patient in a horizontal position.

It is usually not necessary to change the patient's position or to manipulate the feeding tube under fluoroscopic or endoscopic control during insertion. Oral nutritional support may be started, and tube-feeding can be tapered off, when gastrointestinal function is regained.

15.6 Intestinal Absorption Following Burns

Intestinal absorption of nutrients was greatly decreased after severe burn injury. This change may be secondary to systemic disturbance of metabolism, or due to direct action of burn injury on intestine itself. Qin and Xu [34] considered that changes in glucose uptake from the small intestine were not directly caused by scald injury, and were almost certainly secondary consequences of disturbances in electrolyte metabolism and glucose handling by the rest of the body. However, in the experimental study of intestinal absorption of amino acid, Xiao and Jin [35] showed that the amino acid absorption ratio was positively correlated with the activity of $Na^+ - K^+$-ATPase of the small intestine mucosa in both the burn and control groups. They suggested that the decrease in amino acid absorption ratio in the burn group was probably due to the decreased activity of $Na^+ - K^+$-ATPase. It is probable that the impaired intestinal absorption results from both direct action of burn injury and indirect effects including disturbances in electrolyte metabolism, hyperglycemia, and other factors in the intestine.

We [36] investigated the dynamic changes in level of lipid peroxidation products (malondialdehyde, MDA) of intestine and intestinal water, and $Na^+ - K^+$-ATPase activity of intestinal mucosa and the intestinal leucine absorption rate of rats subjected to 30% third-degree burns. We found that the $Na^+ - K^+$-ATPase value of the intestinal mucosa reduced markedly, the wet/dry ratio of intestinal weight and the intestinal MDA content increased significantly, and the in vivo intestinal leucine absorption rate distinctly decreased in untreated burn rats, whereas the intestinal MDA content and wet/dry ratio of intestinal weight significantly decrease and $Na^+ - K^+$-ATPase activity and leucine absorption rate obviously increased in burn rats treated with SOD and CAT. These results strongly suggest that lipid peroxide plays an important role in the impairment of the leucine absorption rate of the intestine after burns, and the edema and reduced $Na^+ - K^+$ ATPase activity of intestinal mucosa resulting from the increased lipid peroxide might play an active role in impairing the intestinal absorption.

The provision of enteral nutritional support would be improved if treatment to increase intestinal absorption especially during the early stage in severe burns was properly instituted.

References

1. Burn Research Institute of the 3rd Military Medical University (ed) (1977) The treatment of burns. People's Health Publisher, Beijing, pp 51–76, 220–226
2. Yang ZJ, Xu WS, Shi JX (eds) (1985) Burn treatment, 2nd edn, Shanghai Science and Technology Publisher Shanghai, pp 169–183
3. Wilmore DW (1979) Metabolic changes in burns, In: Artz GP, Moncrief JA, Pruitt BA (eds) Burns, a team approach. Saunders, Philadelphia, pp 120–131
4. Burdge JJ, Conkright JM, Ruberg RL (1986) Nutritional and metabolic consequences of thermal injury. Clin Plast Surg 13(1): 49–55 (Advances in Burn Care)
5. Pasulka PS, Wachtel TL (1987) Nutritional considerations for the burned patient. Surg Clin North Am 67(1): 109–131
6. Fang ZY, Chen YL, Du FM (1985) Relationship between endocrine changes and clinical course of severe burns. Chin J Plast Surg Burns 1(2): 6–9
7. Shao H, Wang SL, Li Ngao et al. (1989) Effect of lipo-peroxide on hypercatabolism in burned rats. Proceedings of the 2nd Sino-American conference on burn injury and trauma, May 22–25, Beijing, p 243
8. Xie WG, Li Ngao, Wang SL et al. (1989) Tolbutamide and burn hypermetabolism. Proceedings of the 2nd Sino-American conference on burn injury and trauma, May, 22–25, Beijing, p 241
9. Wu J, Shi JQ (1987) An experimental study on the growth hormone cell in the pars distalis of the adenohypophysis after severe burn. Postgraduate symposium of the 3rd Military Medical University II
10. Huang YS, Li Ngao, Yang ZC (1989) Thromboxane A_2 (TXA_2) and prostacyclin (PGI_2) imbalance and its relationship with MSOF in burned patients. Proceedings of the 2nd Sino-American conference on burn injury and trauma May 22–25, Beijing, p 150
11. Jin HS, Chen GJ, Li J (1986) Plasma cortisol and serum thyroxine levels following burn stress. Chin J Plast Surg Burns 2(4): 291–293
12. Tian FQ, Bao JY, Yu FZ (1987) Changes in thyroxin, insulin and blood sugar in burned patients. Chin J Plast Surg Burns 3(4): 262–264
13. Chen YF, Shan KF, Jiang HQ et al (1988) An inquiry into the causes of hypothyroidism in the early stage of serious burns. Chin J Plast Surg Burns 4(2): 92–94
14. Gao XX, Chen WM, Wei LX et al. (1987) The evaluation of determination of Mb, T_3, T_4 by radioimmunoassay in burned patients. Chin J Plast Surg Burns 3(4): 257–258
15. Jn XL, Chen YS (1989) An experimental study of pathological changes and their mechanism of thyroid in rats with severe burns. Postgraduate symposium of the 3rd Military Medical University.
16. Zhai ZJ, Dong YL, Dong Q (1986) Effect of 30% body surface burns on gluconeogenic capacity of rat kidneys. Chin J Plast Surg Burns 2(3): 219–222
17. Xu LS, Wu XQ, Dong YL (1985) Preliminary observation on plasma insulin level and erythrocytic insulin receptor in smoke inhalation injury of dogs. Chin J Plast Surg Burns 1(2): 41–43

18. Xu LS, Wu XG, Dong YL (1986) Changes of the insulin receptor in isolated hepatocytes of burned rats. J Trauma (chin) 2(4): 220–222
19. Xu LS, Wu XG, Dong YL (1988) Research of the insulin resistance in burn rats. Chin J Exper Surg 5(1): 17–18
20. Bessey RW, Watters JM, Aoki TT et al. (1984) Combined hormonal infusion simulates the metabolic response to injury. Ann Surg 200: 264–280
21. Wolfe RR (1985) Glucose metabolism in burn injury: a review. J Burn Care Rehabil 6(5): 408–418
22. Qin ZY, Xu AH (1988) Hyperglycemia in burns. Chin J Plast Surg Burns (1): 54–56
23. Wu JY, Li JY (1987) Hypoglycemia in septicemia of gram-negative bacillus in severe burns. Chin J Plast Surg Burns 3(2): 151
24. Zhang XJ, Shi JX (1986) Preliminary study of muscle protein breakdown. Chin J Plast Surg Burns 2(4): 284–287
25. Wolfe RR, Goodenough RD, Biurke JF et al. (1983) Response of protein and urea kinetics in burn patients to different levels of protein intake. Ann Surg 197: 163–171
26. Rodemann HP, Goldberg AL (1982) Arachidonic acid, prostaglandin E_2 and F_2 influence rates or protein turnover in skeletal and cardiac muscle. J Biol Chem 257(4): 1632–1638
27. Li CL, Yang KQ, Ma JM (1988) An analysis of serum free amino acids in burned patients. Chin J Plast Surg Burns 4(4): 266–268
28. Chen YZ, Zhang GY, Gao LX et al. (1986) A comparative study of free amino acids in serum and blister in burned patients. Chin J Plast Surg Burns 2(2): 109–110
29. Orrawin T, Hidetake M, Alexander JW et al. (1985) Branched chain amino acids in postburn nutritional support. Proc Am Burn Assoc 17: 32
30. Saito H, Orranwin T, Alexander JW et al. (1987) Metabolic and immune effects of dietary arginine supplementation after burn. Arch Surg 122: 784–789
31. Yang Q, Dong YL (1989) Effects of exogenous Na-DL-3-hydroxybutyrate and insulin on skeletal muscle protein metabolism in rats after early severe burn injury. Acta 3rd Milit Med Univ 11(1): 5–9
32. Gottschlich MM, Alexander JW (1987) Review: fat kinetics and recommended dietary intake in burns. JPEN11(1): 80–85
33. Li GL, Wang SL, Li Ngao et al. (1980) Self-made transnasal enteral feeding tube and its administration in 36 cases of burn patients. Chin J Plast Surg Burns 4(4): 298–299
34. Qin ZY, Xu AH (1987) Absorption of glucose from the intestine following experimental seald injury in rats. Burns 13(6): 445–453
35. Xiao LY, Jin XL (1986) Changes of amino acid absorption through small intestines in rats with burn injury. Acta 3rd Miliit Med Univ 8(3): 227–230
36. Li CZ, Li Ngao, Wang SL et al. (1990) The role of intestinal lipid peroxide in reducing the rate of intestinal amino acid absorption in burn rats. Chin J Plast Surg Burns 6(1): 53–56

16 Immunology in Burns

Huang Wen-hua

Immunosuppression of the body defense mechanisms is the consequence of thermal injury and also the main cause of increased susceptibility of the patient to infection, which is a serious complication and the leading cause of death following burns. This may be the reason why burn immunology has become the focus of attention in the field of burn research. Reported clinical observations and experimental work concerning burn immunology, from the early 1970s until now, may be grouped into three categories: (a) effect of thermal injury upon the body defenses, (b) mechanisms of immunosuppression after burn injury, and (c) measures used to modulate the depressed immune defenses of the host.

16.1 Effects of Thermal Injury on the Body Defenses

16.1.1 Cellular Aspects

16.1.1.1 Polymorphonuclear Leukocytes

Polymorphonuclear Leukocytes (PMNs) are one type of phagocytic cell possessing nonspecific immunity. About 1.6×10^7 PMNs/kg body weight per day are produced by bone marrow hemopoietic cells. The reservoir for mature PMNs is located in the bone marrow, in which the number of PMNs is about 20 times that in the peripheral circulation. PMNs are short-lived cells, with a life span of only 10–20 days. They are released into the peripheral blood, where they stay for only 6–8 h before they enter the tissue, where they die 2–3 days later. Although PMNs are short lived, because of their large number, rapid recruitment to the injured tissue, and rapid replenishment from the bone marrow reserve, they still occupy a front-line position in the body defenses by phagocytosing invading microorganisms and removing nectrotic and dead tissue debris. The phagocytosing process of PMNs involves chemotaxis, ingestion, and intracellular killing. These are a series of very complicated biological activities for which the normal functional state of PMNs is required. But following thermal injury, the normal functional state of the PMNs is profoundly disturbed.

Chemotaxis is the directional migration of PMNs as a result of the chemoattractive effect of certain chemotactic factors, including a variety of soluble agents present in the serum and also in the tissue fluid in the inflammatory area, chiefly the split products of activated complement, namely C3a, C5a, C_{567}, and bacterial products. Even PMNs themselves, when activated, may also produce chemoattractants, such as leukotriene B4(LTB4), one of the arachidonic acid metabolites, to attract other PMNs toward the inflammatory site. As soon as PMNs are aggregated to the local area, they are ready to carry out their duty – phagocytosis. However, it has been found that chemotactic movements of PMNs are altered following thermal injury. Zhang and Tan [1], observing the chemotaxis of PMNs by the agarose droplet method, found that the mean of A/B (A, chemotactic mobility; B, random migration) in 49 burned patients was 1.8 ± 0.26, which is significantly lower than that of the control (2.3 ± 0.38) ($p < 0.01$). This low level persisted from the first to the fourth postburn week. They also found that the chemotaxis index of PMNs during severe sepsis, septicemia, or shortly before death was lower than during convalescence ($p < 0.01$). Xu et al. [2], in a study of 46 burn patients, found that the directional movement of PMNs in chemotaxis became markedly retarded in the first two postburn weeks, and recovered after the 3rd week, claiming that the retardation was closely related to the development of septic complications. A total of six patients with persistent low chemotatic migration all developed sepsis and four of them died.

The next step of phagocytosis is ingestion. When in contact with foreign particles, such as bacteria, PMNs will ingest these particles. The ingestion process is facilitated and enhanced by soluble factors present in the serum or tissue fluid, which are named opsonins. Complement C3b and antibodies (immunoglobulins, Igs) are the important and effective ones. Particles, treated with opsonins, will be easily and stably bound to the cell membrane of phagocytes, by which they are finally engulfed. But it has also been found that opsonization is interfered with after burning. Sheng and Tung [3], after an analysis of 36 burned patients, demonstrated that the serum opsonic ability (opsonic index, OI) measured by chemiluminescence (CL) was significantly lowered in burned patients with burns $>35\%$ TBSA (0.69 ± 0.06) compared with that in normal controls (1.05 ± 0.04). The attachment of opsonized particles to the cell membrane is through the close interaction between the opsonins and their appropriate receptors on the surface membrane of the cell. Many kinds of receptors on the cell surface membrane constitute the major structures for communicating with the internal and external environments of the cell. External signals or stimuli (e.g., bacteria) from the extracellular milieu are transported to the cell through the receptors, and the intracellular biological activities (e.g., killing the ingested bacteria) are controlled by the receptors. That is to say, receptors can regulate the cell activity and maintain the balance between the intra- and extra-cellular environments. Thus in phagocytosis the Fc receptor for the Fc fragment of Ig (antibody) and C3b receptor for complement-split product C3b are important for regulating ingestion and killing of bacteria. Huang et al. [4] have found that these receptors were suppressed by thermal injury. Using the rosette formation method they studied both Fc receptor and C3b receptor of PMNs in rats and found that these two receptors progressively decreased in number in the 1st week following scald injury superimposed by wound infection of *Pseudomonas aeruginosa*; particularly the Fc receptor is more intensively interfered with than the C3b receptor. The capacity of bacterial ingestion by PMNs has been studied by many authors [5, 6] in burned patients. The ability of PMNs to phagocytose *Candida albicans* was markedly reduced and closely related with the severity of burns. Jiang et al. [7] observed the capacity of PMNs to ingest *Staphylococcus aureus* in dogs inflicted with inhalation injury with or without body surface burns (30%, 2°–3°) and found that the more severe the injury, the more the impairment of the phagocytosing ability of PMNs. Suppression of the phagocytic functions after injury, including the percentage of phagocytosing cells and phagocytic index (number of bacteria ingested/100 PMNs) was unremarkable in simple inhalation injury, but became pronounced when inhalation injury was combined with body surface burn. However, some authors [8, 9] have denied that there is any marked change in bacterial ingestion of PMNs following thermal injury.

The final step of phagocytosis is intracellular killing or digestion of the engulfed microorganisms. Two patterns of intracellular killing have been demonstrated: anaerobic through the proteolytic activities of lysosome enzymes; and oxygen dependent through the oxidative metabolism of the cell. In the anaerobic pattern, the foreign particle is first enveloped and engulfed into PMNs to form a phagosome inside the cell, and then the lysosome in the cell plasma will fuse with the phagosome to form a lysophagosome, in which proteolytic enzymes originally in the lysosome now come into contact with the ingested particle and destroy it. The oxygen-dependent pattern is the most important intracellular killing process of PMNs. When the cell membrane is disturbed by foreign particles, a series of metabolic changes including increased glycolysis, oxygen consumption, and hexone monophosphate activities will be evoked, resulting in the generation of a group of oxygen-reduced products, such as superoxide anion, hydrogen peroxide, and hydroxyl radical, all of which are powerful bactericidal agents. Hydrogen peroxide, besides its direct bactericidal effect, when combined with myeloperoxidase and in the presence of halide ions (especially Cl^- and I^-), will form a microbicidal system capable of destroying ingested microorganism. Following thermal injury, the intracellular bactericidal ability of PMNs is profoundly suppressed. The bactericidal activity of PMNs as measured by CL in burned patients with burns >35% BSA was lower than that in controls ($1.85 \pm 0.21 \times 10^3$ cpm vs. $3.55 \pm 0.15 \times 10^3$ cpm). Development of sepsis was often associated with a marked lowering of CL. The incidence of sepsis increased to 85.7%, as CL decreased to less than 2×10^3 cpm [3]. Fang et al. [10] observed the microbicidal activity of PMNs by means of the nitroblue tetrazolium (NBT) reduction test in 18 burned patients (>30% BSA), and found that the percentage of PMNs exhibiting the ability to reduce this dye (NBT + cells) was much higher than normal in patients that survived and either normal or subnormal in patients that did not survive. But once sepsis set in or before death, the percentage of NBT + cells increased abruptly. Therefore they proposed that a sudden rise in the reduced percentage of NBT + cells signals the impending occurrence of sepsis. Huang et al. [11], after a study of the oxidative metabolism of PMNs following thermal injury by measuring both

H_2O_2 release and iodination reaction in dogs and rats, demonstrated that early in the first postburn week both the amount of H_2O_2 released and iodine taken up by PMNs gradually but significantly declined, indicating serious impairment of the bactericidal ability of the cells. It might be of interest to note that the release of free oxygen radicals and the proteolytic enzymes from PMNs after burn may be detrimental in that they are capable of causing damage to cells of various organs. This effect may aggravate the already impaired organ functions, and even trigger or accelerate the development of multiple organ failure (MOF) in severely injuried patients.

16.1.2 Macrophages

Macrophages (Mϕ) originate from the bone marrow. When released they enter the blood-stream and become monocytes; they are not mature cells. However, once they have left the circulation and have entered the body tissues, they become resident mature Mϕ, the chief cell population of the mononuclear phagocytic system (MPS, previously called RES). Both morphologically and functionally Mϕ are heterogeneous. Mϕ from different tissues may display divergent characteristics. For instance, compared with alveolar Mϕ, Mϕ of the peritoneal cavity respond very well to chemotactic agents and are also more efficient at rendering antigens immunogenic. Even from same tissue source, Mϕ may exhibit a different functional reactivity. All these characteristics make study of Mϕ difficult and complicated. Different segregation methods, different manipulations, or even different activating processes may yield a particular group of Mϕ which by no means represent Mϕ as a whole. This is why the heterogeneity either due to different stages of maturation or because of the existence of different subpopulations is still unclear. Despite this, however, the characteristics and functions of Mϕ have been widely studied. It is known at least, that Mϕ are important immunocompetent cells participating in both specific and nonspecific immunities, and displaying enhancing or suppressive functions. Therefore, Mϕ play a central role in the regulation of immune response.

In enhancing immune response, Mϕ are phagocytes with nonspecific immunity and play an important role in removing and clearing invading microorganisms; Mϕ are also the accessory cells in specific immunity, relating to the growth and maturation of lymphocytes, as well as processing and presenting antigens to lymphocytes. Wu et al. [12] studied the effects of thermal injury and wound infection on the peritoneal Mϕ in rats through the observation of the reactivities of different surface membrane receptors. In nonspecific immunity, receptors relating to phagocytosis, such as IgG Fc fragments, C3b, or fibronectin, have been studied. Among them, the marked decrease in the reactivity of fibronectin receptor occurring early on the first postburn day was the most prominent change. In contrast, the reactivity of Fc receptor increased after burn, and became significantly different from that of the control on the 7th day postburn. C3b receptor also showed a tendency to increase in reactivity but

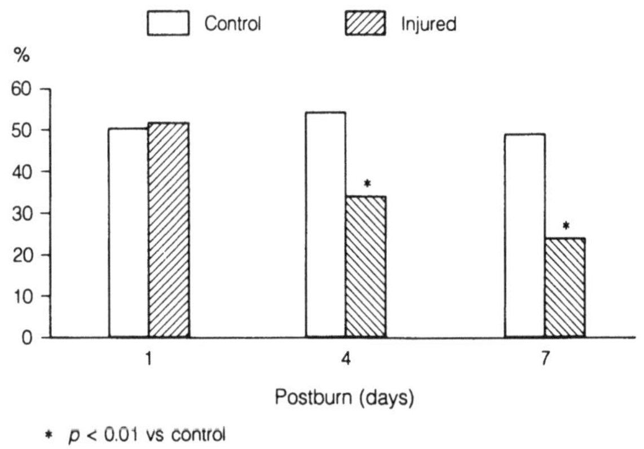

Fig. 16.1. Reactivity of thymocyte receptor of macrophage of injured .rats (% of cluster-forming cells)

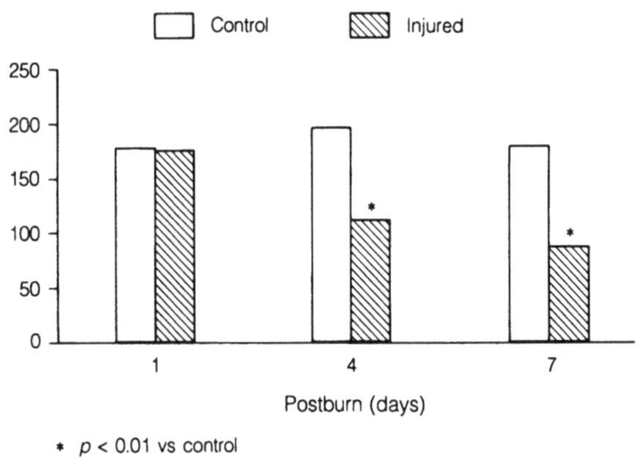

Fig. 16.2. Reactivity of thymocyte receptor of macrophage of injured rats (bound thymocyte/100 cells)

this was not statistically significant. In specific immunity, the thymocyte receptors on the surface of Mϕ are important for the interaction between these two cells. Through this receptor, Mϕ regulate the maturation of lymphocytes and also present antigens to them. In rats following burn and wound infection this receptor showed marked progressive decrese in reactivity during the first postburn week, and its reactivity amounted to only 50% of that of the normal control on the 7th day (F test, $p < 0.01$), indicating that the antigen-presenting function of Mϕ was impaired (Figs. 16.1, 16.2). Kupper et al. [13] also found that the functional defect of T-helper cells was partly due to dysfunction of antigen-presenting cells in thermally injured mice.

In immune response suppression, Mϕ also show inhibiting activity of the lymphocyte response to both mitogens and alloantigens, as well as suppressing the effector phase of natural killer (NK) cell. Fang et al. [14] discovered that the adherent cells of burn patient's peripheral blood inhibited the response of autologous lymphocytes to phytohemagglutinin (PHA). Lahat et al. [15] also found that monocytes interacted with suppressor T cells in the suppression of lymphocyte response to Con A. Suzuki and Pollard [16] observed that spleen Mϕ of burned mice suppressed the production of interferon by spleen lymphocytes.

Macrophages also modulate immune response through synthesis and release of many mediators, such as complement components, fibronectin, prostaglandins, interleukin-1, and colony-stimulating factor. All possess different biological activities. Alterations of these mediators following burn will exert a marked influence on the pathophysiology after burn.

16.1.3 Lymphocytes

Lymphocytes are immunocompetent cells undertaking specific immunity. They are derived from the bone marrow hemopoietic stem cells. During the course of maturation they are divided into two main subpopulations. One is processed by the thymus to become T lymphocyte responsible for cellular immunity, and the other is a B-cell subpopulation, which, when activated, will differentiate into plasma cells serving as antibody-producing cells. In building up the immune response, T and B cells interact with each other, e.g., the production of antibody by B cells is regulated by both helper (Th) and suppressor (Ts) T cells, the main subpopulations of T cells. Under normal conditions, these two subpopulations are kept in balance to control and maintain the specific immunity in the normal functional state.

Following thermal injury, lymphocyte functions are disturbed, and T cell function more so. Zhang et al. [6] and Huang et al. [17] observed that the number (E-rosette-forming cells) and functional response (to PHA) of lymphocytes were markedly reduced in the early postburn period in patients. The degree of reduction and the rate of recovery closely paralleled the size and depth of burn. It was suggested by some authors that the supppression of T cell functions might resullt in an increase in susceptibility of the patient to infection. Shi [18] studied the response of lymphocyte to PHA in 14 burned patients. The results showed that when the area of third-degree burn was greater than 20% BSA, the decrease in response was not only related to the depth of burn, but also closely associated with septic complications. Moss et al. [19] also demonstrated the close correlation between T-lymphocyte function and mortality rate of sepsis following burn injury in mice. The suppressive effect of burn injury on response of splenic cells to PHA was maximal on the 14th postburn day (PBD), while mortality rate of septic challenge by cecal ligation and puncture reached its peak also on the 14th PBD. Recently, many research results have emphasized the significance of interleukin-2(IL-2) production and IL-2 receptor expression of the T cell in establishing and regulating the immune response. Rodrick et al. [20] considered that, although there are multiple immune abnormalities following thermal injury, the most striking and persistent one is the decrease in IL-2 production. Peng et al. [21] observed similar changes in burned rats. IL-2 production declined abruptly and persistently, reaching its lowest level as early as 2 h following burn and maintaining this low level until the end of 10 days with no tendency to recover. Wood et al. [22] found in scalded mice that decreased IL-2 production persisted even when the IL-2-producing cells (mainly T helpers) had returned to normal levels. They suggested that the IL-2 production was vulnerable to the suppressive effect of PGE_2. Besides the production of IL-2, the expression of IL-2 receptors (IL-2Rs) of T cells was also impaired. Teodorczyk-Injeyan et al. [23] found that the expression of IL-2Rs of peripheral blood lymphocytes decreased to 40%–90% of its normal level in immunosuppressed burn patients. Although the number of IL-2Rs might be increased by the administration of exogenous IL-2 to cultured cells in vitro, the affinity of these IL-2Rs was low and nonfunctional. Therefore the proliferative response of lymphocytes would never be restored by exogenous IL-2 in nonsurviving burn patients. It is thus considered that thermal injury affects expression of functional (high-affinity) receptors.

16.1.4 Natural Killer Cells

Natural killer (NK) cells are nonspecific cytotoxic cells, and also play a role in the regulation of immune response. It was reported that NK cells have negative regulation of B cells by inhibiting their activity through affecting the accessory cells, which are cells capable of secreting factors for B-cell proliferation and differentiation, and present antigens to B cells. However, others claimed that NK cells may secrete B-cell growth factor and B-cell differentiation factor and exert positive regulation on B cells. There were also reports that NK cells may present antigen to lymphocytes, thus making themselves accessory cells in the regulation of T-cell function. These results, though divergent, at least indicate that NK cells are an important cell population in the immune system. Following thermal injury the function of this cell population alters. Polacek et al. [24] found that NK cell activity was reduced in the high-risk group of burned patients with or without septic complications. Stein et al. [25] observed that the killing ability of peripheral blood NK cells of burned patients to target cells K562 was only 30% of that of normal persons.

As is well known, red blood cells are gas-exchangers, supplying oxygen and removing carbon dioxide to and from the tissues to provide the optimal environment for living cells and tissues; and blood platelets are important constituents of the blood coagulation system. Nevertheless, both are also members of the immune system, chiefly demonstrating immune adherence activities by virtue of the expression of surface membrane receptors for complement components (C3b). Through these receptors they combine with circulating immune complexes (CICs) and travel to the RES, then where the CICs are finally removed from the body. Because of the large number of RBCs and platelets, it is believed that the vast majority of CICs are eliminated through this route. It was found that the immune-adherent function of RBCs was impaired and the percentage rosette formation with serum (complement)-treated yeast decreased to below normal during a period of 3 ~ 4 weeks postburn follow-up in clinical patients [26] and experimental animals [27], in which the lowest point was found on the sixth postburn day. Guo et al. [28] found that the platelet-adherent activity, determined by agglutination assay using complement (guinea pig serum)-sensitized yeast, was significantly increased at 24 and 48 h postburn in scalded rats, and suggested that this alteration might be one of the factors contributing to the development of disseminated intravascular coagulation (DIC).

16.2 Humoral Aspects

16.2.1 Complement System

As far as the body defense mechanism is concerned, the complement system is a very important and also a very complicated humoral factor. It consists of a group of enzyme-like serum proteins including C1 ~ C9 as well as some initiators and stabilizers such as B factor, D factor, properdin, and also some inhibitors and inactivators such as H factor, I factor, C4-binding protein (C4BP), decay acceleration factor (DAF), and C3b receptor (CR1). Under static conditions, they exist as precursors of enzyme in the serum. Once stimulated they will be activated and convert into a series of components, characterized by a cascading process in which the preceding numbered component acts as an enzyme of the next, proceeding one after the other in a definite order. There are two pathways of complement activation. One is the classical pathway, usually activated by the antigen-antibody complex, C-reactive protein, and so on. The other is the alternative pathway in which they may be activated directly by bacterial products, polysaccharides, zymosan, insulin, etc., not requiring antibody production. Therefore the alternative pathway stands more at the front line of the body defenses than the classical pathway. In the very early phase following thermal injury, the complement system is activated, leading to depletion of complement, which is not beneficial to the body defenses against bacterial invasion. As reported by Haung et al. [29], the total and alternative pathway hemolytic activity decreased in the early postburn period (1–3 days) as observed in 23 cases of burned patients. Recovery of total hemolytic activity was rapid, and approached normal at the end of the first postburn week. But recovery of the hemolytic activity of the alternative pathway was somewhat delayed and remained at a low level for the first 2 weeks, only returning to normal at the end of the 3rd week. This indicated that the alternative pathway was more affected by thermal injury. Furthermore, Huang et al. found that low levels of serum complement were often associated with sepsis and/or a grave prognosis of burned patients. The early depletion of serum complement was also observed

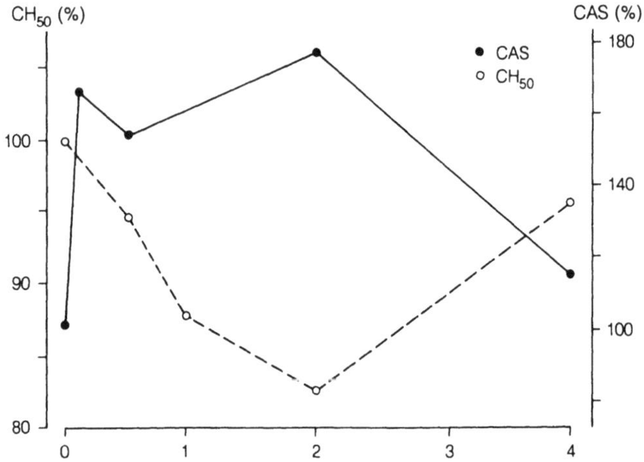

Fig. 16.3. Complement-activating substance (*CAS*) and complement hemolytic activity (*CH50*) (preburn level as 100%) in left ventricular blood

by this group of authors in dogs suffering from severe steam inhalation injury [30]. They explored the mechanism of early depletion by means of enzyme-linked immunosorbent assay (ELISA) using conglutinin as the solid phase to detect large molecular weight substances in the blood, and discovered there was an increase in complement-activating substance in the left ventricular blood as early as 5 min postinhalation injury (Fig. 16.3). These authors claimed that at least one constituent of this large molecular weight substance was IgG, because enzyme-labeled protein A was used as the second antibody in ELISA. They proposed that, when the blood passed through the lung during steam inhalation, plasma proteins were aggregated by heat to form a large molecular weight substance, which might be one of the causes of complement activation, consumption, and finally depletion. Because C4 and B factor are important components of the classical and alternative pathways, respectively, while C3 is the common component of both pathways, Wu et al. [31] selectively studied the changes in complement C3, C4, and B factor in 31 cases of burned patients with burns >30% BSA. They found that C3 and C4 decreased in the first 3 days after burn, and began to recover afterwards. C3 returned to above normal levels about 3 weeks after injury, but recovery of C4 was somewhat retarded. Both C3 and C4 levels were related to size of burn, the larger the size the lower the level. Low levels were often associated with septic complications and/or the death of patients, indicating that the vulnerability of burn patients was increased. There was no marked change in B factor after burn, although the alternative pathway was profoundly interfered with by thermal injury as described above. It seemed that B factor did not participate in this event.

During the course of complement activation, besides the cascade of C1 ~ C9 ending in membrane attack to lyse bacteria or microorganisms, there are several split products of complement, which possess active biological activities closely related to body defense mechanism. C3a and C5a, known as anaphylatoxins, are able to activate the mast cells to secrete histamine, a substance which can cause an increase in vascular permeability and in turn edema formation. Zhou and Ai [32] found in dogs that anaphylatoxin levels in left ventricular blood increased in amount 60 min after steam inhalation, and were significantly higher than levels in controls 60 ~ 120 min after injury. C3a and C5a as well as activated C567 are potent chemoattractants playing important roles in attraction and aggregation of PMNs in the injured and inflammatory area. The aggregated and activated PMNs will release proteolytic enzymes and produce active oxygen radicals. All of these proved to be detrimental to tissues and were also attributed to be important causes of the development of dysfunction of internal organs, especially the lung [33–36].

16.2.2 Fibronectin

Plasma fibronectin (FN) is an opsonic glycoprotein. When foreign particles such as bacteria and tissue debris are opsonized by this glycoprotein, ingestion by Mϕ, especially Kupffer's cells in the liver, is facilitated. Thus FN is closely related to the clearance function of the RES. In traumatized, burned, or septic patients, FN content and its activity in plasma usually decrease, and this decrease is often accompanied by impaired clearance function of the liver. Then foreign particles will accumulate and be deposited in other internal organs to form microemboli or thrombi, which in turn will interfere with the microcirculation and finally result in dysfunction of organs, even resulting in multiple organ failure. The decrease in plasma FN usually parallels the severity of illness in deteriorated patients, and measurement of plasma FN may be used as a parameter to predict outcome in severely ill patients. Huang et al. [37] measured the blood FN activity by agglutination assay with gelatin-coated sheep RBCs in 32 patients with burns >30% BSA, and discovered that in the early postburn period (1st week) there was a marked reduction of plasma FN activity, the degree of which was closely related to the severity of burn. The plasma FN subsequently rose gradually to normal levels. Persistent low levels or further decrease after its return to normal levels usually indicated the occurrence of complications, especially sepsis. Sheng et al. [38] determined plasma FN in 24 burned patients burns with >30% BSA by adopting an immunological quantitative method with anti-FN serum, and found on the 1st and 2nd PBD a significant decrease in plasma FN level in all cases from normal values of 286.94 ± 51.35 μg/ml to 112.56 ~ 185.85 μg/ml and 44.03 ~ 298 μg/ml, respectively, while plasma FN of another nine patients with smaller BSA burns (3%–25%) also determined showed no decrease in early postburn time. Nineteen of the 24 patients survived, and their plasma FN returned to normal levels within 3 ~ 6 days, while plasma FN fell progressively until death in the 5 nonsurvivors.

16.2.3 *Acute-Phase Reactant Proteins*

Acute-phase reactant proteins (APRPs) are a group of plasma proteins. They are so named because the alterations in their blood concentrations are usually associated with acute-phase trauma, burn, or septic infection and also with inflammatory change and/or tissue destruction or necrosis. APRPs include C-reactive protein (C-RP), α_1-acid glycoprotein (α_1-AG), protease inhibitors (e.g., α_1-antitrypsin, α_1-antichymotrypsin, α_2-macroglobulin), transport proteins (e.g., ceruloplasmin, transferrin, haptoglobin, hemopexin, prealbumin), complement components (e.g., C3, C4), blood coagulation proteins (e.g., antithrombin III, plasminogen, fibrinogen), and so on. Most are synthesized and secreted by the liver. Intcrlcukin-1 (IL-1), a mediator of Mϕ, may be one of the regulators of these APRPs.

C-reactive and α_1-AG increase in concentration following traumatic, inflammatory, and/or infectious stimulations. Although the increase is nonspecific, it may be of major importance in the diagnosis and prognosis of the severity of illness. Protease inhibitors, being important plasma proteins in antagonizing the proteolytic enzymes released by activated PMNs and Mϕ, may play protective roles in the prevention of proteolytic digestion of tissues. Among the protease inhibitors, α_1-antitrypsin and α_2-macroglobulin are polyvalent inhibitors against trypsin, chymotrypsin, plasmin kallikrein, thrombin, elastase, etc. As reported by Wu et al. [39], APRP showed pronounced changes following thermal injury in 31 patients with burns >30% BSA. Plasma C-RP, normally at very low levels (0.61 ± 0.18 mg/dl), increased rapidly soon after burn to two fold its normal value on the 3rd PBD. It reached its peak (14.5 ± 3.0 mg/dl) on the 10th PBD and persisted at a high level. Even at the end of the 5th week postburn it was still much higher than normal (10.0 ± 4.2 vs. 0.61 ± 0.18 mg/dl). The changed pattern of α_1-AG was similar to that of C-RP. α_1-Antitrypsin level decreased markedly (189 ± 8 mg/dl) compared with normal values (404 ± 109 mg/dl) on the 1st PBD. Recovery was rapid, reaching and exceeding the normal level on the 3rd PBD. From that time on it persisted at a high level until the end of observation (5 weeks). The increments in C-RP, α_1-AG, and α_1-antitrypsin paralleled the severity of the burn injury. The larger the BSA burned and the percentage BSA third-degree burns, the higher the increments of these three APRPs. The changed pattern of α_2-macroglobulin was different from that of the above three. It was reduced to below normal from the 1st PBD, staying at a low level throughout the 5-week observation period. Changes in these four APRPs were related to development of septicemia, especially the increase in C-RP and α_1-antitrypsin and the decrease in α_2-macroglobulin. These changes may ooccur even 2 days before the onset of septicemia, and were therefore thought to be predictive signs of the onset of septic complications. α_1-AG markedly increased and α_2-macroglobulin markedly decreased in plasma before death, so they were grave signals for the outcome of patients. Dong et al. [40] studied the relationship between plasma C-RP and burn sepsis in 30 cases. Patients were divided into two groups: group A, burns >30% BSA; and group

B, burns <30% BSA. The level of plasma C-RP was much higher in group A ($146 \pm 13\,\mu g/ml$) than in group B ($37 \pm 8\,\mu g/ml$) on the 7th PBD. In group A, 6 out of 14 cases developd septicemia, and plasma C-RP in septic cases increased more markedly ($163 \pm 48\,\mu g/ml$) than that in the nonseptics ($72 \pm 18\,\mu g/ml$). They also found that the plasma C-RP level was significantly higher at 48 h before positive blood culture than 48 h after it turned negative, and suggested that plasma C-RP be used as a parameter for monitoring infection in burned patients.

Transport proteins act as carriers which combine with certain substances to transport them to some parts of the body where the substances are utilized in the metabolism. For instance, haptoglobin combines with hemoglobin during intravascular hemolysis to form the hemoglobin-haptoglobin complex, which is transported from the blood circulation to the liver, and is finally eliminated by the RES. Ceruloplasmin, a carrier for copper, also participates in iron metabolism, and possesses antioxidant properties, inhibiting the peroxidation of liquid caused by free oxygen radicals. Transferrin combines and transports iron. Prealbumin combines and transports thyroxine. Both transferrin and prealbumin are related to the nutritional state of the body; therefore they may be adopted as indices in evaluating the patient's nutrition. Wu et al. [31] analyzed plasma transport proteins in 31 burned patients, finding that haptoglobin decreased immediately after burn, but rapidly increased to above normal levels, attaining a peak (about 400% of normal) on the 10th PBD, and maintaining a high level until the end of the 5th week of observation. Ceruloplasmin, transferring, and prealbumin were all reduced in the early postburn stage. Of these, ceruloplasmin gradually increased after the first postburn week, and reached its normal level in the 2nd week. But transferrin and prealbumin persisted at low levels for the whole course of observation, indicating the presence of malnutrition in burned patients. None of the transport proteins showed evident correlation with septic episodes or death of patients. Reduction of transferrin and prealbumin in burn patients was also observed by other authors [3, 41]. Sheng et al. found that low serum transferrin levels often correlated with a high incidence of septicemia. Xue et al. reported that prealbumin levels in blood were low in the first postburn week but returned to normal at the end of the 2nd week.

16.2.4 Immunoglobulins

Immunoglobulins are plasma proteins produced by B lymphocytes, and they act as antibodies to provide specific humoral immunity. They have been widely studied by many authors [6, 17, 42], especially IgG, IgA, and IgM, in thermal injury. Patterns of change of IgG and IgA are similar, showing a slight decrease in the first postburn week and a rapid return to normal after the 2nd week. IgM shows no remarkable change after burn. None of the immunoglobulins have an obvious relationship with burn size. It seems probable that the specific humoral immunity is not as deeply disturbed as cell-mediated specific immunity thermal injury.

16.3 Mechanism of Immunosuppression Following Burn

As stated above, obviously many aspects of the immune system are affected after burn injury, and the major manifestations are functional suppressions. That is to say, thermal injury brings about acquired immunodeficiency of the body defenses of the victim. The mechanism of development of the acquired immunodeficiency and the causes of immunosuppression are not yet clear, although the presence of suppressive factors in the burned victim's serum and the activation of suppressor cells have been recognized as causes of postburn immunosuppression by many authors.

16.3.1 Suppressive Factors in Serum

In the early 1970s, the presence of substances possessing immunosuppressive activity in the serum of burned patients was proposed. There was a continuous debate until much experimental work and many clinical observations proved their existence. These substances can inhibit the proliferative response of normal lymphocyte to mitogens [43–46], the reaction of mixed lymphocyte culture (MLR) in vitro [47, 48], and delayed hypersensitivity to recall antigens in vivo [49]. They can also suppress the chemotactic response and phagocytic function of neutrophils and macrophages, decrease their oxygen consumption, and lower their oxidative metabolism [11, 43, 50–52]; in addition, they are able to interfere with the clearance rate of the reticuloendothelial system [53].

Although the presence of serum immunosuppressive factors in burn patients is beyond doubt, the origins or sources and chracteristics or properties of these factors are still not clear. Some authors suggested that they arose from burned skin and tissues. Extract of burned skin was toxic to the liver cells and may inhibit the respiratory function of mitochondria of hepatocytes [54–56]; it also increased the mortality of burned mice [57, 58]. Hansbrough et al. [59] discovered that the delayed hypersensitivity response to dinitrofluorobenzene (DNFB) was reduced in normal mice after they were transplanted with burned mouse skin. Schoenenberger et al. [60] has extracted a lipoprotein from burned skin, which could impair the host defense for gram-negative organisms. Nevertheless, many authors claimed that serum-suppressive factors might be the products of abnormal metabolism following thermal injury. Products of arachidonic acid, such as prostaglandin E2 (PGE_2) and leukotriene B4 (LTB_4) were proved to possess suppressive activities, especially PGE_2, which could not only exhibit suppressive effects on immune function, but also activate the suppressor T cells. PGE_2 was confirmed by Ninnemann and Ozkan [61] as one of the immunosuppressive factors of postburn serum. They found that the suppressive activity of postburn

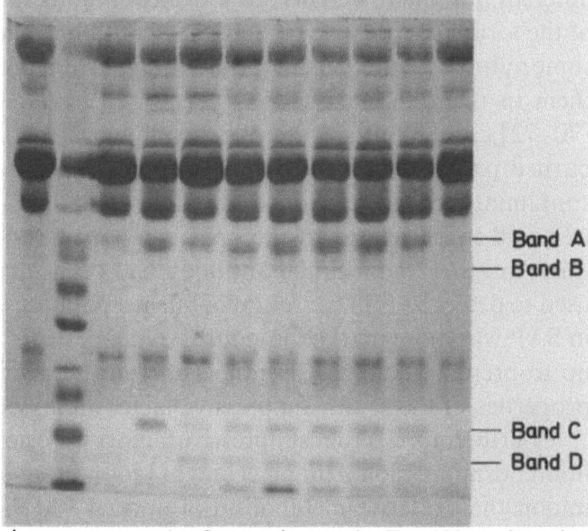

Fig. 16.4. SDS-PAGE (discontinuous system); Separation gel: T = 10%, C = 3%; stacking gel: T = 3%, C = 3%; *lines 1, 3 and 11* (from left to right), normal serum; *line 2*, molecular weight markers; *line 4*, burned serum (2° BSA, 7%, 6 PBD); *line 5*, burned serum (2° BSA, 25%, 15 PBD); *lines 6–10*, burned sera (TBSA 85%, 3° 40% 2, 6, 12, 20, and 27 PBD)

serum was reduced if the serum was treated with anti-PGE_2 antibody or delipidization (PGE_2 as a nonsaturated fatty acid); the serum-suppressive activity reappeared when PGE_2 was added to delipidized serum. It was recently reported that the degradation peptide of complement C1q could inhibit the chemotaxis of PMNs and the mixed lymphocyte reaction (MLR), and also stimulate Ts [62]. Ogle et al. [63, 64] demonstrated that the fluid phase C3b not only lost its opsonic activity but became a suppressive factor in the phagocytosis of PMNs and also in the proliferative response of lymphocytes to mitogens.

Many authors have attempted to separate the suppressive factors from the postburn serum. Huang et al. [65] compared the burned patient's sera (burns > 30% BSA, $n = 38$) with normal sera (pooled sera of 90 blood donors) by SDS-polyacrylamide gel electrophoresis (SDS-PAGE), and found at least four abnormal bands with molecular weights of 44.9, 41.6, 20.2, and 17.1 K present in patient's sera from 2–3 days to 2–3 weeks after burn (Fig. 16.4). Generally, these abnormal bands were not found in normal sera. Various protein analysis methods, such as gel filtration and ion-exchange chromatography, were also used to separate and study the characteristics of the suppressive factors, but their results were conflicting. Many authors reported that the suppressive activity was present in low molecular weight fractions (3–10 kd) [43, 61, 66], which might inhibit the lymphocyte response to mitogen and allogenic antigens in vitro, and increase the mortality when injected into infected mice. Gerner et al. proposed that multiple suppressors were present in postburn serum with different molecular weights [67]. Concerning the properties and characteristics of the serum-suppressive factors, they could be either protein or peptide. While some authors found them in the globulin portion of the serum, others discovered them in the albumin fraction [68, 69]. Recently, Ninnemann and colleagues [70–72] carried out a series of research work, and succeeded in isolating from burned patient serum an immunosuppressive glycopeptide (SAP), a complex-containing protein, carbohydrate, and lipid. The immunosuppressive activity was said to be related to the lipid component, and PGE_2 may contribute to this. Anti-SAP monoclonal antibody had been prepared by these authors and used to detect SAP in the serum of burned patients. They found that the increase in SAP was more marked in nonsurviving patients than in survivors. However, up to present, there has been no conclusive agreement about the sources and properties of the serum suppressive factors following burns.

Furthermore, serum suppressive factors were not the only causes of postburn immunosuppression. Huang et al. [11] found that serum of burned dogs could inhibit the oxidative metabolism of normal PMNs, indicating the presence of suppressive factors in burned serum. But when normal serum was added to burned patient's PMNs, their suppressed oxidative metabolic function could not be completely restored. Loose and Turinsky [51] discovered that when macrophages of burned rats were washed with the cultured in control serum, their suppressed "respiratory burst" response did not return to normal. Donati et al. [73], observing the phagocytosis of *Candida* by PMNs of burned patients, obtained similar results to those above. They suggested that dysfunction of PMNs was partly due to the extrinsic cause, such as the presence of serum suppressive factors, and partly due to the intrinsic defect of the cell itself.

16.3.2 Suppressor Cells

The study of the role of suppressor cells in the mechanism of postburn immunosuppression began in the late 1970s. Miller and Baker [74] observed in 1979 that the monocytes of burned patients, whose lymphocytes showed a reduced response to PHA, may inhibit the response of the normal MLR. They suggested that postburn immunosuppression was at least partly due to the appearance of T-suppressor cells (Ts). Later on many animal experiments and clinical observations demonstrated that lymphocytes of burned victims could depress the immune functions of normal lymphocytes [75, 76]. McIrvine et al. [77] studied the alteration of lymphocyte subpopulations with monoclonal antibodies in 22 burned patients with burns > 30% TBSA, and found inversion of Th/Ts from 1:0.55 to 1:1.4 after thermal injury, reaching its peak on the 5th–7th PBD, and returning to normal at the end of 2 weeks. In eight cases, the ratio of Th/Ts dropped again in the late postburn course, when systemic infection supervened. Changes in these lymphocyte subpopulations coincided with that of the response of these cells to PHA stimulation. A series of experiments were carried out in mice with 30% full-thickness scald by Kupper et al. [78] to study the role of Ts in postburn immunosuppression and infection. The phenotype LY-2^+ subpopulation of murine lymphocytes exhibited suppressive activity. Monoclonal antibody against these subpopulations of cells may inhibit the suppressive action of T lymphocytes of burned mice upon the function of normal lymphocytes. The effect of this T cell population on infection in mice was observed by these authors after ligating and puncturing the cecum. The mortality of the infected mice was 13%. If normal splenic cells were given to the infected mice, mortality was unaltered. But splenic cells of scalded mice would raise the mortality to 90%. When LY-2^+ cells were eliminated from the scalded mouse spleen cells, the mortality decreased to 30%, indicating that T-suppressor cells could inhibit normal immune response, but also aggravate infection.

Besides T-suppressor cells, macrophages also possess subpopulation-exhibiting suppressive activity. Fang et al. [14] reported that adherent cells of mononuclear leukocytes of peripheral blood in burned patients might suppress the mitogenic response of autologous lymphocytes to PHA. A similar result was obtained by Yang and Xu [79] in scalded mice. They found that the adherent spleen cells of scalded mice could inhibit the responses of autologous and isogenic normal lymphocytes to Con A. Suzuki and Pollard [80] demonstrated that suppressive activities were mediated by different cell populations in different postburn periods. They observed the effect of thermal injury upon the production of γ-interferon in mice. The contents of γ-interferon in the serum and the supernatant of splenic cell culture were reduced. Indicating the suppression of production of γ-interferon. Two phases of suppressive activity were shown. The first phase, mediated by adherent cells of the spleen, was observed on the 3rd–7th PBD; and the second, mediated by nonadherent cells of the mononuclear cells, appeared about 3 weeks after injury. Lahat et al. [15] suggested that Ts and suppressive monocytes interacted with each other on mediating suppressive effect on lymphocyte transformation in burned patients.

The relationship between serum suppressive factors and suppressors cells has not yet been thoroughly studied. In light of the time of their appearance following burn injury, the emergence of serum factors was earlier than that of suppressor cells. Campa et al. [81] after an analysis of the responses of lymphocytes to PHA, Con A, and MLR in burned patients, found that the suppressive activity of postburn serum appeared 1–2 days after injury, while activity of Ts appeared later, reaching its peak about 7–8 days postburn. Liu et al. [82] in their experiments found that both serum and splenic cells, taken from scalded mice (3° BSA, 15%) at intervals of 1, 3, 7, and 10 PBD, all showed suppressive effects on immune functions of normal splenic cells as measured by MLR and hemolytic plaque-forming cell (PFC) assays. There were two differences between serum factors and splenic suppressor cells. One was the peak time of suppression, and the other the degree of suppression. The suppressive effect of burned serum reached its peak early on the first PBD with a suppression rate as high as 70% ~ 90%, then gradually declined to 60%–70% on the 10th PBD, while that of the splenic suppressor cells was rather indistinct

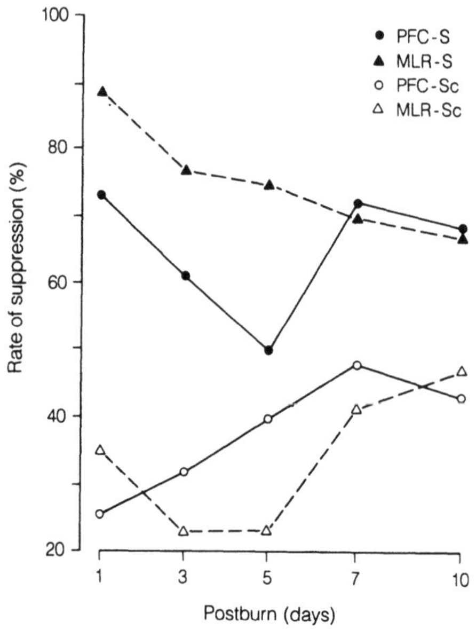

Fig. 16.5. Suppressive efffects of serum and splenic cells of scalded mice on cell-mediated immunity of normal mice. *PFC*, plaque-forming cell; *Sc*, splenic cell; *MLR*, mixed lymphocyte reaction; *s*, serum

at the beginning with a suppression rate of only about 20%–30% on the 1st PBD, but gradually rising to 40%–50% on the 10th PBD. The degree of suppression was higher with serum than cells. The suppression rate of serum was never below and that of the cells never above 50% during the 10-day observation period (Fig. 16.5).

The correlation between the serum factors and suppressor cells may be illustrated by the following fact. As stated above, being one of the important serum suppressive factors, PGE_2 is synthesized and released mainly by macrophages, and it can also activate T-suppressor cells. Therefore, it may be assumed that the mechanism is very complicated during the course of development of postburn immunosuppression. Interactions may exist between cells and cells, serum factors and serum factors, and cells and serum factors.

16.4 Immunomodulation for Postburn Immunosuppression

The significance of postburn immunosuppression to a patient is now becoming more and more understandable. Restoration of the deficient immune functions and rebuilding of the depressed body defense mechanism seem imperative. Measures such as early elimination of eschar and coverage of burn wound, prevention and control of infection, general supportive treatment, and nutritional support are all important and must be conscientiously implemented.

From the immunological point of view, attention should be paid to the restoration of the impaired immune defenses through immunomodulation, which is a subject arousing great interest in both immunologists and clinicians.

16.4.1 Immunoenhancing Agents

16.4.1.1 Thymopentin

Thymopentin (TP-5) is the peptide derivative of thymopoietin, which enhances the differentiation and maturation of T cells and also performs as a regulator of the immune system. Liu et al. [82], studying the suppressive effects of scalded mouse serum and suppressor spleen cells on the function of normal mouse lymphocytes, found that TP-5 might improve the suppressed function of normal lymphocytes to some extent as measured by MLR and PFC in the early postinjury period. Pang and Chen [83], using Con A and LPS as stimulators to observe the T- and B-cell functions in burned mice, also found that an optimum dose of TP-5 might restore the depressed lymphocyte functions following burn. Maghsudi and Miller [84] reported that TP-5 with or without concurrent indomethacin may improve postburn hypoimmunity in scalded guinea pig (burn, 20% ~ 30% BSA), as measured by the antibody-forming cell of the splenic cells in vitro. Waymack et al. [85] reproduced an experimental model of immune function defects in guinea pig with both burn injury and malnutrition, and found that TP-5 could increase the survival rate and prolong survival time in animals with complications of peritonitis, which was induced by burying blood clot containing bacteria in the peritoneal cavity of the burned animal. These authors also discovered that TP-5 might improve the phagocytic function of PMNs and Mϕ in burned guinea pig [86]. Stinnett et al. [87], using a guinea pig model with inoculation of *Pseudomonas aeruginosa* to burn wound, found that when the TP-5 was given before bacterial inoculation the survival rate was raised from 40% to 80% and the survival time prolonged from 6.9 to 11.6 days.

16.4.1.2 C_p-46665

C_p-46665 is a synthetic lipoidal amine with immunomodulating effects by strengthening the ability of phagocytic cells. One dose of CP-46665, given before the inoculation of bacteria on burn wound, improved the survival rate from 50% to 80% and the mean survival time from 8.2 to 12.4 days in burned guinea pig [87]. CP-46665 in a dose of 0.3 mg/kg not only ameliorated the phagocytic function of Mϕ but also enhanced the opsonic activity of serum of burned guinea pig. These improvements may be detected 2 days postburn [86].

16.4.1.3 Corynebacterium parvum

Corynebacterium parvum has been used as an immunoenhancing agent to stimulate Mϕ and the MPS. But its therapeutic effect is still debatable. Stinnett et al. [88] reported that *C. parvum* improved the survival rate of burned dog, and they suggested that it could be used to prevent infection. In contrast, Waymack et al. [89] found that administration of *C. parvum* might result in a higher mortality in burned guinea pig. It seems that the therapeutic results of *C. parvum* were unstable and uncontrollable. It may act as an activator to enhance the function of the MPS, but it may sometimes exhibit suppressive effects. This undesirable result may be mediated by the suppressor population of Mϕ which is induced and activated by *C. pavrum* [90].

16.4.1.4 Other Agents

Besides the above-mentioned agents, others have also been employed in immunoenhancing therapy. Levamisole reduced the incidence of *P. aeruginosa* infection when used in burned patients [91]. ATP-$MgCl_2$ restored the MPS function in scalded rats [92]. Vitamin A reversed the suppressed MLR of scalded mice [93], and vitamin E, when used topically or intraperitoneally, may improve the suppressed cell-mediated immunity as measured by the response to DNFB [94]. Christou et al. [95] recently used Ru 47140 (Biostim) as an Mϕ stimulator and claimed that this drug could improve humoral immunity, as shown by the improved antitetanus antibody production. However, it had no effect on cell-mediated immunity and nonspecific immunity. Lithium carbonate increased the number of PMNs and corrected the chemotaxis deficit, as well as regulating hematopoiesis and promoting the differentiation of hemopoietic stem cells toward the granulocyte series [96–98].

16.5 Inhibitors or Antagonists Against Certain Suppressive Factors and Cells

Ibuprofen, indomethacin, and cyclophosphamide, being proven inhibitors of prostaglandins in animal models, have shown their effectiveness in the reduction of the suppressive activity of scalded mouse serum and splenic cells, restoration of the cell-mediated immunity, inhibition of Ts activity, and correction of the altered Th/Ts ratio [82, 96, 99]. Ibuprofen also prevented an increase in vascular permeability and kept blood vessels patient after thermal injury [100].

Several drugs acting upon the arachidonate cascade had been tried in scalded rabbits as reported by Ichiro [101], including OP-41483 (a derivative of PGI_2), aspirin (cyclooxygenase inhibitor), OKY-646 (thromboxane synthetase inhibitor), and CV-3988 (antagonist against platelet-activating factor). It was claimed that mortality was reduced by using these drugs, and the effects of the former three drugs were better than those of the latter.

Cimetidine is a blocking agent of histamine H_2 receptor. At first, it was used to arrest the development of postburn edema by preventing the change in vascular permeability caused by histamine release [102]. As it was found that it also blocked the H_2 receptor on the T-cell surface, this drug was chosen for treatment of postburn immunosuppression, especially for correction of the altered cell-mediated immunity following burns. Hansbrough et al. [103], through sensitization with DNFB to observe the cell-mediated immunity, found that an optimum dosage of cimetidine restored the cell-mediated immunity in scalded mice, while the H_2-receptor antagonist showed no such effect. These authors also found that cimetidine prevented the decrease in Th/Ts ratio in scalded mice, if the drug was given before the injury [104].

16.6 Elimination of Toxic Materials and Suppressive Factors

Peterson et al. [105] applied cerium nitrate topically in burned mice and claimed that postburn immunosuppression was not present in these animals. They proposed that the improvement of cell-mediated immunity by topical use of cerium nitrate might be due to binding of this drug with toxic substance released from burned tissues, thus preventing the entrance of "toxin" into the general circulation. Similar results were obtained by Luo et al. [106] in their experiments on scalded mice, but they found that the protective effect of cerium nitrate was in inverse proportion to the severity of burn injury. When the cell-mediated immunity, measured by response to DNFB, was suppressed at around 50% of normal in untreated scalded mice, topical use of cerium nitrate brought about the depressed immune response up to normal levels in the treated group. If the severity of burn injury was increased and the immune response reduced to less than 10% of normal, the topical effect of cerium nitrate decreased to an undetectable level. Recently, Wallner et al. [107] observed the effect of topical cerium nitrate on hematopoiesis. They found that this topical agent could neither neutralize the serum-suppressive factor affecting erythropoiesis, nor alter any parameters in evaluating erythrocyte and granulocyte series of hematopoiesis in scalded mice. Munster et al. [108] reported that a low dose of polymyxin B given intravenously to burned patients reversed the suppressed lymphocyte functions and the reduced Th/Ts ratio. They suggested that a small dose of polymyxin B might neutralize the lipopolysaccharide toxicity.

Plasma exchange or plasmaphoresis was considered a reasonable measure for the elimination of toxic or immunosuppressive factors from the burn victim's blood. Results of clinical trials as reported by Ninnemann et al. [109, 110] showed that the MLR of patient's lymphocytes, which was suppressed to 61.9% before exchange therapy, returned to 27.3% after plasma exchange. They regarded this treatment to be beneficial for the restoration of immune functions after burn injury. But McManus [111] found that the reduction in mortality of burned patients by this measure was not obvious, while its complications and side effects could not be ignored.

16.7 Supplement of Reduced and Deficient Components

As stated in the previous section, fibronectin is a glycoprotein possessing opsonic activity and closely related to the phagocytic function of Mϕ as well as the clearance capacity of the MPS. But it decreases to a low level in plasma in the early postburn period and at the moment of septic or other complications. Lanser and Saba [112] reversed the acute decrease of plasma fibronectin (from 341 ± 30 to 98 ± 7 mg/l within 1 h postburn) by administration of pure fibronectin in burned rats with moderate sepsis. Doke et al. [113] tried plasma exchange therapy with frozen fresh plasma in 11 burned patients. The plasma fibronectin level was increased from 91 ± 69 to 204 ± 127 μg/ml, but was still lower than normal. Frozen fresh plasma also supplies complement which has been depleted in the early postburn period, such as plasma proteins and immunoglobulins.

16.8 Traditional Chinese Drugs

Many traditional Chinese drugs can function as immunomodulators to restore lymphocyte proliferative response to mitogen, to enhance natural killer cell activity, to regulate immune response, and also to provide several bactericidal and virustatic properties. Many authors have reported good results in treating certain malignant tumors, pernicious anemia, the decrepitude of old age, and several refractory infections in China. Recently, Traditional Chinese Medicine have also been used to treat burn injury. Zhu [114] reported that Radix Acontiti praeparata maintained the peritoneal macrophage phagocytic function of burned animals at nearly normal levels when given subcutaneously, while in untreated animals phagocytic activity was reduced, reaching its nadir at 16 h postburn. Ginsenoside had been tried by You et al. [115] as a therapeutic agent in treating lung edema in rabbits inflicted with inhalation injury. One dose of 25 mg/kg ginsenoside was given 15 min postinjury. Results showed that the reduction in arterial oxygen partial pressure was somewhat less than in the untreated control group, although the difference was not statistically significant. Lie et al. [116] found that *Lonicera japonica* Thumb and *Astragalus membranaceus* (Fischo) Bge may restore the suppressed T-cell response to Con A and the ability of IL-2 production of splenic cells in scalded mice; especially the latter could raise the IL-2 production ability up to 150% of normal (Figs. 16.6, 16.7).

From the above review, it may be seen that studies on immunomodulation and the attempt to restore acquired immunodeficiency after thermal injury remain in the experimental stage. There may be a long way still to go before definite benefits can be gained clinically. Vigorous efforts should be made to elucidate the complexity of mechanisms causing postburn immunosuppression, and to search for measures to prevent the rapid decrease in immunosuppression as well as to rebuild the reduced body defense mechanisms after burn injury.

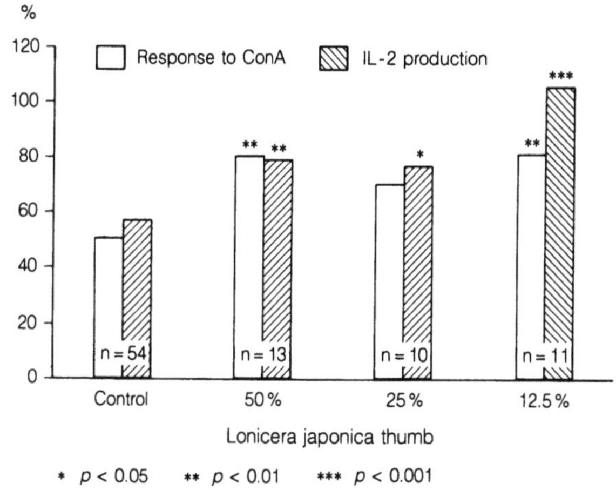

Fig. 16.6. Effects of *Lonicera japonica* thumb on cell-mediated immunity of scalded mice

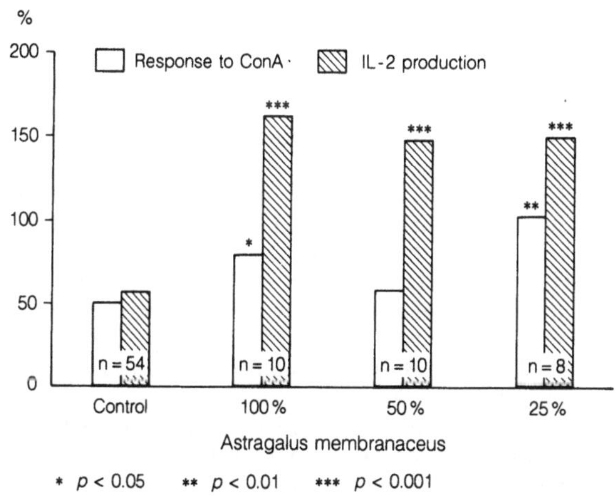

Fig. 16.7. Effects of *Astragalus membranaceus* on cell-mediated immunity of scalded mice

References

1. Zhang CW, Tan WY (1982) Clinical observations of chemotactic response of neutrophils in burned patients. Chin Med J 62: 569–579
2. Xu OZ, Xu YP, Shi JX et al. (1983) Study of chemotaxis of neutrophils and its relationships with burn infection in thermally injured patients. Chin J Surg 21: 134–137
3. Sheng ZY, Tung YL (1987) Neutrophil chemiluminescence in burned patients. J Trauma 27: 587–595
4. Huang WH, Wu JZ, Hu ZX et al. (1985) Effect of thermal injury on functions of neutrophils in scald rats with wound infection, through observation on the changes of IgG-Fc receptor and C_3b receptor of the cells. Chin J Exp Surg 2: 128–130

5. Guo ZR, Sheng ZY, Zhu ZM et al. (1982) Changes of phagocytic function of leukocytes in burned patients. Chin J Surg 20: 417–420
6. Zhang ML, Liu ZY, Zheng GY et al. (1981) Changes in several immune functions in burned patients. Beijing Med 3: 201–203
7. Jiang KY, Li A, Huang WH et al. (1984) Kinetic observation on severe inhalation injury in dogs during the period of 14 days postinjury. In: 3rd Military Medical College (ed) Symposium of burns and plastic surgery, pp 131–139
8. Alexander JW, Wixson D (1970) Neutrophil dysfunction and sepsis in burn injury. Surg Gyherol Obstet 130: 431–438
9. Palder SB (1984) Polymorphonuclear leukocyte function in the burned patients. Proc 16th Ann Meeting ABA, no 147
10. Fang ZY, Xiang XE, Sun JL (1980) The clinical significance of NBT reduction assay in severely burned patients. Acta Acad Med 2nd Milit Med Coll 3: 62–64
11. Huang WH, Li A, Wu JZ et al. (1986) Experimental observation of microbicidal activity of PMN by measuring the response of oxidative metabolism following thermal injury. Acta Acad Med 3rd Milit Med Coll 8: 203–208
12. Wu JZ, Huang WH, Hu ZX et al. (1986) Observation of the effects of burns and wound infection on peritoneal macrophage functions in rats, through the changes of reactivities of cell membrane receptors. Chin J Plast Surg Burn 2: 128–131
13. Kupper TS, Green DR, Dusum SK et al. (1985) Defective antigen presentation to a cloned T helper cell by macrophages from burn mice can be restored with interleukin 1. Surgery 98: 199–206
14. Fang PY, Shi JX, Yang ZJ et al. (1984) Effect of peripheral glass-adherent cells on the PHA induced autologous lymphocyte transformation in burned patients. Shanghai J Immunol 4: 218–223
15. Lahat N, Hornstein L, Moscona AR et al. (1985) Monocyte suppressor function in burns: T cell-monocyte interaction in mediating suppression. Immunol Lett 9: 43–47
16. Suzuki F, Pollard RB (1982) Mechanism of the suppression of IFNr responsiveness in mice after thermal injury. J Immunol 129: 1811–1815
17. Huang WH, Li A, Hu ZX et al. (1982) Observation of kinetic changes of serum immunoglobulin, lymphocyte transformation on E-rosette forming cell assay in burned patients. Chin Med PLA 17: 10–13 8:15
18. Shi JX (1985) Burn immunology. In: Yang ZJ et al. (eds) Treatment of burns, 2nd edn. Shanghai Scientific Tech Press, Shanghai, pp 121–145
19. Moss NM, Jordan A, Rodrich ML et al. (1986) Correlation between T-lymphocyte function and mortality from sepsis after burn injury. Surg Form 37: 93–94
20. Rodrick ML, Wood JJ, Grbic JT et al. (1986) Defective IL-2 production in patients with severe burns and sepsis. Lymphokine Res 5 [Suppl 1]: s75–s80
21. Peng DZ, Huang WH, Li A et al. (1988) Observation of kinetic changes of stress hormones and immune functions of splenic cells in burned rats. Master's thesis. Burn Res Inst, 3rd Milit Med Coll 1988
22. Wood JJ, Grbic JT, Rodrick ML et al. (1987) Suppression of interleukin-2 production in an animal model of thermal injury is related to prostaglandin synthesis. Arch Surg 122: 179–184
23. Teodorczyd-Injeyan JA, Sparkes BG, Mills GB et al. (1987) Impaired expression of IL-2 receptor (IL-2R) in the immunosuppressed burned patients: reversal by exogenous IL-2. J Trauma 27: 180–187
24. Polacek V, Jira M, Fara M et al. (1985) NK activity in severe burn injury. Proceedings of the 1st Sino-American conference on burn injury 1985, no 76
25. Stein MD, Gamble DN, Klimpel KD et al. (1984) Natural killer cell defects resulting from thermal injury. Cell Immunol 86: 551–556
26. Chen YL, Guo F, Fang ZY et al. (1988) The clinical significance of changes of immune function of RBC in burn patients. Chin J Plast Surg Burn 4: 277–278

27. Lin HY (1986). Experimental study of changes of immune adherence function of RBC after burns. Proc 11th Meeting Burn Plast Surg PLA, p 78
28. Guo F, Chen YL, Han FY (1985) Changes of immune adherent activity of blood platelets following thermal injury in rats. Shanghai J Immunol 5: 275–277
29. Huang WH, Li A, Hu ZX et al. (1984) Kinetic changes of serum total and alternative path-way hemolytic activities of complement and concentrations of C_3 in burn patients. Acta Acad Med, 3rd Milit Med Coll 6: 61–66
30. Huang WH, Li A, Jiang KY et al. (1984) Preliminary exploration of the mechanism of early decrease of serum complement activity in steam inhalation injured dogs. Shanghai J Immunol 4: 214–217
31. Wu JZ, Huang WH, Li A et al. (1988) Changes and clinical significance of serum complement components and carrier proteins in burned patients. J Trauma (Chin) 4: 12–15
32. Zhou SZ, Ai YL (1982) Preliminary study of kinetic change of plasma anaphylatoxin of left ventricular blood of steam inhalation injured dogs. Acta Acad Med, 3rd Milit Med Coll 4: 66–72
33. Li Ao (Ngao), Jiang KY, Yang ZC et al. (1987) Roles of some inflammatory mediators in the pathogenesis of early pulmonary edema in steam respiratory burns. Chin Med J 100: 132–141
34. Xie BF, Li A, Yang ZC et al. (1988) Kinetic changes of balance between elastase-anti-protease in early smoke inhalation injury in rabbits. Symp Burn Plast Surg, 3rd Milit Med Coll 1988, pp 178–189
35. Liu XS, Li A, Yang ZC et al. (1988) Role of active oxygen metabolites of neutrophils in smoke inhalation injury in dogs. Symp Burn Plast Surg, 3rd Milit Med Coll 1988, pp 225–234
36. Feng ZM, Li A, Yang ZC et al. (1988) Role of radicals in pathogenesis of smoke inhalation injury in rats. Symp Burn Plast Surg, 3rd Milit Med Coll 1988, pp 190–196
37. Huang WH, Huang XY, Li A (1986) Preliminary observation of the relationship between the measurement of plasma fibronectin and the changes of burn patients' condition. Chin J Surg 24: 222–224
38. Sheng ZY, Xu SH, Jia XM et al. (1987) Changes in plasma fibronectin level in burns patients. Burns 13: 114–117
39. Wu JZ, Huang WH, Feng SZ et al. (1986) Changes and clinical significance of certain acute phase reactant proteins following thermal injury. J Trauma (Chin) 2: 207–210
40. Dong YL (1986) Burn infection and changes of C-reactive protein. Proc 11th Burns Plast Surg PLA 1986, p 132
41. Xue LB, Wang SY (1988) Kinetic observation on serum prealbumin in burned patients. Chin J Plast Surg Burns 4: 142–143
42. Guo ZR, Sheng, Jia XM (1982) Changes of immunoglobulins in burned patients. Beijing Med 4: 86–88
43. Hakim AA (1977) An immunosuppressive factor from serum of thermally traumatized patients. J Trauma 17: 908–919
44. Constantian MB (1978) Association of sepsis with an immunosuppressive polypeptide in the serum of burn patients. Ann Surg 188: 209–215
45. Ninnemann JL et al. (1979) Thermal injury-associated immunosuppressions: occurrence and in vitro blocking effect of post-recovery serum. J Immunol 122: 1736–1741
46. Gu XM, Shih TS, Yang CC et al. (1983) Changes in lymphocyte response to PHA and serum immunosuppressive activity after thermal injury. Burns 10: 86–91
47. Ninnemann JL, Condie JT, David SE et al. (1982) Isolation of immunosuppressive serum components following thermal injury. J Trauma 22: 837–844

48. Ninnemann JL, Stockland AE (1984) Participation of prostaglandin E in immunosuppression following thermal injury. J Trauma 24: 201–207
49. Wolfe JHN, Wu AVO, Connor NE (1982) Anergy, immunosuppressive serum and impaired lymphocyte blastogenesis in burn patients. Arch Surg 117: 1266–1271
50. Loose LD, Turinsky J (1979) Macrophage dysfunction after burn injury. Infect Immun 26: 157–162
51. Loose LD, Turinsky J (1980) Depression of the respiratory burst in alveolar and peritoneal macrophages after thermal injury. Infect Immun 30: 718–722
52. Pearson G, Nakamura M, Heck E et al. (1981) Impaired oxygen consumption activity of neutrophils by inhibitor (s) in burn sera. JBCR 2: 208–211
53. Loegering DJ (1983) Reticuloendothelial depressing substance and burn injury in animals and patients. J Trauma 23: 111–115
54. Kremer B, Allgower M, Graf M et al. (1981) The present status of research in burn toxin. Intensive Care Med 7: 77–87
55. Aoyama H, Suzuki K, Izawa Y (1982) Mitochondrial-toxic activity in burned human skin: relation to severity of burn and period after burn. Burns 9: 13–16
56. Chen ZR, Chen YS, Meng XM et al. (1986) Disturbance of respiratory function of mitochondria of hepatocytes in rats following combined radiation-burn injury. J Trauma (Chin) 2: 7–11
57. Holder IA (1983) "Metabolic" factors in thermal injury: role of nucleic acid. Burns 9: 350–354
58. Rosenthol SR (1982) Burn toxin and its competition. Burns 8: 215–219
59. Hansbrough JF, Zapata-Sirvent R, Peterson V et al. (1984) Characterization of the immunosuppressive effect of burned tissue in an animal model. J Surg Res 37: 383–393
60. Schoenenberger GA, Burkhardt F, Kalbever F et al. (1975) Experimental evidence for a significant impairment of host defence for gram-negative organism by a specific cutaneous toxin produced by severe burn injury. Surg Gynecol Obstet 141: 555–561
61. Ninnemann JL, Ozkan AN (1989) Definition of a burn injury-induced immunosuppressive serum component. Proc 16th ABA 1984, abstract no 1
62. Ninnemann JL, Ozkan AN (1987) The immunosuppressive activity of C_{1q} degradation peptides. J Trauma 27: 119–122
63. Ogle CK, Ogle JD, Alexander JW (1984) Inhibition of bacterial clearance in the guinea pig by fluid-phase C_3b. Arch Surg 119: 57–60
64. Ogle CK, Ogle JD, Johnson C et al. (1987) Inhibition of lymphocyte proliferation by fluid-phase C_3b as influenced by macrophage. Arch Surg 122: 234–238
65. Huang WH, Hu ZX, Huang XY et al. (1989) Abnormalities of serum proteins following thermal injury. Burns 15: 11–14
66. McIrvine AJ, Walfe JHN, Collins K et al. (1983) Fetal infection in mice after injection of immunosuppressive serum fraction from surgical patients. Br J Surg 70: 558–561
67. Garner WD, Prager MD, Baxter CR (1981) Multiple inhibitors of lymphocyte transformation in serum from burned patients. JBCR 2: 97–101
68. Feng SJ, Kong LW, Gu XM et al. (1987) Preliminary isolation and characterization of serum suppressive factors following thermal injury in swine. Chin J Plants Surg Burn 3: 47–50
69. Yang WZ (1983) Preliminary isolation of serum components processing immunosuppressive activity in burned rabbits. Master's thesis. Biochem Dept 2nd Shanghai Med Coll 1983
70. Ozkan AN, Ninnemann JL (1985) Circulating mediators in thermal injuries: isolation and characterization of a burn-injury induced immunosuppressive serum component. JBCR 6: 147–151

71. Ozkan AN, Ninnemann JL, Sullivan JJ (1986) Progress in the characterization of an immunosuppressive glycopeptide (SAP) from patients with major thermal injuries. JCBR 7: 388–397
72. Ozkan AN, Ninnemann JL (1987) Reversal of SAP-induced immunosuppression and SAP detection by a monoclonal antibody. J Trauma 7: 123–126
73. Donati L, Lazzarin A, Signorini M et al. (1983) Preliminary clinical experience with the use of immunomodulators in burns. J Trauma 23: 816–831
74. Miller CL, Baker CC (1979) Changes in lymphocyte activity after thermal injury, the role of suppressor cells. J Clin Invest 63: 202–210
75. Keane RM, Munster AM, Birmingham W et al. (1982) Suppressor cell activity after major injury: indirect functional assays. J Trauma 22: 770–773
76. Jacobson BK, Kupper TS, Baker CC (1984) Immunosuppression following surgical excision and synergeneic grafting in major thermal injury. Proc 16th Am Burn Assoc 1984, abstract no 109
77. McIrvine AJ, O'Mahony JB, Saporoschetz I et al. (1982) Depressed immune response in burn patient. Use of monoclonal antibody and functional assay to define the role of suppressor cells. Ann Surg 196: 297–304
78. Kupper TS, Baker CC, Ferguson TA et al. (1985) A burn induced Ly-2 suppressor T cell lowers resistance to bacterial infection. J Surg Res 38: 606–612
79. Yang L, Xu BX (1987) Influence and possible role of adherent cells to autologous lymphocyte response to Con A in scald mice. Master's thesis. Microbiol Dept, Ji-nan Med Coll 1987
80. Suzuki F, Pollard RB (1987) Suppressor cells generated in mice late after thermal injury. J Trauma 27: 379–383
81. Campa M, Benedettini G, DeLibero G et al. (1982) The suppressive activity of T-lymphocyte and serum factors in burned patients. Burms 8: 231–239
82. Liu X, Huang WH, Li A et al. (1986) Observation on the changes of immune functions after scald and the suppressive activities of spleen cells and serum of scald mice. Master's thesis. Burn Res Inst, 3rd Milit Med Coll 1986
83. Pang XL, Chen ZR (1987) Immunological alterations of burned mice and the effect of immunomodulators. Master's thesis. Dept Radiat Med, 3rd Millit Med Coll 1987
84. Maghsuki M, Miller CL (1984) The immunomodulation effect of TP-5 and indomethacin in burn induced hypoimmunity. J Surg Res 27: 133–138
85. Waymack JP, Miskell P, Gonce SJ et al. (1984) Immunomodulators in the treatment of peritonitis in burned and malnourished animals. Surgery 96: 308–314
86. Waymack JP, Gonce SJ, Miskell P et al. (1985) Mechanism of action of two new immunomodulators. Arch Surg 120: 43–48
87. Stinnett JD, Loose LD, Miskell P et al. (1983) Synthetic immunomodulators for prevention of fatal infection in a burned guinea pig model. Ann Surg 198: 53–59
88. Stinnett JD, Alexander JW, Morris MJ et al. (1981) Improved survival in severely burned animals using intravenous *Corynebacterium parvum* vaccine post injury. Surgery 89: 237–242
89. Waymack JP, Miskell P, Gonce SJ et al: Synthetic immunomodulators for the correction of burn immune deficits. Proc 16th ABA annual meeting 1984, abstract no 148
90. Holdon HT, Herberman RB (1985) Modulation of immunity by macrophage. In: Mitchell MS (ed) The modulation of immunity. Pergamon, Oxford pp 35–79
91. Mazzoleni F, Chiarelli A, Corsano A et al. (1981) Burn-induced immunological modifications. Preliminary results with levamisole. Acta Chir Plast 23: 74–81
92. Chaudry IH, Kupper TS, Schleck S et al. (1982) Impairment of RE function following thermal injury and its restoration with ATP-MgCl administration. Circ Shock 9: 297–305
93. Fusi S, Kupper TS, Green DR et al. (1984) Reversal of postburn immunosuppression by the administration of vitamin A. Surgery 96: 330–335

94. Rundus C, Peterson VM, Zapata-Sirvent R et al. (1984) Vitamin E improves cell mediated immunity in the burned mouse: a preliminary study. Burns 11: 11–15
95. Christou NV, Zakaluzny I, Marshall JC et al. (1988) The effect of the immunomodulator Ru41740 (Biostim) on the specific and non-specific immunosuppression induced by thermal injury or protein deprivation. Arch Surg 123: 207–211
96. Hansbrough J, Peterson V, Zapata-Sirvent R et al. (1984) Postburn immunosuppression in an animal model II. Restoration of cell-mediated immunity by immunomodulating drugs. Surgery 95: 290–296
97. Perez HD, Kaplan HB, Goldstein IM et al. (1980) Reversal of an abnormality of polymorphonuclear leukocyte chemotaxis with lithium. Clin Immunol Immunopathol 16: 308–315
98. Gallicchio VS, Chan MG (1980) Modulation of murine pluripotent stem cell proliferation in vivo by lithium carbonate. Blood 56: 1150–1152
99. Zapata-Sirvent R, Hansbrough JF (1985) Postburn immunosuppression in animal model III. Maintenance of normal splenic helper and suppressor lymphocyte subpopulations by immunomodulating drugs. Surgery 97: 721–729
100. Ehrlich HP (1984) Promotion of vascular patency in dermal burns with ibuprofen. Am J Med 77(1A): 107–113
101. Ichiro O (1986) The effect of the drugs which affect the arachidonate cascade upon experimentally burned rabbits. 7th Int Cong Burn Injuries 1986, abstract no A239
102. Yoshioke T, Monafo WW, Ayvazian VH et al. (1978) Cimetidine inhibited burn edema formation. Am J Surg 136: 681–685
103. Hansbrough JF, Zapata-Sirvent R, Bender EM et al. (1985) Prevention of suppressed cell-mediated immunity in burned mice with histamine-2 receptor antagonist drugs. J Surg Res 39: 150–156
104. Zapata-Sirvent R, Hansbrough JF, Bartle EJ et al. (1986) Prevention of post traumatic alteration in lymphocyte subpopulations in mice by immunomodulating drugs. Arch Surg 121: 116–122
105. Peterson VM, Hansbrough JF, Wang XW et al. (1985) Topical cerium nitrate prevents postburn immunosuppression. J Trauma 25: 1039–1044
106. Luo ZH, Huang WH, Li A et al. (1988) Effect of topical cerium nitrate on cell-mediated immunity in scald mice. Symp Burn Plastic Surg, 3rd Milit Med Coll 1988, pp 277–281
107. Wallner SF, Vautrin R, Katz J (1987) The effect of topical agents on hemopoiesis following thermal injury. studies on an animal model. Burns 13: 259–265
108. Munster AM, Winchurch RA, Thupari JN et al. (1986) Reversal of postburn immunosuppression with low dose polymixin B. J Trauma 26: 995–998
109. Warden GD, Ninnemann JL, Stratta RJ et al. (1984) The effect of exchange therapy on postburn lymphocyte suppression. Surgery 96: 321–329
110. Ninnemann JL, Stratta RJ, Warden GD et al. (1984) The effect of plasma exchange on lymphocyte suppression after burn. Arch Surg 119: 33–38
111. McManus WF (1984) Is there a role for plasma phoresis/exchange transfusin in the treatment of the septic burn patients? J Trauma 24 [Suppl. 9]: s137–s138
112. Lanser ME, Saba TM (1983) Correction of serum opsonic defects after burn and sepsis by opsonic fibronectin administration. Arch Surg 118: 338–342
113. Doke M, Hunt JL, Purdue GF et al. (1985) Effect of plasma exchange therapy on circulating fibronectin in burn patients. JBCR 6: 239–242
114. Zhu LQ (1984) Effect on extract of Radix acontiti praeparata on the phagocytic function of peritoneal macrophages in mice. Paper presented on 10th Burn Plast Surg Meeting, PLA
115. You ZY, Yang ZC, Jiang KY et al. (1986) Experimental observation of therapeutic effect of ginsenoaide and ketoprofen on pulmonary edema in smoke inhalation injury. Symp Burns Plast Surg, 3rd Milit Med Coll, 1986, pp 202–206

116. Liu X, Huang WH, Li A et al. (1989) Restoration of suppressed immune functions with immunomodulators of Chinese traditional and Western medicines in scald mice. Proceedings of the 2nd Sino-American conference on burn injury and trauma 1989, no 52

17 Pediatric Burn Injury

Yang Zong-chen and Li Ngao

Burn constitutes one of the most commonest causes of accidental injury. Of burned patients, over one-half are children. Fortunately, approximately 90% of the burn injuries suffered by children are minor and can be treated in the outpatient department, only 10% of them requiring hospitalization. Most burn injuries in children are scalds, especially in children between the age of 1 and 3 years, and flame burns are seen more commonly in children over the age of 3 years. In our institute, 1225 out of 4641 burn patients were under 12 years of age. Of these patients, 507 (41.4%) were under the age of 3 years, and 905 (73.9%) were suffered from flame burns. Burns resulting from flame are usually caused by matches and stoves. Most involve ignition of clothes. Scalds occur predominately in the kitchen usually as a result of spilling of hot liquid from a container which the child has pulled down from a table, or when the child has run into somebody carrying a container. Bathtub scalds are also frequent.

17.1 Initial Evaluation

The burn injury is evaluated to determine how the emergency treatment is to be carried out and the necessity of admission into hospital. Though a number of things must be done immediately, it is always imperative to take a brief history, including the details of when, where, and how the injury happened, and what was the burning agent. Details of the site of the accident are important, which may suggest the occurrence of smoke inhalation and/or associated injury. The patient's past disease history, tetanus immunization status, and drug allergies must be ascertained.

The first decision is whether to hospitalize and to administer an intravenous infusion. The size, depth, and location of the burns are the most important determinants. It is generally convenient to categorize burn injury into minor, moderate, and severe. The extent of injury is determined not only from the total surface area burned, but also from the depth of injury. Minor burns include partial-thickness burns of less than 10% TBSA and full-thickness burns of less than 2% TBSA. Patients with minor burns are usually treated as outpatients as represent approximately 90% of patients with burns seeking medical treatment. Moderate burns involve 10%–30% TBSA, and full-thickness burns less than 10% TBSA. These patients should be hospitalized. Minor burns affecting special areas, such as the face, neck, hands, and feet also require hospitalization. If there is any question as to whether a burned child can be managed adequately at home, it is better to hospitalize the child for a few days. Children with minor to moderate injury may be treated in a general hospital, but those children with severe burns in excess of 30% TBSA are probably best managed in a burn unit, or a burn center.

17.2 Emergency Management

At the scene of the injury, airway patency should first be ensured, and any smoldering clothing removed. If chemical injury is suspected, irrigation with copious amounts of water should be performed. First aid objectives are to alleviate pain, to prevent wound contamination, and to transport the victim safely to a hospital. The application of cold water to minor burns can be helpful in reducing pain, and is effective in limiting not only the extent but also the depth of burn, provided it is applied within several minutes after injury. [1]. The burns should be covered with a clean, dry, sheet. Topical ointment should not be applied before the patient arrives at a medical facility. Oxygen should be administered and the patient taken to the nearest hospital facility. Patients with extensive burns should not be given water during transportation because of the hazard of aspiration and water intoxication. A 2-year-old girl with a flame burn involving 35% TBSA was admitted to our institute 20 h after the injury. About 500–600 ml water was given during transportation. The child arrived in a comatose state with deep breathing, severe edema, and epileptiform seizures. Her serum sodium level was as low as 106 mEq/l. She died 3 h after admission. At autopsy, severe brain edema and cerebellar hernia were found. In severe burns, intravenous fluid therapy should be initiated early, especially in those who cannot reach a medical facility within 1 h.

17.3 Fluid Resuscitation

An understanding of how the child differs from the adult in the body fluid balance will greatly assist in meeting the fluid needs of the burned child. In adults, the extracellular fluid volume constitutes about 20% of body weight and about one-half the volume of intracellular fluid. In infancy, the extracellular fluid accounts for approximately 50% of the total body weight. This figure drops to 35% in a young child. However, the electrolyte concentrations of extracellular fluid alter very little with growth. The plasma bicarbonate and sodium concentrations are somewhat lower in a child than in an adult. In an infant, the normal plasma chloride level is 110 mmol/l, while in an adult it is 100 mmol/l. The blood volume in infants is relatively greater, accounting for about 10% of the total fluid volume, or approximately 80 ml/l body weight, than that in adults, which is about 55–70 ml/kg. It should also be emphasized that the infant the ability to excrete concentrations of urine greater than 800 mOsm is less and the metabolic rate in proportion to weight is higher than in adults. The higher metabolic rate may result in higher insensible and renal water loss.

Table 17.1. Formula for estimation of fluid replacement

First 24 h postburn:	
Electrolyte-containing fluid	1 ml/kg % TBSA
Colloid-containing fluid	0.5 ml/kg % TBSA
Electrolyte-free water	Varying with body weight and age

Fluid replacement should be initiated with the administration of an isotonic electrolyte solution, such as lactated Ringer's solution, while more precise calculations for resuscitation are underway. A polyethylene catheter should be inserted, in preference to a needle, in a vein of an unburned extremity if it is available. The principles of aseptic technique and sterile dressing must be strictly followed to prevent the septic complications resulting from the intravenous catheter, which have been noted to be very common in burned patients with colonized wounds. It is necessary to ascertain the body weight of the patient and the extent of burn injury, so that the amount of fluid to be replaced can be accurately estimated. Several programs of fluid resuscitation have been proposed that are based on the body weight and the extent of burn injury. Our formula is outlined in Table 17.1

Half amount of the fluid to be replaced should be administered during the first 8 h, one-fourth during the second 8 h, and one-fourth during the third 8 h period. Adjustment of the amount and the rate of administration should be made to ensure an urinary output of 1 ml/kg/h during the first 48 h. The other popular regimen in use is the Parkland formula, which estimates the fluid lost within the first 24 h to be 4 ml/kg % TBSA for older children, and 3 ml/kg % TBSA for young children. However, all these regimens are calculated on the basis of experience obtained in adult patients. These estimates are found to be relatively inaccurate for the resuscitation of children with extensive injuries, who frequently appear to require significantly more fluid, depending upon the depth of burn and the extent of the body surface area involved [2]. The discrepancy was attributed to the fact that children generally have a greater body surface area in relation to their weight compared with adults, and consequently standard adult formulas do not adequately meet the fluid loss in children. The recommendations for initial resuscitation in children with major burn injuries have undergone significant revisions during the past few years.

Some authors suggest that fluid resuscitation in children is best based on body surface area by utilizing the formula of 500 ml/m^2 burned area and 2000 ml/m^2 total body surface area for maintenance fluid volume to be given over the first 24 h [3]. Controversy exists over the use of hypertonic salt solutions and also the supplemental use of colloids in children [4–7]. Authors who advocate the use of hypertonic saline believe that intravascular expansion can be obtained by removing water from the cellular space. But there are a number of complications after the infusion of hypertonic salts. Not infrequently, hypernatremia, hyper-osmolarity, and intercellular dehydration can become severe problems, particularly in children, and cerebral hemorrhage may also occur [8]. This makes use of this form of resuscitation hazardous except in very expert hands. The administration of colloids in children with severe burns now seems to have gained widespread acceptance, and appears to decrease the total fluid requirement [9, 10]. Intravascular protein loss has been shown to decrease the colloid osmotic pressure of plasma. The most recent animal studies have shown that protein loss is most marked during the first 6–8 h postburn. Colloids should be instituted from 8 to 24 h postburn, after which children may tend to retain sodium. So at this time it may be appropriate to change the Ringer's lactate to 0.5% normal saline in 5% glucose. Generally, one-half to three-fourths of the amount given in the first postburn day is needed to the second 24 h following burn. After 24 h, as the capillary permeability has returned to normal, and protein molecules are more likely to be retained, it may be beneficial to administer plasma or albumin, particularly if the hematocrit is in excess of 45%. No matter what formula is used, the adequacy of resuscitation must be assessed by a series of clinical parameters. The reliable method of judging the adequacy of fluid replacement is by careful hourly monitoring of urinary output. Hourly urinary flow is comparatively an accurate reflection of renal blood flow and thus of cardiac output. Since measurement of urinary output is so important, all children with burns at least larger than 15% TBSA should have a urinary catheter placed. An adequate urinary flow is about 1 ml/kg per hour. While the measurement of hourly urine flow is probably a reliable guide to the adequacy of fluid replacement, a more accurate guide would be a serial measurement of cardiac output. However, it is not always possible or necessary to measure cardiac output. Some physiological parameters in addition to urinary flow may be used to estimate the adequacy of cardiac output. They include such considerations as maintaining vital signs at normal levels, a clear sensorium, a normal blood pH, and a rapid response of capillary refilling with normal arterial blood gases. Vital signs vary according to age. Pulse rate should be kept at around 120 beats/min with a systolic blood pressure of 60–70 mm Hg in the newborn age group. Pre-school-age children usually have a pulse rate of about 100 beats/min and a blood pressure of 100/60 mm Hg. In the majority of cases, these clinical parameters are employed to guide the fluid resuscitation. In only very complicated cases is monitoring of the central venous pressure, pulmonary artery pressure, and pulmonary arterial wedge pressure required. Children rarely have preexisting cardipulmonary disease, and the additional risk of placing a Swan-Ganz catheter is frequently unnecessary [11].

After the first 48 h postburn, diuresis will occur, provided fluid resuscitation and cardiac output are adequate. Most patients gain as much as 20% of their basal body weight in association with fluid resuscitation. Losses from diuresis and increased wound evaporation will bring the patient back to basal body weight in the succeeding 5–7 days. During this phase, body weight as well as serum sodium concentration and osmolality are good guides to fluid replacement. Water loss from evaporation must be replaced after the first 48 h to prevent dehydration by administering 1–2 ml free water/kg/% TBSA/24 h; or fluid is replaced according to the following formula: 3750 ml/m^2 burned area plus

1500 ml/m^2 total body surface [12]. The sodium requirement will be low after 48 h; usually 50 mEq sodium and 20–30 mEq potassium/day are given. A solution containing two-thirds 5% glucose and one- third normal saline with 20–30 mEq potassium added to each liter of the solution is preferred.

Oral fluid administration is begun in most cases on the second postburn day. To begin with homogenized milk is given by continuous drip via a nasogastric tube every hour. The amount of milk given depends on the patient's tolerance, which is evaluated by measuring hourly the residual fluid in the stomach. The majority of children will tolerate large amounts of oral fluid, particularly milk, to satisfy daily maintenance needs and the additional requirement due to loss from evaporation. Usually it takes a slightly larger amount of oral feeding than intravenous infusion to replacc cvaporative losses. The sooner the patient weaned from intravenous therapy the better. Ideally, by the end of 48 h oral fluid administration should replace intravenous therapy. When the child is able to take food voluntarily, a liquid diet is given, and it is gradually advanced to a regular diet with supplements.

17.4 Nutrition

The nutritional management of any patient with a major thermal injury is critically important. Hypermetabolism, increased glucose flow, and severe protein and fat wasting are characteristics of the response to major burns. Metabolic requirements increase substantially in relation to the size of burn wound and may reach 200% of the normal resting energy expenditure (REE), if 60% or more of the body surface area is involved [13]. Pediatric patients are a poor risk from a nutritional standpoint because of their high basal metabolic requirement, relatively larger surface area in proportion to body weight, and lower endogenous caloric reserves [14].

The hypermetabolic response is temperature sensitive but not temperature dependent. The ambient temperature must be maintained at 28°C–33°C to minimize the metabolic expenditure of maintaining a core temperature and to provide greater comfort.

Glucose kinetics in burn patients are abnormal. Glucose tolerance curves obtained during the shock phase are diabetic like with an elevated fasting glucose level and a decreased rate of disappearance. Daily nitrogen loss varies from 25 to 30 g/m^2 per day at the height of the hypermetabolic response between the 7th and 17th postburn days [15].

The energy requirement has been found to be approximately 25 kcal/kg plus 40 kcal % TBSA/day, or the daily maintenance calorie requirement can be estimated on the basis of 1800 kcal/m^2 TBSA/day, the daily calories required for the burn itself amounting to 2200 kcal/m^2 TBSA. The protein demands can be met by supplying 3–5 g protein/kg. In addition, some polyunsaturated fats should be provided to prevent essential fatty acid deficiency. Vitamins with increased amounts of vitamin C, and potassium, zinc, and magnesium are also required. Recent studies indicate that an increase in protein intake to higher levels may be beneficial to children with major thermal injuries. Significant improvements in both mortality and morbidity are achieved by increasing dietary protein from 16% to 23% of the total calorie intake [16]. Another important metabolic factor is the optimum calorie: nitrogen (N) ratio. It is suggested that any patient with a burn greater than 10% TBSA should receive a dietary regimen based on a non protein kcal:N ratio of 100 or more in order to achieve a positive nitrogen balance [16]. In order to obtain a better understanding of nutritional status, daily body weight is measured and the serum albumin is monitored weekly. Nitrogen balance studies are not necessary, or can be calculated from the nitrogen intake minus the nitrogen output.

The protein: nitrogen ratio is 6.25:1. The daily nitrogen output can be estimated by summing up the losses from urine, skin, and intenstine. Urine nitrogen loss can be determined from a 24 h urine sample. Nitrogen losses through the skin and intestine amount to approximately 2 g/day in smaller burns and up to 10 g/day in extensive burns during the autolytic phase.

The quality as well as quantity of protein used to replace the protein losses has a direct influence on survival rate. Enternal nutritional support is superior to supplying calories and protein by the intravenous route. The oral route is the most effective method of supplying calories and protein. If patients are unable to take adequate amounts of food by mouth, nasal tube feeding of any sort may be required. Freshly prepared feedings at body temperature given continuously are best tolerated. Tube feedings should also be low in osmolality, ranging between 300 and 700 mOsm. They should contain no more than 1 cal/ml. Sometimes night tube feeding is required in addition to regular meals and diet supplement in daytime. Intravenous hyperalimentation should be restricted because of the potentially increased incidence of sepsis. However, in those patients with superior mesenteric artery syndrome or paralytic ileus, enteral nutrition should be discontinued, and parenteral hyperlimentation via the central venous route is indicated. In some instances, peripherally administered isotonic mixtures of amino acids, glucose, vitamins, and fat emulsion may meet the demand. In both peripheral and central parenteral hyperalimentation, a strict aseptic technique and changing the intravenous sites every 3 days are essential in order to prevent septic thrombophlebitis. Insulin supplementation is usually required when sufficient calories are given, and 1 unit/kg body weight insulin may be required per day. In the presence of an inexplicable febrile course, the catheter should be removed and its tip cultured.

The loss of albumin from burn wound in the form of exudate continues beyond the first hours until the wound is healed, and it becomes exacerbated if heavy bacterial colonization of the wound takes place. Impairment in the synthesis of plasma protein in the liver and occasionally protein losses via the urinary gastrointestinal tract magnify the plasma protein deficiency. In the absence of septicemia, the administration of 10–20 g albumin, or an equivalent amount of plasma, per square meter body surface burned per week, in three divided doses, suffices to maintain serum albumin levels between 2 and 4 g/dl and the plasma colloid osmotic pressure greater than 15 mmHg [12].

It has been demonstrated that thermal injury to the skin may result in immediate destruction of red blood cells circulating through the burned area, and actually a large number of red cells are partially damaged with a diminished life span. In the preponderance of plasma loss during the shock phase, most patients initially exhibit polycythemia. Anemia may be obvious usually after 3–7 days. Therefore the blood replacement is needed during the 3rd–5th day after burn. The usual dose is 10 ml/kg body weight administered over a 3- to 4-h period. During the period of wound debridement and skin grafting, repeated transfusion may be required.

17.5 Treatment of Infection

Burn wound surface provides a warm protein-laden growth medium for microorganisms, whether they are exogenous or endogenous in origin. They will quickly grow and spread throughout the wound. While it is unrealistic to try to prevent the burn wound from being colonized, however, control of the microbial flora is achievable. Many prophylactic topical agents are being used. Topical therapy is essentially the same as that used in adult patients. These include 0.5% silver nitrate, mafenide acetate, nitrofurazone, povidone-iodine, silver sulfadiazine, gentamicin ointment or cream, and mycostatin. It is important to realize that no single agent is totally effective against all burn wound microbes. Therefore, the use of topical agents should be guided by an in vivo test or in vivo results. Silver sulfadiazine is the topical agent of first choice. Absorption of silver from the burn wound scarcely ever occurs, but approximately 10% of the sulfur-group will be absorbed. Transient leukopenia, occurring after the first few days of application, was found in about 5% of patients treated with silver sulfadiazine [17]. Usually the leukopenia spontaneously disappears when the drug is discontinued. Silver sulfadiazine may be reapplied when the white blood cell count returns to a normal range. Mafenide is a very effective broad-spectrum bacteriostatic agent. It is rapidly absorbed from the burn wound and must be reapplied in some cases. It seems to cause inhibition of epithelial regeneration. Mafenide is also a strong carbonic anhydrase inhibitor and may lead to metabolic acidosis which is compensated for initially by hyperventilation and reduction of the P_aCO_2. It has been found to be relatively safe if it is applied to burn wounds of less than 20% TBSA.

Systemic sepsis remains the major cause of death in burned patients. Antibiotic prohylaxis, initially with penicillin G, reduced early mortality from group β-hemolytic streptococcal sepsis. However, new pathogens have been emerging, first *Staphylococcus aureus*, then gram-negative organisms, and finally fungi and viruses. The value of prophylactic systemic antibacterial therapy in the care of burn patients is still debatable. Routine prophylalctic administr-ation of penicillin in the immediate postburn period is no longer practised. This is because β-hemolytic streptococcus infection is now uncommon in burn patients and can be treated easily if it occurs. Specific systemic antibiotic therapy should be instituted early when bacterial invasion is confirmed by the discovery of organisms from the bloodstream or by the presence of a typical clinical picture of septicemia. Frequent bacterial surveys including cultures of exudates, various secretions, excretes, and blood should be performed to guide the use or selection of antibiotics. If necessary, quantitative bacteriological analysis of burn wound biopsies should be performed. Intravenous catheters, which are a common possible source of infection, should also be frequently checked. Besides, an epidemiological survey of the bacterial flora residing in the burn ward is also important. Usually, there is a definite lapse of time between colonization of a burn wound and clinical infection. Routine culturing of a patient and frequent monitoring of changes in unit microflorae will allow ample time to select appropriate narrow-spectrum agents to decrease rate of growth or eliminate potentially troublesome organisms [18]. The same procedures will facilitate the selection of a systemic antimicrobial agent once the responsible pathogen in the septic patient is identified. No single antibiotic will be adequate in all cases over a period. In order to ensure that the level of a systemic antibiotic is adequate, it is imperative that frequent determinations of serum levels be made and the dosage schedule be adjusted accordingly.

17.6 New Techniques of Burn Wound Management

The aims of burn wound management in children are similar to those for adults. Several new techniques have been reported to have particularly utility in pediatric burn injury. The ultimate solution of the restoration of the function of the skin and the ultimate protection of the body from burn wound pathogens can only be achieved by wound coverage with viable skin. Up to present, excision of all deep burn wounds, either deep partial or full- thickness burns, has become the treatment of first choice if the patient can stand the stress of surgery [19].

The primary excision should be undertaken as ealry as possible following resuscitation and restoration of physiological balance. In extensive burns, early maximal reduction of the burn surface area is the aim, but the operation should be staged over a period of several days and priority is usually given to those burn areas easily excised and grafted. However, preservation of function of particular areas, such as the hands and neck, should be considered and these areas excised first. Third-degree burns are best excised down to the fascia. Sequential tangential excision is generally performed for deep second-degree burns. There may be significant bleeding and adequate blood replacement must be available. Excised burn wounds are covered immediately, if possible, with split-thickness autografts. Doner sites for autograft in small burns are seldom a problem. However, in patients with large-area burns, difficulty arises because of the scarcity of available donor sites. In China, the extensive excision wound is first covered with a large sheet of fenestrated allograft. In the fenestrations small pieces of autografts are transplanted. If the distance between autografts is less than 1 cm, and each autograft has an area of not less than 0.25 cm^2, the allograft will be replaced slowly and unnoticeably by the gradual coalescence of the expanding autograft. In cases where donor areas are available, meshed autograft in a ratio of 1:4 or 1:3 with an onlay of a meshed allograft in a ratio of 1:2 has been used with good results [20]. This technique has markedly improved the survival rate of burn injury in children. Herndon reported that the LD_{50} in pediatric burn patients between 1981 and 1985 in his institute reached 93% [21]. In order to achieve temporary coverage of extensive burn wound until sufficient autograft is available for coverage, biological dressings or artificial skin have been used. They are currently used as [22]: (a) immediate (within 16 h) coverage of fully debrided superficial second-degree burn, (b) coverage of granulation of excised wound between crops of autograft, (c) as a test graft prior to autograft application, and (d) after debridement of granulating wound with patches of necrotic tissue still adherent to the wound surface.

17.7 Airway Care

One of the priorities in the management of the burn patient is airway care. In the case of infants and young children, even a minor airway compromise may be risky. Therefore endotracheal intubation should be performed in any patient with inhalation injury and in those individuals with deep face and neck burns that will subsequently develop edema and hypoxia, resulting in respiratory insufficiency [23]. Elective intubation is far simpler and safer than attempting to establish an emergency airway in the presence of edema and hypoxia. However, tracheostomy is indicated in cases of prolonged tracheal intubation (longer than 3 days), excessively profuse secretions, difficult airway management, and/or when prolonged assisted ventilation is required. Since tracheostomy has been shown to be associated with frequent complications in the form of pneumothorax, pneumonia, and tracheitis, it should be used only when necessary. In infants and children the tracheal incision should be made through the fourth and fifth tracheal cartilage rings. This level is selected to avoid suprasternal collapse in the event of inadvertent detachment of the tracheostomy tube [24]. Erosion of the posterior wall of the trachea can also be prevented by a lower tracheostomy. Since the upper airway is more angulated in children than in adults, children are more susceptible to this complication when tubes made of silastic or less-irritating plastic substances are used. Scrupulous aseptic technique must be observed in the management of the airway in terms of suctioning; and maintenance of humidifiers and frequent bacteriological surveillance is imperative.

If burn is associated with inhalation injury, care of the airway is even more important. Mortality is higher than in patients with cutaneous burn alone. However, the incidence of inhalation injury is somewhat lower in children than in adults because most burn injuries are scalds. Acute asphyxia due to oxygen consumption by the fire is a common cause of early death so does carbon monoxide poisoning. In the case of inhalation injury, edema is caused by smoke, in which there is a number of toxic gases, including aldehydes, sulfur and nitrogen oxides, and hydrochloric acid, which produce pathological changes in the respiratory tract. The most important changes are pulmonary edema and atelectasis. Pulmonary edema is primarily a result of increased capillary permeability. Early qualitative changes in surfactant as well as airway obstruction by pseudomembranous casts are the causes of atelectasis. In patients suspected of having inhalation injury, treatment should begin at the scene of the fire. Inhalation of high concentrations of oxygen will counteract the effects of carbon monoxide and speed its clearance. Endotracheal intubation should be employed to provide a patent airway at the first hint of impending obstruction from soft-tissue edema. Positive pressure ventilation is beneficial during the period of pulmonary edema [25]. Humidification of inhaled air as well as endotracheal suction and lavage to remove casts of sloughed mucosa are frequently necessary.

References

1. Sorensen B (1967) First aid in burn injuries: treatment at home with cold water. Med Treat 4: 1199–1202
2. Mason AD (1980) The mathematics of resuscitation: 1980 presidential address, American Burn Association. J Trauma 20: 1015–1020
3. Carvajal HF (1973) Acute management of burn in children. South Med J 68: 129–131
4. Galdwell FT, Bowser BH (1979) Critical evaluation of hypertonic and hypotonic solution to resuscitate severely burned children: a prospective study. Ann Surg 189: 546
5. Goodwin CW, Maguire MS, MaManus WF et al. (1983) Prospective study of burn wound excision of the hand. J Trauma 23: 510–517
6. Reaves LE, Antonacci AC, Shires GT (1983) Fluid and electrolyte resuscitation of thermally injured patients. World J Surg 7: 566–572
7. Stratta RJ, Warden GD, Saffle JR et al. (1983) Plasma exchange therapy during burn shock. Curr Surg 40: 429–432
8. Fimberg L (1959) Pathoger.esis of lesions in the nervous system in hypernatremic status. Pediatrics 23: 40–45
9. Demling RH (1983) Improved survival after massive burns. J Trauma 23: 179–184
10. Monafo WW, Halverson JD, Schechtman K (1989) The role of concentrated sodium solutions in the resuscitation of patients with severe burns. Surgery 95: 129–135
11. Holzman BH, Scott GB (1981) Control of infection and technique of isolation in the pediatric intensive care unit. Pediatr Clin North Am 28: 703–721
12. Herndon DN, Thomoon PB (1985) Treatment of burns in children. Pediatr Clin North Am 32(5): 1311–1332
13. Harmel RP, Vane PW, King DR (1986) Burn care in children: special consideration. Clin Plast Surg 13: 95
14. Solomon JK (1981) Nutrition in severely burned child. Prog Pediatr Surg 14: 63–79
15. Sorof HS, Pearson E, Artz CP (1967) An estimation of nitrogen requirement for equilibrium in burn patients. Surg Gynecol Obstet 112: 159–172
16. Alxander W, Machillan BG, Stinnet JD et al. (1980) Beneficial effects of aggressive protein feedings in severely burned children. Ann Surg 192: 505–517

17. Chan CK, Jarrett F, Moylan JA (1976) Acute leukopenia as an allergic reaction to silver sulfadiazine in burn patients. J Trauma 16: 395–396.
18. Wilkin TJ, Bennett JE (1980) The use of systemic antibiotics in the treatment of burns. Surg Gynecol Obstet 151: 404
19. Burke JF, Quinby WC, Bondoc CC (1976) Primary excision and prompt grafting as routine therapy for the treatment of thermal burns in children. Surg Clin North Am 56: 477–494
20. Herndon DN, Gore D, Cole M et al. (1987) Determinants of mortality in pediatric patients with greater than 70% full-thickness total body surface area thermal injury treated by early total excision and grafting. J Trauma 27(2): 208–212
21. Herndon DN, Lemaster J, Benid S et al. (1986) The quality of life after major thermal injury in children: an analysis of 12 survivors with 80% total body surface 70% third degree burns. J Trauma 26(7): 609–619
22. Pruitt BA, Curreri PW (1971) The use of homograft and heterograft skin. In: Polk HC, Stone H (eds) Contemporary burn management. Little Brown, Boston, p 399–417
23. Cudmore Re, Vivori E (1981) Inhalation injury to the respiratory tract in children. Prog Pediatr Surg 14: 33–61
24. MacMillan BG, Frienberg DL (1982) Special problems of pediatric burn patients. In: Hummet RP (ed) Clinical burn therapy, a management and prevention guide. Wright PSG, Boston, p 468
25. Mathru M, Venus B, Rap TLK et al. (1983) Noncardiac pulmonary edema precipitated by tracheal intubation in patients with inhalation injury. Crit Care Med 1: 804–806

18 Rehabilitation in Burns

Tang Sheau-shi

The main topic of this chapter is the management of scars following thermal injury. Scar overgrowth may result in deformity and disabling complications, such as contracture of tendon and dislocation of joints. Collagen formation and contraction start before burn wound closure and progress for a year or more until the scar completely matures. Although scar tissue may mature and soften naturally, the deformity as a result of contracture during the scar overgrowth stage is permanent. In most instances, later plastic surgery cannot be avoided. The purpose of treatment is to minimize the contracture deformities and the functional loss secondary to scar overgrowth with rehabilitation techniques. Maximum functional activity should be restored, and optimal conditions for later plastic surgery should be the aim. A favorable outcome may then be obtained.

18.1 Mechanism of Scar Formation

Healing of deep burn wound involves a series of complicated histological, biochemical, and immunological dynamic procedures. During burn wound healing, the excessive deposit of fibrin and collagen may induce hypertrophic scar, which can be divided into overgrowth stage and maturation stage. The overgrowth stage varies individually. If this stage is only several weeks long, there is a nonhypertrophic scar. But if it continues for several months or even 3 or 4 years, hypertrophic scar will be formed [14].

The imbalance between collagen synthesis and its lysis, large amounts of abnormal mucopolysaccharide production, and myofibroblast overgrowth are the causes of hypertrophic scar formation.

Collagen is a type of hard and nonactive protein. Under normal conditions, its turnover is very slow and only in the process of wound healing does the production of collagen from fibroblast increase. In addition, several physical, chemical, and biological factors and several inflammatory mediators released by neutrophils or macrophages may activate the fibroblast to synthesize more collagen [5]. The amount of collagen synthesized in hypertrophic scar is twice that in normal mature scar. The percentage of type III collagen increases to 33% from the original 25% [7]. In normal skin, the collagen is decomposed slowly and completely. However, scar collagen turns over rather more rapidly after trauma because of the presence of abundant collagenase in the wound. Collagen antibody can be found in burn wound or serum from healed burn patients, which inhibits collagenase activity and reduces the level of collagenase required by collagen absorption and the degradation process. [2, 13]. Furthermore, in hypertrophic scar, collagen fibers are in a thick envelope of abnormal mucopolysaccharide, which hinders the hydrolytic action of collagenase, resulting in incomplete breakdown of collagen. Majno (1971) was the first to identify a type of contractible fibroblast in the process of healing. Gabbiani and Majno (1972) called this type of cell myofibroblasts [6]. The presence of smooth-muscle-like bundles in cellular plasma of these cells is the main cause of contracture and deformity [3]. In an open wound, the number of myofibroblasts increases progressively while the percentage of fibroblasts decreases. At 6 days postburn, the percentage of myofibroblasts in granulation tissue reaches 46% and that of fibroblast is 54%. One year after burn, however, the percentage of myofibroblasts in active hypertrophic tissue is as high as 96% but that of fibroblast is only 4%. With maturation of the scar, the percentage of myofibroblasts decreases [1]. Myofibroblast contraction bends collagen bundles in its vicinity, so that the distance from one end to another shortens and the bundles entwine with one another to form nodular whirl-like structures, making the surface of the scar uneven. Some harder components of stroma in burn scar, such as sulf-cartilagin A and 4-sulf-cartilagin B, increase greatly, replacing sulf-cartilagin B and keratosulfate [11]. Enclosure of collagen by the harder stroma may increase the consistency of the collagen mass, and forms a protective sheath to prevent collagen from decomposition by collagenase. During the scar overgrowth stage, the capillaries also overgrow to meet the high-oxygen requirement of collagen anabolism. Therefore, there is an abundant of capillary network with thick walls and occluded or partially occluded lumens due to contraction of the endothelium, all of which produce an outer appearance of congestion of the scar. When scar tissue matures, the number of capillaries decreases, lumen occlusion disappears, and the scar color turns to pale [9].

18.2 Control of Hypertrophic Scar

Prevention or control of scar overgrowth and contracture is based on the fact that scar tissue can be transformed under mechanical pressure. It is found that pressure therapy and splinting are effective for the control or prevention of scar hypertrophy and contracture formation. Other auxiliary treatments include functional exercises, psychiatric treatment, and iontophoresis of Chinese herbal drugs.

18.2.1 Pressure Therapy

During convalescence from burn, patients will usually flex their joints to ease the pain, and contractures are aggravated. Deformities due to contracture in all joints will certainly ensue if it is not corrected. Therefore, the correct pressure,

Table 18.1. Relationship between time of starting pressure therapy and duration of treatment

Duration of treatment (months)	Time of starting pressure-therapy (months postburn)			Cases
	3 months	4–6 months	6 months	
3–6	26			26
7–17	54	2		56
13–18	10	2		12
> 18	1		1	2
Total	91	4	1	96

which is equal but opposite to the force produced by flexion of the joints, should be applied for at least 6 months to maintain a good functional position in all joints. With this technique, the scar maturity can be accelerated and the scar overgrowth stage can be shortened significantly (Table 18.1).

18.2.1.1 Elastic Bandage

Elastic bandage is manufactured from an elastic fabric or a fabric incorporated with rubber. It exerts a pressure of 10–15 mmHg on each layer. Elastic bandage is most suitable for use on extremities with unhealed deep burn areas or on joints which need splinting. With this elastic bandage, a wrapping of two to three layers is indicated on the extremities and three to four layers on the trunk. If the contracture is located at the axilla, the upper arm should be maintained in 90° of abduction and 10° of anterior flexion (to prevent the shoulder joint from anterior dislocation). A semicircular-shaped sponge should be placed in the armpit, and a figure-of-eight bandage made [10].

18:2.1.2 Elastic Garments

At the Burn Center of Reijing Hospital, which is affiliated to Shanghai Second Medical University, various types of eleastic garments for the face, trunk, pelvic region, hand, and foot have been used to treat 789 cases of burn-scar hypertrophy from 1982 to 1988. Therapeutic effects were systematically observed in 96 cases. It was shown that wearing an elastic garment is an effective method for treating burn scar hypertrophy. In order to apply effective pressure, each patient should be measured individually. Figures 18.1–18.4 show the method of measurement. The elasticity of the elastic fabric is greater in the longitudinal direction than in the horizontal direction. A suitable degree of elasticity is desirable so that effective pressure can be exerted without any uncomfortable feelings. The edges of the face mask, trunk garment, trousers, gloves, and socks should exceed the scar area. On

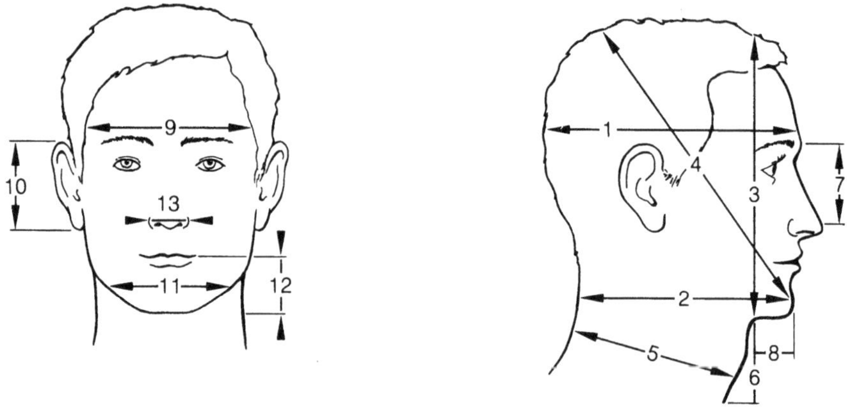

Fig. 18.1. Elastic facial mask. *Numbered lines* represent the sites for measurement for making a facial mask. The openings on the facial mask should be correctly located over the mouth, nostrils, eyes, and ears

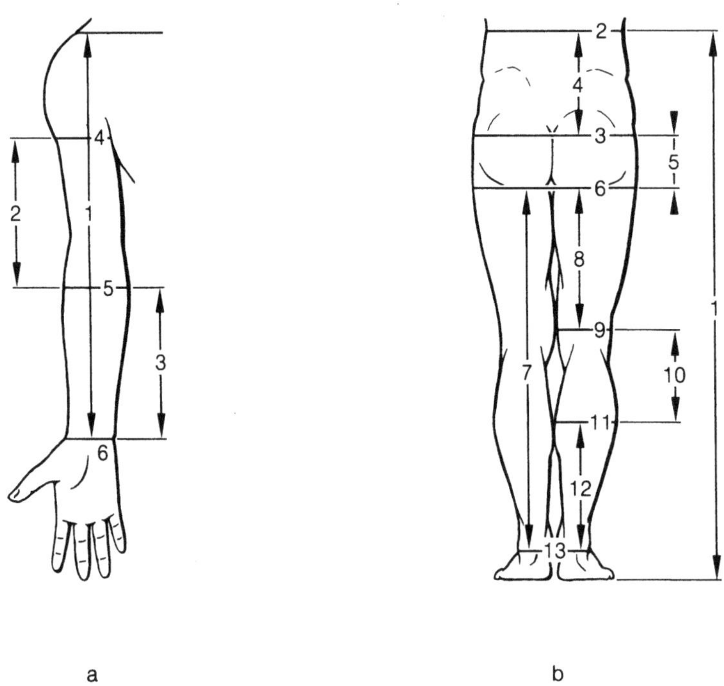

Fig. 18.2 a, b. Measuring lines for making an elastic sleeve and trouses. **a** Measurement for an elastic sleeve has been performed. **b** Measurement for elastic trousers. For the estremities, measurements of the circumference must be made especially in patients in whom excision down to the fascia has been performed

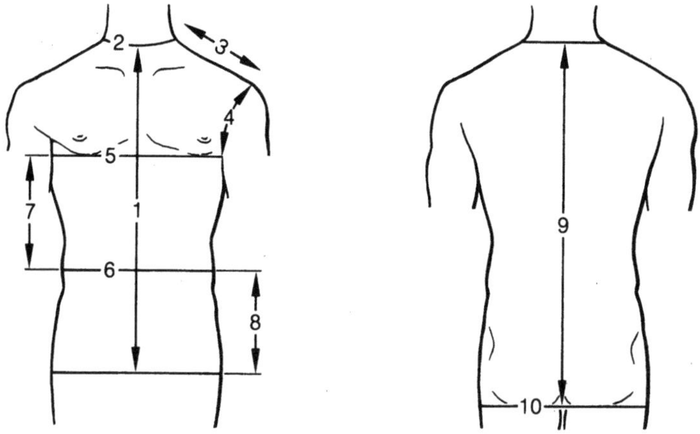

Fig. 18.3. Measurements for an elastic trunk garment

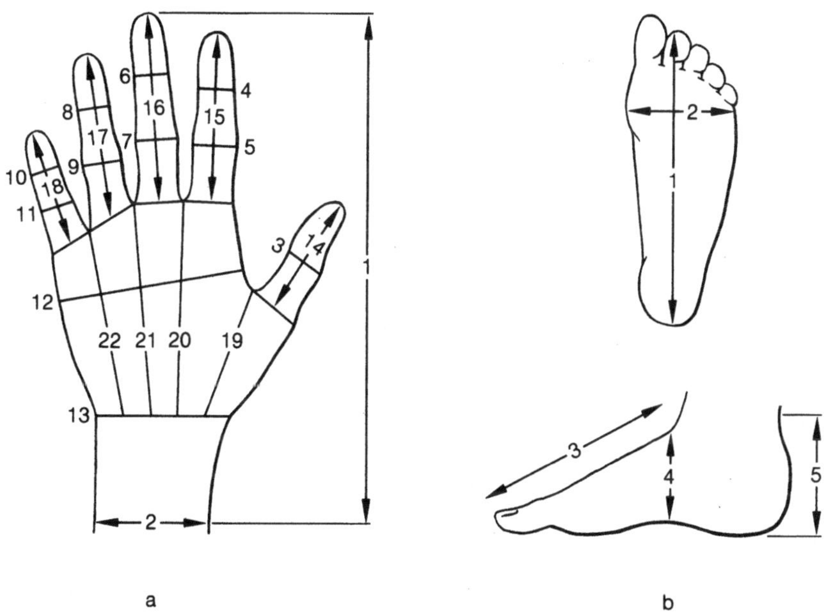

Fig. 18.4. a Measurements for elastic gloves; b measurements for elastic socks

a face mask, openings should be made for the ears, eyes, nostrils; and mouth. Two sets of such garments should be prepared for cleaning.

The time of starting pressure therapy is closely related to the treatment results. In a follow-up study, in 91 cases of 96 burn patients who wore Jobst pressure garments within 3 months after burn, 80 patients had completely

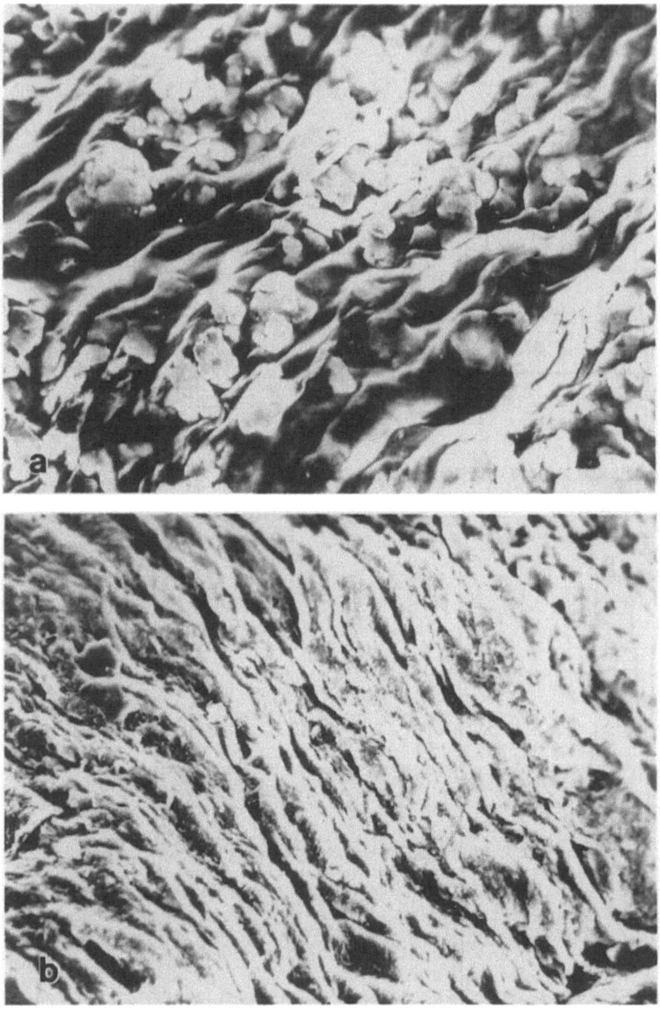

Fig. 18.5 a, b. Biopsies of scar tissue were take in three patients before and after pressure therapy (Jobst garments) using the electronic scanning microscopic technique. **a** Collagen nodules and round cell infiltration before pressure therapy. **b** Collagen fibers are thinner and H-arranged in a direction parallel to that of the skin surface after 6-month pressure therapy

matured scar within 1 year. In 26, the maturing process took only 3–6 months, because in the early phase of burn wound healing collagen nodules in the scar tissue are not as firmly coherent, so that their reformation by mechanical pressure is much easier. Samples of scar tissue were taken in from three patients before and after pressure therapy and studied with the electronic scanning microscopic technique. It was shown that the collagen nodules in the scars disappeared after treatment for 6 months. The collagen fibers were rearranged in a direction

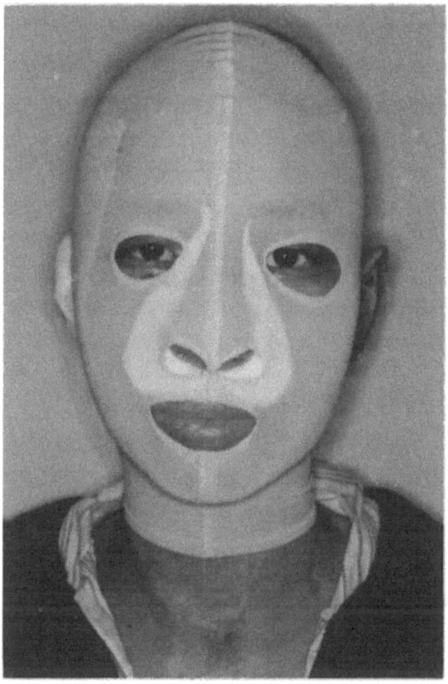

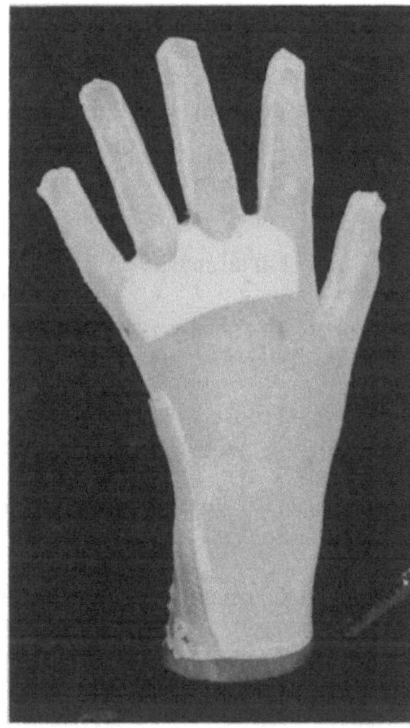

Fig. 18.6 (*left*). Polyethylene sponge padding is applied to the concavity between the nose and mouth before the elastic fiscial mask is used

Fig. 18.7 (*right*). Polyethylene sponge padding used in the web space, with an elastic glove

parallel to that of the skin surface. The number of cells decreased significantly (Fig. 18.5). Recently closed wound very easily suffers from blistering, abrasion, and even ulceration after pressure garments are worn because the epidermic layer is very thin. If it is delayed or has to be stopped due to ulceration, scar hypertropy will reappear, and the pain will become aggravated. Unbearable pain and itching in the scar areas produced by rewearing of pressure garments may prevent this treatment from being reused. For this reason, if the pressure garment has to be taken off due to ulceration, an elastic bandage should be applied to continue the pressure therapy.

The therapeutic effect of pressure therapy is better in the extremities than on the flat anterior and posterior surfaces of the trunk and depressed areas such as the webs and the area around the nose and mouth. According to Laplace's law, the pressure applied to spherical surface is inversely proportional to the radius of the sphere. Pressure garments may exert more effective pressure on a surface with a smaller spherical radius than on a surface with a larger spherical radius. Therefore, padding with a 0.6-cm-thick polyethylene sponge should be used on the flat or depressed area to reduce the spherical radius, so that better therapeutic effects of pressure therapy can be obtained [4] (Figs. 18.6, 18.7, Table 18.2).

Table 18.2. Application of elastic garments and TPI at 48 sites in 32 cases and their therapeutic effects

Sites	Types of elastic garment	Sites with plastic pad	Cases[a]	Therapeutic effects	
				Excellent	Effective[b]
Mouth	Facial mask	Area surrounding mouth	5	3	2
Nose		Two sides of nose	10	8	2
Elbow	Sleeve	Elbow fossa	5	5	
Hand	Glove	Webs	10	7	
Thigh	Trousers	Anterior thigh	1	1	
Popliteal fossa		Popliteal fossa	3	3	
Ankle	Socks	Anterior ankle	3	3	
Foot		Dorsal metatarsal toe	3	3	
Chest	Garment	Anterior thorax (0.6 cm of two layers)	2	2	
Abdomen	Trousers	Left abdomen	2		2
Buttock	Trousers	Buttock	2		2
Wrist	Glove	Dorsal wrist	2	2	

[a] In 32 patients, plastic pads were applied at 48 sites, over 2 sites for each case.
[b] The symptoms were cleared, with maturation of the scar still incomplete.

Pressure therapy may retard the skeletal growth of children, especially in infants below 2 years old. Prolonged pressure of a face mask or mandibular sling may result in chin recession or retardation of mandible growth, resulting in malocclusion. An elastic garment may also result in a thinner extremity than its counterpart and abnormal development of the thoracic cage. Of these complications, the incidence of mandibular retardation is the greatest (Table 18.3). On the flexion aspect of a joint, the pressure garment may form creases, which may produce abrasions of the scar tissue when the joint moves. Ulcers may form when infection sets in. Therefore, a pad of polyethylene sponge should be placed between the scar surface and the elastic garment. Because the skin of the scar is very thin, the patient is advised to wear silk stockings underneath the pressure garment to facilitate the application of the latter and to reduce undue friction [12]. Professional guidance and follow-up from medical workers specialized in burn surgery are required to obtain a favorable effect and to prevent complications.

Table 18.3. Complications from wearing elastic garments

Types of elastic garment	Mandible recession	Backward contraction	Reduced circumference of extremities			Sites of ulceration		
			0.3 cm	0.8 cm	1.0 cm	Elbow	Popliteal	Metatarso-Phalangeal
Mandibular sling	2							
Facial mask		1						
Sleeve			1	1	1	1		
Trousers					1		3	
Socks								1

18.2.1.3 Splinting

There are many thermoplastic materials which can be used to fabricate splints. Thermoplastic splints are used for effective prevention of scar contracture. The deformity formed within 3 months after burn can be easily corrected by the mechanical force of splinting because the overgrowth of collagen nodules in the scar has not reached its peak and they are still relatively loose. For this reason, it is better to apply the splinting as early as possible, certainly no later than 3 months after burn. As early splinting will have a favorable effect, as soon as the burn wound is healed, a thermoplastic splint should be applied to maintain all the joints in their positions.

Neck. The splint should be placed on the anterior aspect of the neck to maintain a hyperextension position. If the scar is located on one side, the head should bend to the contralateral side so that the scarring area can be kept in a stretched position.

Elbow and Knee. The splint should be placed on the anterior aspect of the elbow or knee to maintain a full extension position.

Hands. The wrist is supported in a position of 15° extension. The metacarpophalangeal flexion is 70°. The proximal and distal interphalangeal joints are in a position of full extension. The thumb is in the position of opposition and radial abduction.

Shoulder. The optimal position is 90° of abduction and external rotation.

Ankle and Foot. The optimal position is 90° dorsiflexion and 0° inversion; the toes are all in the extension position.

Transisopentadiene (TPI) is pliable. When immersed in water at 72°–77°C, it becomes soft and can be readily cut and molded into any forms as desired. It hardens when cooled. If the water temperature is higher than 80°C, TPI becomes sticky and can be used to make a dynamic splint. With splinting treatment satisfactory effects have been obtained in 71 sites in 55 patients who were suffering from joint deformities due to scar contracture. These regions include hand, neck, mouth, elbow, knee, shoulder (axilla), and toes (Tables 18.4, 18.5). Before treatment, ten patients were suffering from neck deformity due to scar contracture. They are unable to raise their head. The mandibulocervical angle disappeared and even the lower lip was everted. After 3–6 months of splinting treatment, the angle reappeared, the neck length returned to normal, raising the head became possible, and eversion of the lower lip was corrected without resorting to plastic surgery. Two patients with deep facial burn developed a microstomia deformity, which admitted only one finger. After dilatation with a thermoplastic dilator, it admitted three fingers. Deep burn of the hand may cause edema due to compromise in venous return after prolonged immobilization, or

Table 18.4. Deformities in 40 hands of 26 patients: results of treatment

Deformities	Number	Conditions after treatment	Evaluation	
			Excellent	Effective
Claw hand	6	Claw-like deformity corrected and thumb can move to a position of opposition	4	
		Claw-like deformity partially corrected; flexion of MCP joints; thumb in incomplete abduction and opposition		2
Deformity with less severity	33	Both appearance and function completely restored	31	
		90° flexion of MCP joints; thumb in complete abduction and opposition		2
Flexion contracture	1			1

Table 18.5. Deformities and conditions after treatment of 23 sites in 22 patients

Deformities	Cases	Conditions after treatment	Evaluation	
			Excellent	Effective
Elbow:				
90°–180° flexion; limitation in both flexion and extension	9	180° extension, 90° flexion	9	
Shoulder:				
30°–45° abduction	3	90° abduction	3	
Knee:				
150°–160° of flexion	7	180° extension, 90° flexion;	6	
		160° extension, 90° flexion		1
Ankle:				
10°–15° dorsiflexion	4	Neutral position	4	

due to the removal of superficial veins and lymphatics in surgical operations. Organization of the edema fluid may contribute to stiff joints and hinder functional exercises. With the use of a thermoplastic splint to fix the joints in a proper position, edema can disappear completely within 3 days, and the stiff joints become lossened again. A much more favorable effect can be obtained if the splinting treatment is combined with finger traction and an elastic bandage to fix the splint. The postburn contracture deformity of the hand and neck cannot be effectively corrected with an elastic bandage or garments only. A thermoplastic splint is necessary. The joint deformities should be corrected step by step, especially in the neck and hand. For example, for a neck contracture, the thermoplastic splint is first made to conform with the deformity. Two to 3 days later, it is gradually extended until the mandibulocervical angle gradually reappears, and the mandible returns to the normal position. For the hand, it is immersed in warm water for 15 min at first, and passive exercise is given at the same time to relieve the joint stiffness. Then a wrist splint is applied to maintain a full extension position or 10° or 15° dorsiflexion. The metacarpophalangeal joints are in full extension or slight flexion and the interphalangeal joints with flexion contracture and thumb with adduction deformity can only be corrected to a limited extent to avoid pain and compromise of the venous return. The splint is changed at intervals of 2–3 days so that the correction is made progressively but persistently, until the proper position of the joints is completely restored. Overcorrection may cause tissue damage and should be avoided. For major joints of the extremities, wrist joint, and metatarsal joints, the deformities can be corrected after two to three revisions of the splints. If the deformity has corrected whereas the scar has not yet matured, interruption of treatment will cause recurrence of the contracture deformity. Therefore the splints should be worn day and night except for functional exercises or for cleansing.

Transisopentadiene thermoplastic splint is nontoxic, does not cause hypersensitivity, is nonageing, and can be cleansed and sterilized. However, it is not porous. The newly healed scar tends to form blister due to friction, or a bedsore may even form due to pressure when the TPI splint is applied. So it is necessary to pad the splint with one to two layers of gauze, and to clean the splinted area every day.

18.3 Physical Therapy and Functional Exercises

In the patients with extensive burn, the range of joint motion is limited because of scar contracture. The limited joint movements are also due to edema, pain, apprehension, or being confined to bed for a long time. So, it is necessary to encourage the patients to do active exercises early. As soon as the wound is closed, hydrotherapy (local areas or whole body) combined with active exercises should be started. After bathing, some hygroscopic creams, such as 1% tannic acid cream and urea cream, can be applied to the scar surface. Massage is then performed. After that, the patient is dressed with an elastic bandage and fitted with a splint or elastic garment. All these methods are helpful for scar maturation.

Ultrasound ion conduction with a solution of galla sinensis may significantly relieve several of the symptoms associated with scar tissue such as pain, itch, and congestion, and accelerate the scar-softening process. Three to four treatments may abate itch to varying degrees. Ten days constitutes one therapeutic course.

Usually three to four successive therapeutic course are required and may be combined with pressure therapy. The latter is essential to prevent hypertrophy of scar and other symptoms when the treatment is over.

A rehabilitation program of deep burn is carried out mainly at home. Cooperation from the patient and family, as well as guidance from the burn specialist, is critical in achieving an optimal therapeutic response [8]. After starting the treatment, close observation should be continued for several weeks or months. It is very difficult for younger children to be cooperative in this therapeutic process and the results are usually therefore not as good as those in adults.

References

1. Baur PS (1982) Myofibroblasts: their antitàchments and consequences in human burn wounds granulation tissues and scars. J Burns Care Rehabil 3: 214–219
2. Baur PS, Larson DL, Stacey TR et al. (1976) Ultrastructural analysis of pressure-treated human hypertrophic scars. J Trauma 16: 958–967
3. Baur PS, Barrott B, Linares HA et al. (1978) Wound contractions, scar contractures and myofibroblasts: a classical case study. J Trauma 18: 8–22
4. Cheng JCY (1984) Pressure therapy in the treatment of post-burn hypertrophic scar – a critical look into usefulness and fallacies by pressure monitoring. Burn 10: 154
5. Chvapil M (1980) Zinc and other factors of the pharmacology of wound healing. In: Hunt JK (ed) Wound healing and wound infection. Appleton century Crofts, New York, pp 135–149
6. Gabbiani G, Majno G (1972) Dupuytren's contracture: fibroblast contraction – an ultrastructural study. Am J Pathol 66: 131–138
7. Jackson DS (1980) The biochemical basis of repair. In: Hunt TK(ed) Wound healing and wound infection. Appleton Century Crofts, New York, pp 32–44
8. Johson CL, O'shanghanessy EJ, Ostergren G (eds) (1981) Burn management. Raven, New York, pp 5–16, 48–90
9. Kischer CW, Shetlar MR (1979) Microvasculature in hypertrophic scars and the effects of pressure. J Trauma 19: 757–764
10. Laeson DL, Abston S, Evans EB et al. (1971) Techniques for decreasing scar formation and contractures in the burned patient. J Trauma 11: 807–823
11. Larson DL, Baur PS, Linares HA et al. (1975) Mechanism of hypertrophic scar and contracture formation in burn. Burns 1: 119–127
12. Leung KS, Cheug JCY, Ma GFY, Clark JA et al. (1984) Complications of pressure therapy for post-burn hypertrophic scars. Burn 10(6): 434–438
13. Linares HA, Larson DC (1978) Proteoglycans and collagenase in hypertrophic scar formation. Plast Reconstr Surg 62: 589–593
14. Pruitt BA (1979) The burn patient. II. Late care and complication of thermal injury. Curr Probl Surg 16: 77–83

Subject Index

MIX
Papier aus verantwortungsvollen Quellen
Paper from responsible sources
FSC® C105338

If you have any concerns about our products,
you can contact us on
ProductSafety@springernature.com

In case Publisher is established outside the EU,
the EU authorized representative is:
Springer Nature Customer Service Center GmbH
Europaplatz 3, 69115 Heidelberg, Germany

Printed by Libri Plureos GmbH
in Hamburg, Germany